INTRODUCTION TO
HUMAN ANATOMY

CARL C FRANCIS

Department of Anatomy
Case Western Reserve University
Cleveland, Ohio

ALEXANDER H. MARTIN

Department of Anatomy
University of Wisconsin
Madison, Wisconsin

SEVENTH EDITION

With 401 illustrations, including 32 in
color, and a Trans-Vision® insert on
human anatomy containing 15 full-color
plates by Ernest W. Beck

THE C. V. MOSBY COMPANY
SAINT LOUIS   1975

Seventh edition

Copyright © 1975 by The C. V. Mosby Company

All rights reserved. No part of this book may be reproduced
in any manner without written permission of the publisher.

Previous editions copyrighted 1949, 1954, 1959, 1964, 1968, 1973

Printed in the United States of America

Distributed in Great Britain by Henry Kimpton, London

Library of Congress Cataloging in Publication Data

Francis, Carl C 1901-
    Introduction to human anatomy.

    Bibliography: p.
    Includes index.
    1. Anatomy, Human. I. Martin, Alexander,
1932-   joint author. II. Title.
[DNLM: 1. Anatomy. QS4 F818i]
QM23.2.F7 1975   611   75-2455
ISBN 0-8016-1646-8

GW/CB/B 9 8 7 6 5 4 3 2 1

To the memory of

T. Wingate Todd

a pioneer in the teaching of Living Anatomy

PREFACE
TO SEVENTH EDITION

Anatomy is a dynamic science, incorporating ongoing research. Because of such investigations, anatomical concepts are constantly changing, and although the structure of many organs may not be altered markedly, the functions ascribed to several systems, particularly endocrine, cardiovascular, and nervous, are still being elucidated. We have updated the textbook to reflect such new developments as well as to reflect suggestions and criticisms from faculty and students who have used the text in the past.

Developmental considerations have been included when deemed necessary, and alterations in function have also been utilized to develop the concept of integration between structure and function.

The changes in both space and context will, we believe, enhance the study of anatomy. It is our sincere hope that the popularity of the textbook will continue.

CARL C FRANCIS
ALEXANDER H. MARTIN

PREFACE
TO FIRST EDITION

This textbook is an attempt to present in the smallest possible compass the essential facts of human anatomy. Stress has been laid on the function of each part and on the integration of each tissue and organ of the body.

BNA terminology has been used as the official source throughout the text, but synonyms in common use have been indicated.

Miss Helen Williams, artist of the Department of Anatomy, drew almost all the illustrations. Her meticulous work, constructive criticisms, and suggestions have been invaluable in compiling the book.

I wish also to acknowledge my indebtedness to my colleagues within the Department of Anatomy, particularly to Dr. Samuel W. Chase and to Mr. M. V. Anders.

CARL C FRANCIS

CONTENTS

NEWHAM SCHOOL OF NURSING,
FOREST GATE HOSPITAL,
FOREST LANE,
LONDON, E7 9BD.

xi

INTRODUCTION TO
HUMAN ANATOMY

CHAPTER 1

THE BODY AS A WHOLE

Anatomy is the science of the structure of the body. Although the primary concern of anatomy is with structure, structure and function should always be considered together. Moreover, by means of surface anatomy, emphasis should be placed on the anatomy of the living body.

The cell is the basic structural unit of the body. Our life cycle begins with the fusion of a maternal cell, or ovum, and a paternal cell, or spermatozoon, in a process known as fertilization. The egg cell, or ovum, is one of thousands that develop in the ovaries of the woman. From birth until puberty the egg cells are immature and are encased in separate tiny sacs in the ovary. At puberty the sacs begin to swell as one after another the eggs begin to ripen. Once every 28 to 30 days, one, or occasionally more, of the egg cells is released in a process called ovulation. Shortly after ovulation the fingerlike fimbriae on the lateral end of the uterine (fallopian) tube sweep the egg into the lumen of the tube (Fig. 1-1).

The sperm cells, which contain the male hereditary material, are produced in threadlike tubes in the testes. Like the egg cells, the sperm cells begin to mature at puberty. When sperm cells are deposited in the female reproductive tract, they pass through the uterus and into the uterine tubes propelled mainly by the contraction of the muscular wall of these organs. Concurrent release of an ovum can result in fusion of the germ cells, an event, fertilization, that normally occurs in the lateral third of the uterine tube. Soon after this union the fertilized cell, now called a zygote, begins a series of rapid cell divisions termed cleavage. With each division, cell size becomes smaller.

I

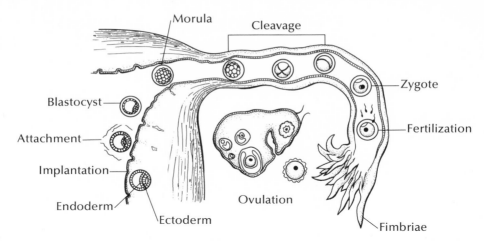

Fig. 1-1. Schematic representation of early development of the conceptus.

The large number of new cells collectively has the appearance of a mulberry and is known as the morula. As cell division continues, the morula is passed down the uterine tube by rhythmic contractions of the tube as well as by ciliary movement. About the time the morula enters the uterine cavity, it consists of an inner cell mass surrounded by a peripheral layer of cells, the trophoblast. Fluid from the uterine cavity enters the morula, and eventually the mulberry-shaped group of cells becomes hollow with the majority of the cells (the inner cell mass) located at one side of the hollow ball, now known as the blastocyst. Approximately seven days after ovulation, implantation of the blastocyst begins in the wall of the uterus.

At this point in development, definite cell differentiation occurs. On the surface of the inner cell mass, facing the cavity of the blastocyst, a single layer of flattened cells, the endoderm, appears. The remaining cells of the inner cell mass form the ectoderm. A third layer of cells, the mesoderm, forms later between the ectoderm and endoderm. These three layers of cells, called the germ layers, are the forerunners of the various specialized cells that will make up the body organs. The ectoderm, or outer layer, will become the covering of the body, or skin, as well as the central nervous system. The endoderm, in a sense, lines the inner surface of the body and forms the lining of the digestive and respiratory tracts. The mesoderm provides tissues for the lining of the body cavities, for the muscles, for parts of the skeleton, for the cardiovascular and lymphatic systems, as well as for the so-called "packing tissue," or mesenchyme.

The prenatal growth of the developing child may be divided into three main periods. (1) The preembryonic period extends from fertili-

2

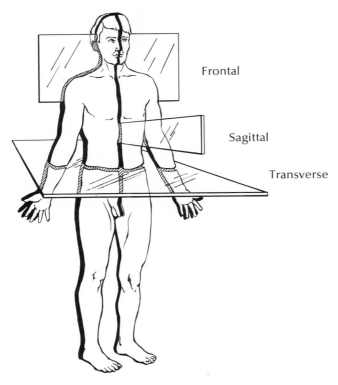

Frontal

Sagittal

Transverse

Fig. 1-2. Human body in the anatomical position with three planes of section represented.

zation to the formation of the germ layers or from one to two weeks, inclusive. (2) The embryonic period extends from the third to eighth week and is a time of rapid growth and differentiation. All of the major organs of the body are laid down during the embryonic period, and during this time, almost all congenital anomalies become apparent. (3) The fetal period extends from nine weeks until birth and is characterized by growth and development of the organ systems established during the embryonic stages. After birth the baby continues to grow and develop; some of the changes occurring during childhood will be discussed in the chapters on the skeletal and nervous systems.

In this book the types of cells that the body uses as building material will be described first. A group of similar cells specialized to perform a certain function is called a tissue. Several tissues unite in a definite pattern to perform a given function, thus forming organs, and a group of organs constitutes a system. The systems will be discussed in detail one by one. The skeletal, articular, and muscular systems work together to produce movement. The nervous system secures information from the environment and regulates body functions. The circulatory, digestive, and respiratory systems are essential for the digestion of food and the maintenance of life. The urinary system provides a constant internal chemical milieu by excreting waste material. The reproductive system is necessary for the perpetuation of the species. The integumentary system, or the skin, is a protective covering as well as an organ of excretion. Finally, the endocrine system correlates and adjusts the body functions into one harmonious whole.

Studying anatomy is much like learning a foreign language. One must first build a vocabulary of anatomical terms, and since anatomy is a descriptive science, the terms must be used correctly. To avoid confusion anatomists have adopted the convention of referring all descriptions to what is known as the "anatomical position." It is the position of an erect body, feet together, eyes looking straight ahead, arms by the sides, and palms of the hands facing forward. All descriptive accounts, oral or written, must refer to this position (Fig. 1-2).

In the description of anatomical structures, many terms are necessary, and constant reference should be made to the glossary. Some general terms will be used very frequently and should be thoroughly understood at the beginning.

Planes of body

The body or any part thereof may be divided along certain planes. These may be defined as follows:

1. *Sagittal, median,* or *longitudinal:* a plane vertical to the ground dividing the structure into right and left halves.
2. *Frontal* or *coronal:* a plane vertical to the ground dividing the structure into anterior and posterior portions.
3. *Transverse, horizontal,* or *cross:* a plane parallel to the ground dividing the structure into upper and lower parts.

Directional terms

Directional terms usually occur in pairs and are as follows:

1. *Superior* or *cephalic:* toward the head or the upper part of a structure; the superior extremity includes the arm, forearm, and hand.
2. *Inferior* or *caudal:* away from the head or toward the lower end of a structure; the inferior extremity includes the thigh, leg, and foot.
3. *Anterior: ventral* or *front;* the sternum or breast bone forms part of the anterior chest wall.
4. *Posterior: dorsal* or *back;* the posterior portion of the skull is the back or occipital portion. In human anatomy the terms anterior and posterior are used in preference to ventral and dorsal because man walks erect.

5. *Medial:* toward the midline of the body; the medial side of the arm is the side nearest the chest wall.
6. *Lateral:* away from the midline of the body; the eyes are lateral to the nose.
7. *Proximal:* toward the trunk or beginning of a structure; the wrist is proximal to the hand.
8. *Distal:* away from the trunk or the source of a structure; the foot is distal to the ankle.
9. *Central:* toward the center; the brain belongs to the central nervous system.
10. *Peripheral:* away from the center; the nerves of the hand are part of the peripheral nervous system.
11. *Deep:* away from the surface; the humerus is in the depth of the arm.
12. *Superficial:* near the surface; the superficial fascia lies just under the skin.
13. *Median:* in the middle of a structure; the median nerve is situated in the central part of the upper extremity. Median is not the same as medial.
14. *Intermediate:* between two other structures; the intermediate cutaneous nerve of the thigh is between the medial and lateral nerves.

Man belongs to the class of animals known as mammals, but he has certain features that clearly distinguish him from other mammals. Some of these distinctive human characteristics are as follows:

1. The brain and brain case of man are much larger relatively than those of the vast majority of mammals and are actually larger than those of many mammals of greater bulk. The average size of an adult human brain is about 1,500 cc, and that of an adult gorilla is about 510 cc.
2. The human face is smaller than the brain case. Man has the same number of teeth as a gorilla, but the teeth are smaller and closer together. The nasal bones and bridge of the nose are more prominent in man. Human nostrils are pointed inferiorly; ape nostrils are pointed anteriorly. Man alone has a chin.
3. The spinal column in an adult human is S-shaped, with curves convex anteriorly in the cervical and lumbar regions and concave anteriorly in the thoracic and sacral regions. In man the head is well balanced on the spinal column, therefore the neck muscles are less developed, and the neck is slender.
4. Man is the only animal in which the thumb can, in the fullest sense, be opposed to the other digits, and man's entire hand is

5

extremely mobile and capable of very delicate finger movements.

5. The thorax in man is flattened from anterior to posterior and is, therefore, relatively broad and flat.

6. The pelvic girdle is broad, and the muscles that attach the lower extremity to the trunk are well developed to maintain man's erect body posture. The buttocks are a characteristic human structure. The muscles of the calf of the leg in man are likewise large in comparison to those of other primates.

7. The great toe is not opposable in man but is opposable in the ape. The foot bones of man are arranged in arches that assist in absorbing the shock of walking.

8. In the adult human the lower extremities are longer than the upper extremities. This is due largely to an increase in the length of the femora.

REVIEW QUESTIONS

1. What is the basic unit of structure of the human body?
2. Distinguish between a fertilized ovum, an embryo, and a fetus.
3. Distinguish between a sagittal plane, a coronal plane, and a horizontal plane.
4. Distinguish between a cell, a tissue, an organ, and a system.
5. Name five organ systems and give one function of each.
6. Define briefly each of the following directional terms: superior, inferior, anterior, posterior, medial, and lateral.
7. Give five distinctive human characteristics.
8. Describe the anatomical position.

CHAPTER 2

CELLS AND TISSUES

Cells are the vital units that make up all the tissues of the body. **CELLS**
Tissues in turn are specialized to perform a particular function
or functions. Organs are composed of several tissues arranged to fulfill
the special functions of the organ.

Cells vary greatly in size and shape due, in part, to their activity.
Therefore, it is impossible to describe a typical cell. However a conventional cell, illustrating features that are present in cells generally,
as well as various types of cells are depicted in Figs. 2-1 and 2-2 and
in Plate XII of the Trans-vision insert. The conventional cell is surrounded by a cell membrane containing a fluid called cytoplasm, within which is a small denser mass, the nucleus. The nucleus contains
the apparatus for maintaining the genetic makeup of cells, and the
cytoplasm is specialized to express other properties of protoplasm,
such as absorption, assimilation, conductivity, contractility, respiration, secretion, and phagocytosis.

The nucleus is limited by a well-defined nuclear membrane. Within each nucleus there may be one or more distinct masses, the nucle-
oli, which stain with acid dyes. In each nucleus are numerous bits of
blue staining matter called chromatin granules, which reflect the portions of the thin, extended chromosomes that stain with basic dyes.

The structures and bodies in the cytoplasm are of two main types:
(1) organelles, which are living specialized structural parts of the cytoplasm, and (2) inclusions, which are accumulations of nonliving material such as food—carbohydrate, fat, and protein; secretion granules and globules; and pigments.

Organelles include mitochondria, which are believed to be sites
where the cells produce energy; endoplasmic reticulum, tubules, on

7

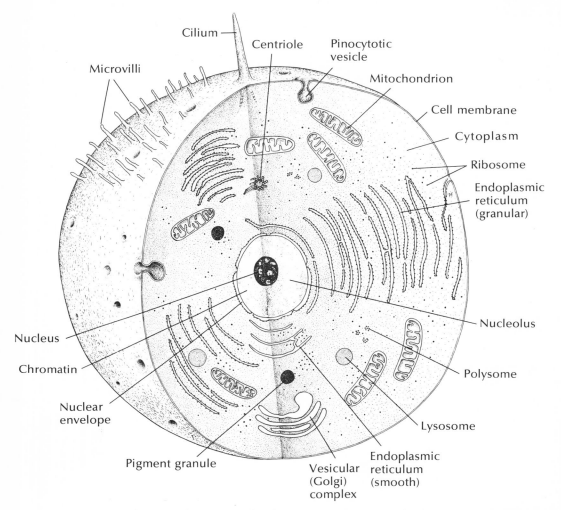

Fig. 2-1. The standard cell, showing the organelles that are common to all cells. See text for a discussion of each. (From DiDio, L. J. A.: Synopsis of anatomy, St. Louis, 1970, The C. V. Mosby Co.)

the surface of which proteins are synthesized and in which proteins are transported to the golgi complex, which "packages" substances before secretion; lysosomes, baglike structures that contain digestive enzymes; centrioles, which play a part in spindle formation and polarization of the spindle fibers during cell division; ribosomes, tiny bodies of RNA in which protein synthesis occurs; and fibrils, most pronounced in muscle cells, which are concerned with contractility.

Cells reproduce by a process called cell division, or mitosis. Mitosis is a continuous process that has been arbitrarily divided into five

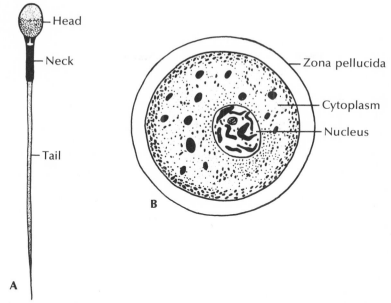

Fig. 2-2. Reproductive cells. **A,** Spermatozoon. **B,** Ovum.

stages. These stages as well as events that occur during the process are depicted in Table 1.

Tissues may be divided into four major categories in which there are many subtypes.

TISSUES

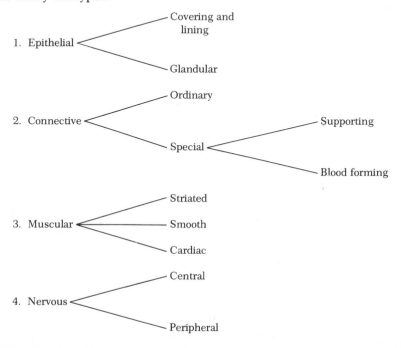

9

Table 1. Mitosis

Interphase	Prophase	Metaphase	Anaphase	Telophase
1. Period between divisions	1. Chromosomes condense	1. Chromosomes align on the spindle along the "equator" of the cell	1. Sister chromosomes separate and move toward poles	1. Chromosomes unwind
2. Chromosomes are thin, extended threads	2. Nuclear membrane disappears			2. Nuclear membrane and nucleolus reform
3. Each parent centriole is paired with a smaller daughter centriole	3. Nucleolus breaks down			3. Constriction occurs around center of cell
4. Chromosome (DNA) replication occurs	4. Centrioles move apart			4. Each daughter cell has same genetic material as parent cell
5. Centrioles begin to separate	5. Connections are made between chromosomes and centrioles			
6. Spindle starts to form				

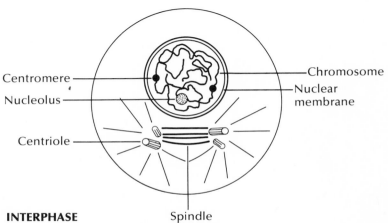

Centromere

Nucleolus

Centriole

Chromosome

Nuclear membrane

Spindle

INTERPHASE

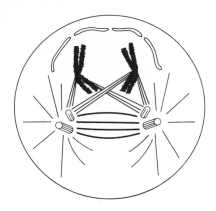

PROPHASE

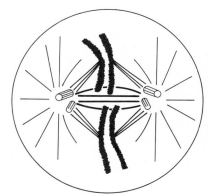

METAPHASE

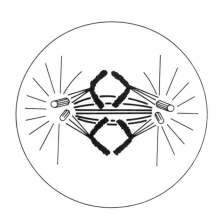

ANAPHASE

TELOPHASE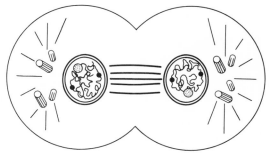

11

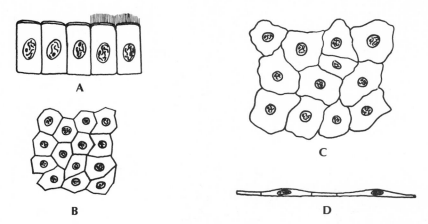

Fig. 2-3. Various types of simple epithelium. **A,** Simple columnar epithelium in cross section. **B,** Simple columnar epithelium, surface view. **C,** Simple squamous epithelium, surface view. **D,** Simple squamous epithelium in cross section.

Epithelial tissue

Epithelium performs three functions: (1) protection, (2) selective absorption, and (3) secretion. It covers the body surface, lines the body cavities, forms the inner lining of the vascular and lymphatic systems, and forms the glandular portion of secretory organs.

Simple epithelium consists of a single layer of cells resting upon a thin layer of amorphous material, the basement membrane. The cells may be flat and scalelike, forming simple squamous epithelium, or they may stand side by side forming simple cuboidal or columnar epithelium. Squamous epithelium that lines blood vessels and lymphatics is called endothelium; that lining the body cavities (pleural, pericardial, and peritoneal) is known as mesothelium. Cuboidal cells are of about equal height and width, whereas columnar cells are tall and thin. Columnar cells may undergo certain modifications. The free surface of each cell in certain areas of the respiratory system (from nasal cavity to bronchioles) as well as in the uterus and uterine tubes develops cilia, which look like fine hairs. These cilia, beating in harmony, move mucus along the respiratory tract and in the uterine tubes, help to move the egg cell toward the uterus. Pseudostratified epithelium consists essentially of columnar cells that are crowded closely together thereby distorting their rectangular form. Not all of the cells reach the free surface of the epithelium, but all have a portion touching the basement membrane (Fig. 2-4).

Stratified epithelium consists of two or more layers of cells. Stratified squamous epithelium is found on surfaces exposed to friction, abrasion, and extremes of temperature; such surfaces are the skin,

12

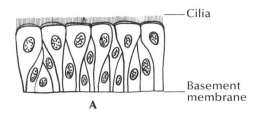

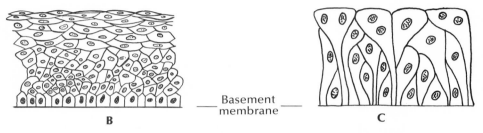

Fig. 2-4. Various types of stratified epithelium. **A,** Pseudostratified, ciliated, columnar epithelium. **B,** Stratified squamous epithelium. **C,** Transitional epithelium.

lips, inside of mouth, esophagus, pharynx, and anal canal. The outer layers of such epithelia are being constantly thrown off and renewed by the growth of deeper layers. Transitional epithelium is a stratified epithelium in which the surface cells have an elongated pearlike shape. This type is found along the urinary tract. The cells of this epithelium possess to an unusual degree the ability to change position by sliding over each other. If the viscus they line, for example, the urinary bladder, is distended, the epithelium is reduced to three or four layers. When the viscus is empty, the cells heap up forming several layers between basal and surface cells.

A membrane is usually defined as a sheet of tissue that lines or covers a body surface and is composed of epithelium or connective tissue. Mucous membrane lines cavities and passageways open to the exterior, such as the respiratory and digestive tracts. Serous membrane, pleural, pericardial, and peritoneal, lines the closed body cavities. Synovial membrane is found within joint cavities, bursae, and tendon sheaths. Cutaneous membrane is a term used to refer to the skin. The word membrane is also used to describe various definite sheets of connective tissue that separate spaces or connect structures such as the interosseous (see Fig. 4-12) or thyrohyoid membranes.

Glands. In areas where secretion is needed over and above that　　13

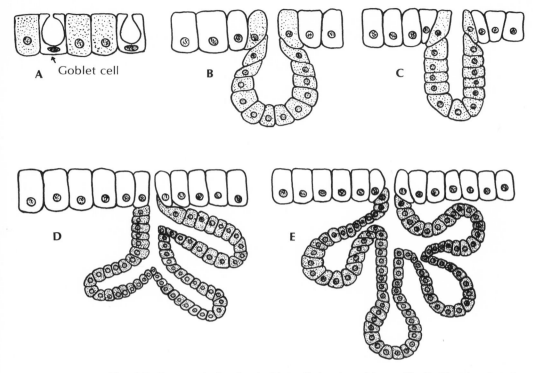

Fig. 2-5. Types of glands. **A,** Unicellular (a goblet cell). **B,** Simple alveolar (saccular). **C,** Simple tubular. **D,** Compound tubular. **E,** Compound alveolar.

which can be provided by cells of a membrane, epithelial cells specialize to provide secretion. Such glands are classified as exocrine or endocrine. Exocrine glands secrete out of the body, and endocrine glands secrete into the body. Both varieties are located within the connective tissue substance of the body, therefore exocrine glands must have a duct to convey their secretion to the surface. Exocrine glands may be classified according to the form of their duct and may be simple or compound tubular, alveolar or tubuloalveolar (Fig. 2-5). Since endocrine glands secrete directly into the substance of the body (capillaries), they are often called "ductless glands." Certain glands, such as liver and pancreas, have both exocrine and endocrine functions.

Certain epithelial cells are specialized for the reception of sensory stimuli. These cells are found in the taste buds of the tongue, in the olfactory area of the nasal cavity, and in the rods and cones of the retina. Epithelium that receives sensory stimuli and transmits nervous system impulses is frequently called neuroepithelium. Epithelial cells also give rise to the reproductive cells, sperm and ovum, which form in the testis or ovary, respectively.

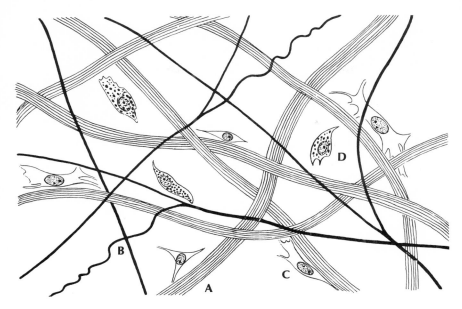

Fig. 2-6. Areolar connective tissue. *A,* Collagen fiber; *B,* elastic fiber; *C,* connective tissue cell; *D,* macrophage with ingested granules.

Connective tissue

The second of the basic tissues, the most abundant and widespread in the body, is called connective tissue because it connects the other tissues together and to the skeleton. The skeleton is built of a special kind of connective tissue and, as we will see, another kind of connective tissue, the hemopoietic, produces the cells of the blood.

Connective tissue has a connecting and supporting role because certain connective tissue cells produce material, intercellular substance, that occupies a position between the cells. The intercellular substance, nonliving and possessing various degrees of strength, may consist of fibers or an amorphous ground substance. Some fibers are composed of a white organic compound, collagen, and others are composed of elastin, which gives a yellowish appearance to the tissue.

Connective tissue may be subdivided into the following categories: (1) loose ordinary (areolar), (2) dense fibrous, (3) adipose, (4) cartilage, (5) bone, (6) hemopoietic, and (7) reticuloendothelial.

Loose ordinary (areolar) connective tissue is so called because it is stretchable and found widely throughout the body. Areolar tissue, a combination of cells (fibroblasts), collagen, and a few elastic fibers embedded in a soft matrix, forms the basis of the subcutaneous tissue and extends almost everywhere in the body. There is no sharp demarcation between loose and dense ordinary connective tissue, and one type commonly merges with the other (Fig. 2-6).

15

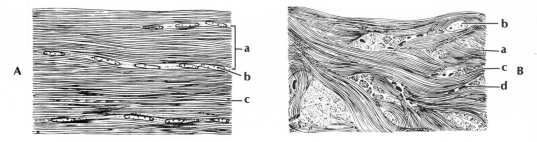

Fig. 2-7. Dense connective tissue. **A,** Parallel arrangement as in a tendon; *a*, collagen fiber; *b*, connective tissue cell; *c*, fibril. **B,** Matted arrangement as in the dermis of the skin; *a*, collagen fiber; *b*, connective tissue cell; *c*, fibril; *d*, elastic fiber.

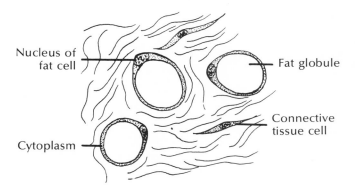

Fig. 2-8. Fat cells.

Dense ordinary connective tissue consists mainly of fibers, either collagen or elastin, and relatively few cells (Fig. 2-7). Examples of the dense form (collagen), which is very resistant to a pulling force, are periosteum, aponeuroses, muscle sheaths and tendons, ligaments, organ capsules, and dura mater, the outer meningeal layer.

If there are many elastic fibers, yellow tissue results that has the property of stretching easily and of returning to its original form when released. Certain ligaments of the vertebral column, the ligamenta flava, as well as the walls of large arteries, such as the aorta, have an abundance of elastic tissue.

Adipose tissue represents a specialized kind of loose connective tissue characterized by the presence of a great many fat cells filling in the interspaces between the fibers (Fig. 2-8).

Cartilage. The cells of cartilage (chondrocytes) appear as islands in a dense noncellular translucent substance called the matrix. The cells are usually spheroidal and occur singly or in small groups, and

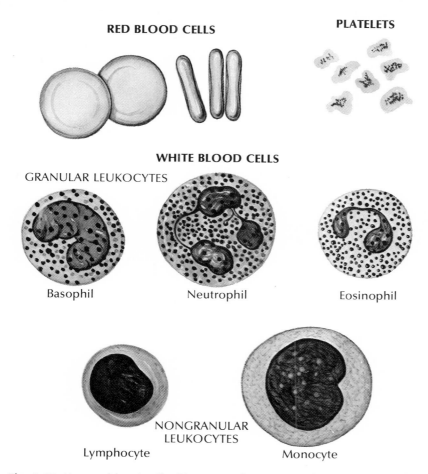

RED BLOOD CELLS

PLATELETS

WHITE BLOOD CELLS

GRANULAR LEUKOCYTES

Basophil   Neutrophil   Eosinophil

NONGRANULAR
LEUKOCYTES

Lymphocyte   Monocyte

Fig. 2-12. Human blood cells. There are close to 30 trillion red blood cells in the adult. Each cubic millimeter of blood contains from 4.5 to 5.5 million red blood cells and an average total of 7,500 white blood cells. (From Anthony, C. P., and Kolthoff, N. J.: Textbook of anatomy and physiology, ed. 8, St. Louis, 1971, The C. V. Mosby Co.)

tive tissue containing many small blood vessels. Within the meshes of connective tissue there are a few fat cells and some mature red and white cells, but these are greatly outnumbered by immature blood cells having a great variety of form, size, and staining reaction.

Lymphatic tissue is found in the lymph nodes and in the spleen. These organs are described in the chapter on the lymphatic system. When a lymph nodule is actively producing new cells, it is large, and each follicle is packed with a tremendous number of lymphocytes of all sizes. When inactive, a lymph nodule is smaller, and the lymphocytes are less numerous, particularly in immature forms.

Lymph. Lymph is similar in composition to blood plasma. It contains a very small number of cells, mainly lymphocytes (Fig. 2-12). It is usually clear, but the lymph contained in the lymphatics from the small intestine appears milky because of fat globules that have been absorbed from the food. Therefore, these lymphatics are called lacteals, and the contained lymph is called chyle.

Reticuloendothelial tissue. Reticular tissue is composed of a loose mesh of very fine fibers that are best demonstrated histologically by impregnation with silver. This tissue is always associated with endothelium.

There are certain scavenger cells called macrophages, and they are found in the reticular tissue framework of lymph nodes and spleen; in the lining cells of the sinusoids of the liver, adrenal gland, and hypophysis; and in the outer covering of blood capillaries.

Some of the macrophages arise from cells in areolar connective tissue, others from the monocytes of blood and probably from the lymphocytes, and some from cells of reticular tissue. These cells, macrophages, have the ability to take up small particles of foreign substance and colloidal dyes. In the lung, they ingest particles of dust. In the spleen and liver, they pick up worn-out erythrocytes. In lymph nodes, they frequently contain any substance that has found its way into the lymph. They tend to increase in areas of local inflammation and are one of the defense mechanisms mobilized by the body to combat infections. In the liver, they are called Kupffer cells. All of the macrophages and the reticular tissues are grouped together as the reticuloendothelial system.

Muscle, tendon, and ligaments

Muscle. Muscle, the contractile tissue of the body, is composed of units that have the power of contraction under stimulation. Muscles under the control of the will, such as those of the limbs, are known as voluntary; the others, such as those of the digestive and cardiovascular systems, are involuntary. Muscles used in walking, writing, and speaking fall into the voluntary category and are also known as skeletal muscles. These are also called striated muscles because the cytoplasm of the cells has fine transverse bands microscopically visible in longitudinal sections. In striated muscles the individual cells, known as fibers because of their elongated shape, lie in parallel lines with their nuclei found on the surface of individual fibers. Each fiber is a long cylinder and usually contains several round or oval nuclei located at the periphery. The fibers are arranged in compact bundles separated by fine connective tissue sheaths. These fine sheaths are septa extending into the muscle from an outer connective tissue sheath that invests the entire muscle (Fig. 2-13).

22

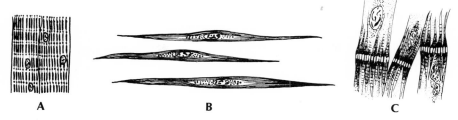

Fig. 2-13. Muscle. **A,** Section of striate fibers. **B,** Smooth muscle cells. **C,** Section of cardiac muscle, fibers artificially separated.

The muscles of the stomach, intestines, and blood vessels belong to the group of involuntary muscles over which there is no direct conscious control. They are also called nonstriate or smooth muscles because their cytoplasm has no transverse striations. Cardiac muscle fibers anastomose with each other, and the nuclei are found in the central portion of the fibers.

Smooth muscle cells are long and fusiform; the nucleus is located in the central part of the cell. In the walls of hollow viscera, smooth muscle bundles may be disposed in longitudinal, circular, or oblique coats, or they may be interwoven. The stomach has three coats: longitudinal, circular, and oblique; the intestine has two coats: longitudinal and circular. In the uterus the muscle bundles are interwoven.

Tendon. Most muscles secure an attachment to bone by means of tendons. These are compact parallel bundles of dense white connective tissue. However, certain muscles are attached directly to bone.

Ligaments. Ligaments attaching bone to bone are composed of white fibrous connective tissue, but the arrangement of the fiber bundles is irregular, and the tissue is usually sheetlike in form.

Nerve tissue

In the brain and spinal cord, in addition to nerve cells or neurons, there are many supporting cells collectively called neuroglia. The neuroglia, of various sizes and shapes, are characterized by small oval nuclei and long branching processes that are closely interwoven. Special staining methods are required to demonstrate these cells properly.

Nerve cells, or neurons, are specialized for the conduction of impulses from one part of the body to another. A neuron consists of a cell body and its processes. The cell body contains a nucleus and a surrounding mass of cytoplasm. The processes (afferent) that bring impulses to the cell body are called dendrites, and the process (efferent) that conducts impulses away from the cell body is called the axon. In newer terminology the term dendrite is restricted to the dendritic zone or receptor membrane of a neuron. Impulse conduction is always

23

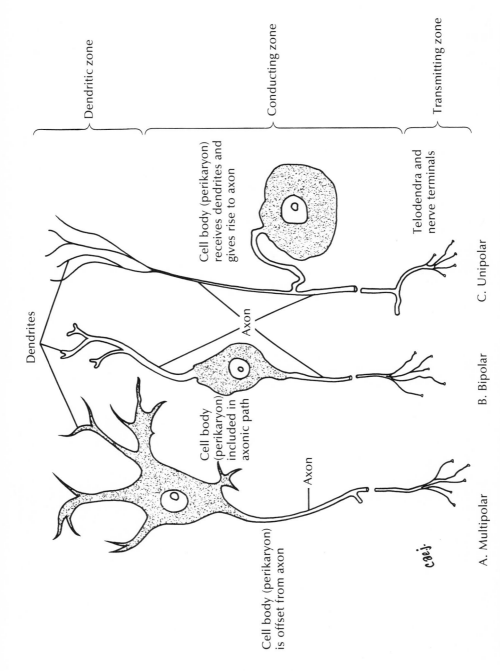

Fig. 2-14. Main types of nerve cells. Perikarya are tracings from photographs. (From Minckler, J.: Introduction to neuroscience, St. Louis, 1972, The C. V. Mosby Co.)

away from the dendritic zone and toward the cell body and is carried by a process designated as an axon. In the dorsal root ganglia, the cytoplasmic process extending towards the periphery is now known as a peripheral axon, and the process extending toward the central nervous system is called the central axon (Fig. 2-14). Neurons may be divided into three main categories based on the number of processes arising from the cell body: (1) unipolar are found exclusively in sensory ganglia, which are collections of sensory neurons located outside the central nervous system, and have one T-shaped process formed by fusion of dendrite and axon near the cell body, (2) bipolar have one axon and one dendrite and are characteristically found in the specialized sensory systems of vision, audition, and olfaction, and (3) multipolar form the majority of neurons and have one axon and more than one dendrite (Fig. 2-14).

A nerve trunk is composed of bundles of nerve processes, afferent and efferent, surrounded by a sheath of connective tissue. Many nerve processes have a sheath of fatty substance called myelin, a very effective insulator. The myelin is constricted at regular intervals along

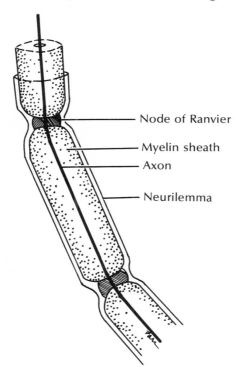

Node of Ranvier

Myelin sheath

Axon

Neurilemma

Fig. 2-15. Diagram of an axon and coverings. (From Anthony, C. P., and Kolthoff, N. J.: Textbook of anatomy and physiology, ed. 8, St. Louis, 1971, The C. V. Mosby Co.)

25

the axon forming the nodes of Ranvier. Although neurophysiology is beyond the scope of this book, it can be stated that in myelinated fibers, depolarization occurs only at the nodes; thus, the impulse or wave jumps from node to node, a phenomenon called "saltatory conduction." This type of conduction allows the speed of an impulse to be increased, since depolarization need only occur at the nodes of Ranvier to propagate a nerve impulse (Fig. 2-15).

Outside the myelin sheath is a second sheath, the neurilemma, which is a thin delicate membrane. The ends of the axons have no sheath. Some thin axons have a neurilemma but no myelin sheath, although in the autonomic nervous system, some axons are completely devoid of any sheath and are called "naked axons."

SUMMARY OF CELL REPRODUCTION

There is considerable variation in the ability of cells to produce new cells. It has been pointed out that blood cells are replaced constantly. All types of epithelium are renewed rapidly. Supporting tissues are replenished, and this is especially evident in repair following injury. Voluntary muscle increases in size (hypertrophy) in response to increased exercise, but an increase in number of cells (hyperplasia) does not occur. There is little, if any, increase in the number of nerve cells after birth.

In tumor formation there is an increase in the number of cells, but this is not a response to the healthy needs of the body. The new cells are usually abnormal in size, shape, and content.

REVIEW QUESTIONS

1. Name three organelles that can be seen in a cell and give one function for each.
2. Name four tissues.
3. Give one location in the body for each of the following epithelia: simple squamous epithelium, stratified squamous epithelium, simple columnar epithelium, and transitional epithelium.
4. How are exocrine and endocrine glands distinguished?
5. Where would you find each of the following: mucous membrane, serous membrane, and synovial membrane?
6. Describe briefly dense fibrous connective tissue. Give one location.
7. What is the distinguishing type of cell in adipose tissue?
8. What is the distinctive characteristic of yellow elastic connective tissue? Give one location in the body where it is found.
9. Distinguish between a cartilage and a bone lacuna.
10. Define perichondrium.
11. What is red marrow? Where is it found in an adult?
12. What is yellow marrow?
13. What are the distinguishing features of voluntary, smooth, and cardiac muscle?
14. What is the difference between the axon and a dendrite of a nerve cell?
15. Name five kinds of cells in blood.
16. How many red and white cells are normally present in one cubic millimeter of blood?
17. What cells are formed in myeloid tissue?
18. What is the difference between hypertrophy and hyperplasia?

26

HUMAN ANATOMY

FULL-COLOR PLATES WITH SIX IN TRANSPARENT

"TRANS-VISION"® SHOWING STRUCTURES OF THE HUMAN TORSO

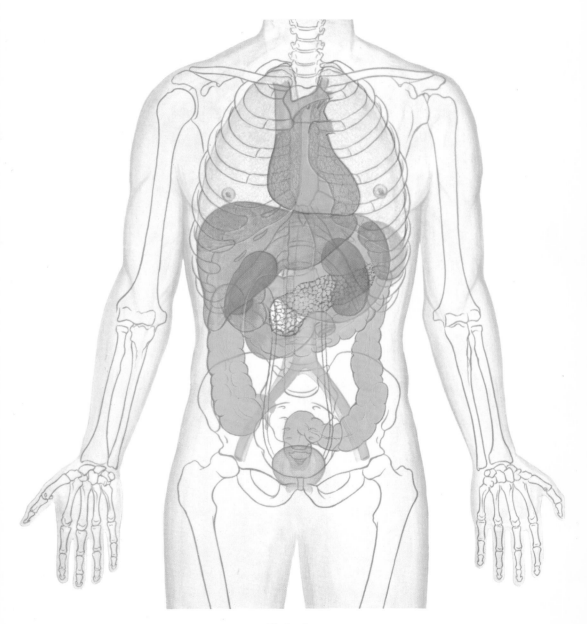

Plate I

ERNEST W. BECK, medical illustrator

in collaboration with
HARRY MONSEN , Ph.D.
Professor of Anatomy, College of Medicine, University of Illinois

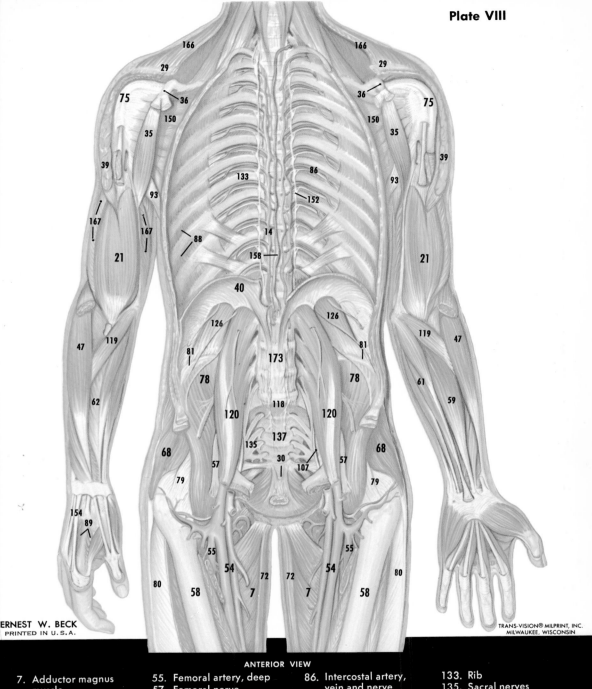

Plate VIII

ANTERIOR VIEW

ERNEST W. BECK
PRINTED IN U.S.A.

TRANS-VISION® MILPRINT, INC.
MILWAUKEE, WISCONSIN

Plate IX

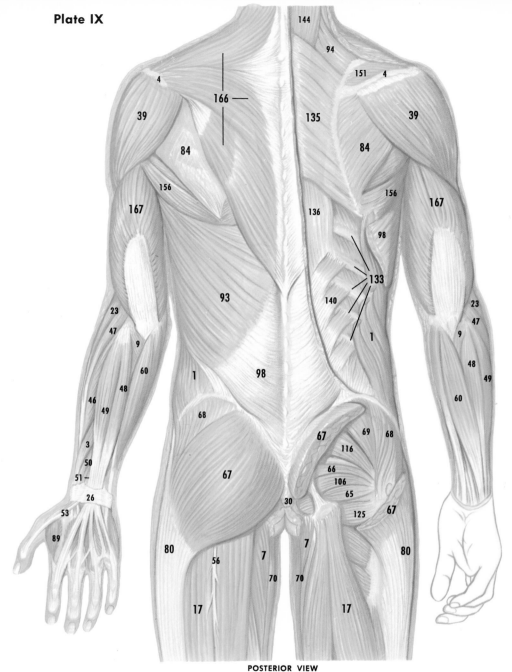

POSTERIOR VIEW

1. Abdominal oblique muscle, external
3. Abductor pollicis longus muscle
4. Acromion process of the scapula
7. Adductor magnus muscle
9. Anconeus muscle
17. Biceps femoris muscle
23. Brachioradialis muscle
26. Carpal ligament, dorsal
30. Coccyx
39. Deltoid muscle
46. Extensor carpi radialis brevis muscle

47. Extensor carpi radialis longus muscle
48. Extensor carpi ulnaris muscle
49. Extensor digitorum communis muscle
50. Extensor pollicis brevis muscle
51. Extensor pollicis longus muscle
56. Femoral cutaneous nerve, posterior
60. Flexor carpi ulnaris muscle
65. Gemellus inferior muscle

66. Gemellus superior muscle
67. Gluteus maximus muscle
68. Gluteus medius muscle
69. Gluteus minimus muscle
70. Gracilis muscle
80. Iliotibial tract
84. Infraspinatus muscle
89. Interosseous muscle, dorsal
93. Latissimus dorsi muscle
94. Levator scapulae muscle
98. Lumbodorsal fascia

106. Obturator internus muscle
116. Piriformis muscle
125. Quadratus femoris muscle
133. Ribs (VII-XII)
135. Rhomboideus muscle
136. Erector spinae muscle
140. Serratus posterior inferior muscle
144. Splenius capitis muscle
151. Supraspinatus muscle
156. Teres major muscle
166. Trapezius muscle
167. Triceps brachii muscle

Plate X

BONES AND SINUSES OF THE SKULL

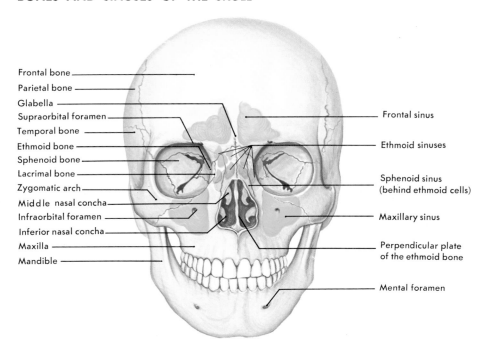

Frontal bone

Parietal bone

Glabella

Supraorbital foramen

Temporal bone

Ethmoid bone

Sphenoid bone

Lacrimal bone

Zygomatic arch

Middle nasal concha

Infraorbital foramen

Inferior nasal concha

Maxilla

Mandible

Frontal sinus

Ethmoid sinuses

Sphenoid sinus
(behind ethmoid cells)

Maxillary sinus

Perpendicular plate
of the ethmoid bone

Mental foramen

HEMISECTION OF THE HEAD AND NECK

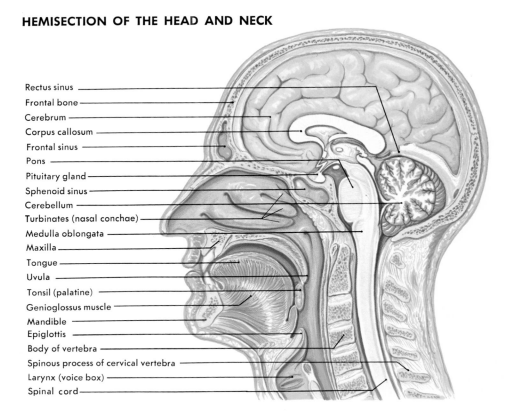

Rectus sinus

Frontal bone

Cerebrum

Corpus callosum

Frontal sinus

Pons

Pituitary gland

Sphenoid sinus

Cerebellum

Turbinates (nasal conchae)

Medulla oblongata

Maxilla

Tongue

Uvula

Tonsil (palatine)

Genioglossus muscle

Mandible

Epiglottis

Body of vertebra

Spinous process of cervical vertebra

Larynx (voice box)

Spinal cord

Plate XI

ANATOMY OF THE EAR

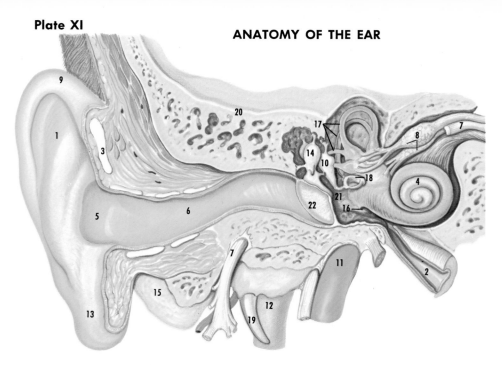

1. Anthelix	7. Facial nerve	12. Internal jugular vein	18. Stapes (stirrup)
2. Auditory tube	8. Ganglia of the vestibular nerve	13. Lobe	19. Styloid process
3. Cartilage	9. Helix	14. Malleus (hammer)	20. Temporal bone
4. Cochlea	10. Incus (anvil)	15. Mastoid process	21. Tympanic cavity
5. Concha	11. Internal carotid artery	16. Round window	22. Tympanic membrane (eardrum)
6. External acoustic meatus		17. Semicircular canals	

ANATOMY OF THE EYE

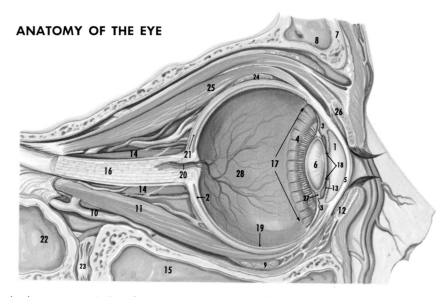

1. Aqueous chamber	8. Frontal sinus	15. Maxillary sinus	22. Sphenoid sinus
2. Choroid	9. Inferior oblique muscle	16. Optic nerve	23. Pterygopalatine ganglion
3. Ciliary muscle	10. Inferior ophthalmic vein	17. Ora serrata	24. Superior oblique muscle
4. Ciliary processes	11. Inferior rectus muscle	18. Pupil of the iris	25. Superior rectus muscle
5. Cornea	12. Inferior tarsus	19. Retina	26. Superior tarsus
6. Crystalline lens	13. Iris	20. Retinal artery and vein	27. Suspensory ligament
7. Frontal bone	14. Lateral rectus muscle	21. Sclera	28. Vitreous chamber

Plate XII

SCHEMATIC BODY CELL

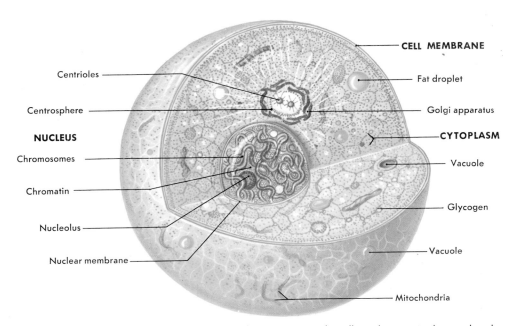

Centrioles —
Centrosphere —
NUCLEUS
Chromosomes —
Chromatin —
Nucleolus —
Nuclear membrane —

CELL MEMBRANE
Fat droplet
Golgi apparatus
CYTOPLASM
Vacuole
Glycogen
Vacuole
Mitochondria

Every living cell, regardless of its shape or size, has three main parts: the cell membrane, cytoplasm, and nucleus. Together they constitute protoplasm. Billions of such cells as shown above make up the tissues of our bodies.

TYPES OF CELLS

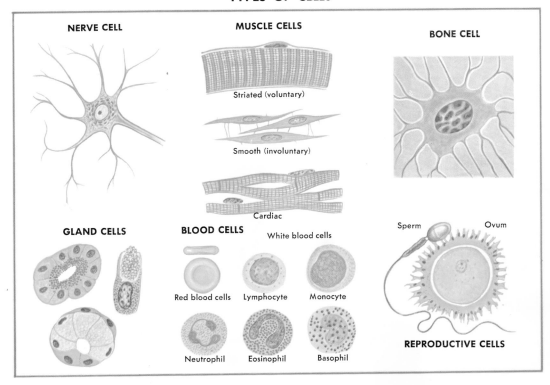

NERVE CELL

MUSCLE CELLS

Striated (voluntary)

Smooth (involuntary)

Cardiac

BONE CELL

GLAND CELLS

BLOOD CELLS

White blood cells

Red blood cells   Lymphocyte   Monocyte

Neutrophil   Eosinophil   Basophil

Sperm   Ovum

REPRODUCTIVE CELLS

Plate XIII

SKELETON

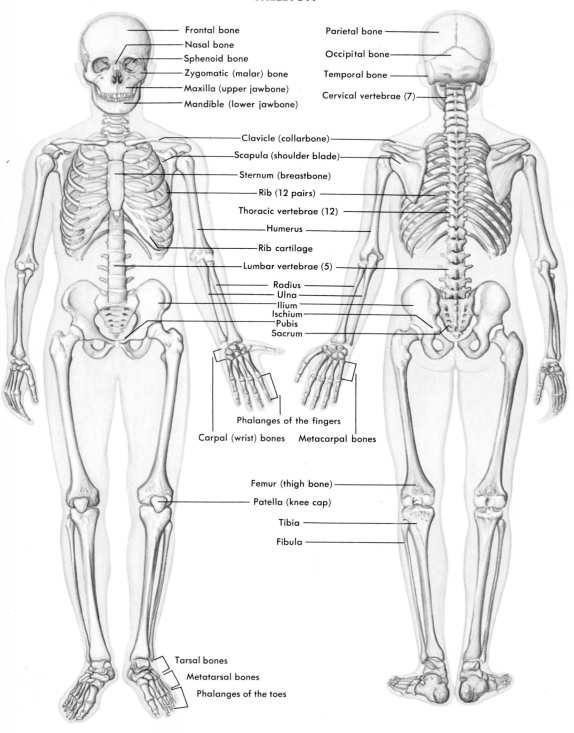

Frontal bone

Nasal bone

Sphenoid bone

Zygomatic (malar) bone

Maxilla (upper jawbone)

Mandible (lower jawbone)

Parietal bone

Occipital bone

Temporal bone

Cervical vertebrae (7)

Clavicle (collarbone)

Scapula (shoulder blade)

Sternum (breastbone)

Rib (12 pairs)

Thoracic vertebrae (12)

Humerus

Rib cartilage

Lumbar vertebrae (5)

Radius

Ulna

Ilium

Ischium

Pubis

Sacrum

Phalanges of the fingers

Carpal (wrist) bones

Metacarpal bones

Femur (thigh bone)

Patella (knee cap)

Tibia

Fibula

Tarsal bones

Metatarsal bones

Phalanges of the toes

Plate XIV

FEMALE PELVIC ORGANS

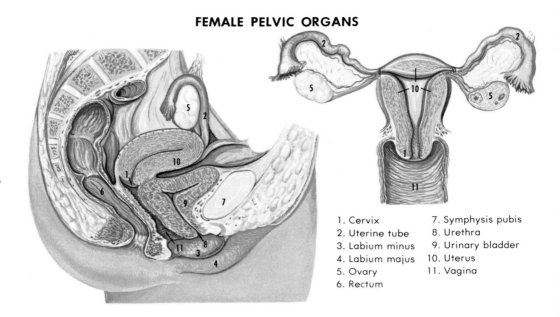

1. Cervix	7. Symphysis pubis
2. Uterine tube	8. Urethra
3. Labium minus	9. Urinary bladder
4. Labium majus	10. Uterus
5. Ovary	11. Vagina
6. Rectum	

MALE PELVIC ORGANS

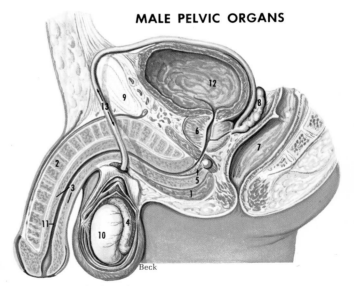

Beck

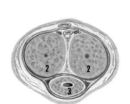

SECTION THROUGH PENIS

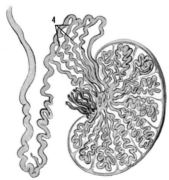

**SCHEME OF DUCT ARRANGEMENT
IN THE TESTIS AND EPIDIDYMIS**

1. Bulb of urethra	7. Rectum
2. Corpus cavernosum	8. Seminal vesicle
3. Corpus spongiosum	9. Symphysis pubis
4. Epididymis	10. Testis
5. Duct of bulbourethral	11. Urethra
gland	12. Urinary bladder
6. Prostate gland	13. Ductus deferens

Plate XV

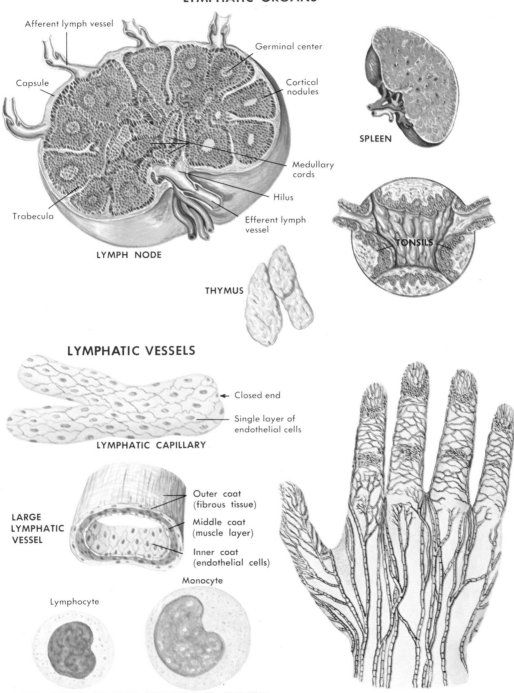

LYMPHATIC ORGANS

Afferent lymph vessel

Germinal center

Cortical nodules

Capsule

SPLEEN

Medullary cords

Hilus

Trabecula

Efferent lymph vessel

TONSILS

LYMPH NODE

THYMUS

LYMPHATIC VESSELS

Closed end

Single layer of endothelial cells

LYMPHATIC CAPILLARY

Outer coat (fibrous tissue)

Middle coat (muscle layer)

LARGE LYMPHATIC VESSEL

Inner coat (endothelial cells)

Monocyte

Lymphocyte

FREE CELLS OF THE LYMPHATIC SYSTEM

LYMPHATICS OF THE HAND

CHAPTER 3

THE SKELETON

The skeleton, composed normally of 206 bones and associated cartilage, is the rigid framework of the body (Plate XIII, Transvision). There are two main subdivisions of the skeleton: (1) the axial, which includes the bones of the head, neck, and trunk and (2) the appendicular, which includes the bones of the extremities. In addition, seedlike bones called sesamoids are found near the attachment of certain tendons of hand, foot, and knee. The patella, or kneecap, found in the quadriceps tendon anterior to the knee joint, is the largest sesamoid bone. In the sutures of the skull, discrete ossicles of varied size and shape, called sutural or wormian bones, are occasionally found.

Besides providing support, the skeleton performs four other important functions: (1) protection: the skull and vertebral column protect the central nervous system, the rib cage protects heart, lungs, liver, and spleen, and the bony pelvis guards the female organs of reproduction; (2) attachment of muscles: body position and movement are determined by the contraction of muscles, which change the relation of one bone to another; (3) hemopoiesis: the red bone marrow is a blood-forming organ; and (4) mineral storage: bones serve as storage sites, especially for calcium (99% of body calcium is found in bone).

Bones may be classified according to their shape, for example:

1. *Long bones:* humerus, femur, radius, ulna, tibia, fibula, and phalanges. Long bones with associated musculature form a system of levers that provides for locomotion and prehension.
2. *Short bones:* carpals, tarsals. Short bones are found where compactness and limited motion are required.

27

3. *Flat bones:* cranial bones, such as parietal, frontal, occipital, and temporal, as well as ribs, scapulae, and sternum. Flat bones confer protection and provide a broad area for muscle attachment.
4. *Irregular bones:* vertebrae, sphenoid, ethmoid, mandible, sacrum, and coccyx. Irregular bones protect against compressive forces.

Bones may also be classified on the basis of their *development.* The first evidence of the skeleton in the human embryo is a thickening of the mesenchyme at the sites of future bones and cartilage. About the sixth week in utero, some of the mesenchymal cells differentiate into chondroblasts and lay down a cartilage matrix. Further growth results in the formation of a cartilage model for a major portion of the skeleton, a process called endochondral ossification.

In a limited region, namely the skeleton of the cranial vault and face, the mesenchymal cells lay down a fibrous tissue membrane as the foundation for future bone formation. In these areas the cartilaginous phase is absent, and the process is called intramembranous ossification. Between the sixth and eighth weeks of fetal development, centers of ossification appear in the central area of the membrane, and bone formation radiates out toward the periphery. At birth, appreciable areas at the margins of the cranial vault bones are still membranous (Figs. 3-1 and 3-2). These areas of incomplete ossification are called fontanelles. The largest, the anterior fontanelle, is in the midline between the two parietal bones and the frontal bone. Between the

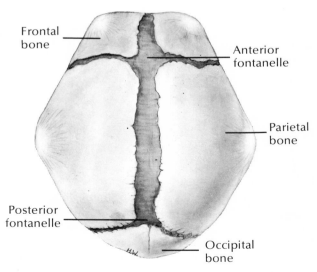

Frontal bone

Anterior fontanelle

Parietal bone

Posterior fontanelle

Occipital bone

Fig. 3-1. Skull at birth, superior view. (Male, term fetus.)

parietals and the occipital bone is a smaller area called the posterior or occipital fontanelle. At birth, since much of the brain case is still membranous, the skull may be molded into various irregular shapes during delivery. These irregularities usually disappear during the first few months of life. A physician may secure samples of blood from an infant by passing a hypodermic needle through the anterior fontanelle into the superior sagittal venous sinus, which lies in the midline just below the vault of the skull.

Let us now return to a discussion of the cartilage model and outline the events by which cartilage is replaced by bone, a process called endochondral ossification. At approximately the end of the second month of fetal life (seventh to eighth week) the cartilage cells located at the center of the diaphysis (shaft) of future long bones and in the body of irregular bones hypertrophy; the matrix becomes calcified, and the cells die. An osteogenic mesenchymal bud, consisting of blood vessels, bone-forming cells (osteoblasts), and primitive marrow cells, penetrates into and breaks up the cartilages in these areas, and bone is laid down on the framework of the calcified cartilage. This constitutes a primary ossification center (Fig. 3-3). It is important to appreciate that the cartilage is not converted into bone but is replaced by bone. Ossification extends in both directions within the shaft of long bones and radiates outward toward the periphery of irregular bones. In man at the time of birth the shafts of long bones and the bodies of some irregular bones are ossified, although the ends, epiphyses, of

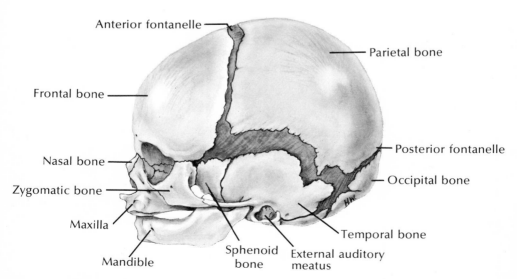

Fig. 3-2. Skull at birth, lateral view. (Male, term fetus.)   29

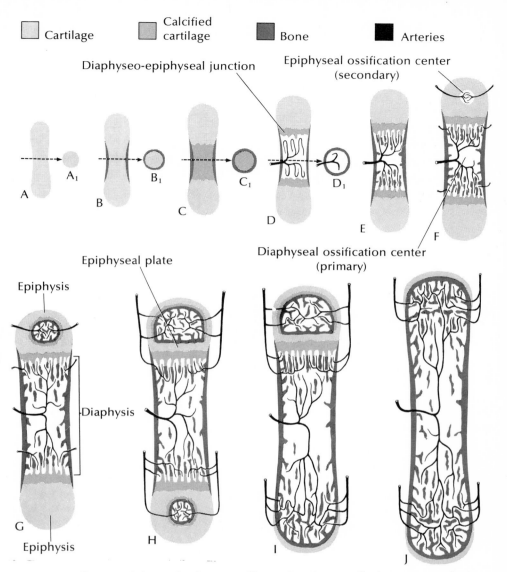

Fig. 3-3. Schematic diagrams illustrating intracartilaginous or endochondral ossification and the development of a typical long bone. A to J are longitudinal sections, and A_1 to D_1 are cross sections at the levels indicated. **A,** Cartilage model of the bone. **B,** A subperiosteal ring of bone appears. **C,** Cartilage begins to calcify. **D,** Vascular mesenchyme enters the calcified cartilage. **E,** At each diaphyseo-epiphyseal junction there is a zone of ossification. **F,** Blood vessels and mesenchyme enter the upper epiphyseal cartilage. **G,** The epiphyseal ossification center grows. **H,** A similar center develops in the lower epiphyseal cartilage. **I,** The lower epiphyseal plate is ossified. **J,** The upper epiphyseal plate ossifies, forming a continuous bone marrow cavity. When the epiphyseal plates ossify, the bone can no longer grow in length. (Modified after Bloom and Fawcett, 1968; from Moore, K. L.: The developing human, Philadelphia, 1973, W. B. Saunders Company.)

long bones and the margins and processes of irregular bones remain cartilaginous.

Just before birth, during the ninth fetal month, a second phase in the ossification of the skeleton begins. It consists of a process similar to the establishment of the primary ossification center that now occurs in the cartilaginous ends of the long bones and in the margins and processes of irregular bones. This new bone formation is called secondary ossification, and a particular bone may have one or more such secondary centers. They appear progressively throughout the skeleton from approximately the time of birth to the fifteenth to twentieth year of life. However, during the growing period of the individual the epiphyses are not completely ossified. A narrow strip of cartilage remains between the shaft and the ends of long bones and between the body and the margins of irregular bones. This strip is known as the epiphyseal cartilage or plate, and it plays a significant role in bone growth.

There is no growth of bone tissue per se. There is interstitial growth in cartilage, but there is no interstitial growth of bone because of the mineralization of the interstitial tissue. Such growth is the unique role of the epiphyseal plate or cartilage. Continuous proliferation of cells in the midregion of the epiphyseal plate produces new tissue and increases the length of the bone. Concomitantly there is maturation and replacement of the newly formed cartilage at the edges of the plate, predominately on the diaphyseal (shaft) side. This is the mechanism by which long bones increase in length without an apparent increase in the width of the epiphyseal cartilage. A similar process increases the size of irregular bones. When the individual reaches his mature stature, growth of the epiphyseal cartilages ceases. However, replacement of the cartilage by bone continues and soon the epiphysis and the diaphysis are fused by bone (Figs. 3-4 to 3-10).

The periosteum performs an equally significant role in bone formation. Its inner layer (osteogenic) is made up largely of osteoblasts that lay down bone in a manner much like the growth rings of a tree. There is no intermediate cartilage formation; this is another example of intramembranous ossification and accounts for the major portion of the adult long bone.

Two other phenomena that must be included as essential to an understanding of bone growth are (1) the relative amount of growth at the proximal and distal epiphysis of a long bone and (2) the maintenance of the characteristic shape and proportions of bone during the growing period.

One might assume an equal contribution to the growth of a bone from each epiphysis. This is not so. The proximal and distal epiphy-

3 MONTHS

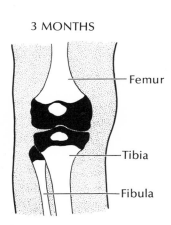

Femur

Tibia

Fibula

Fig. 3-4

1 YEAR

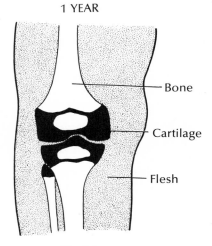

Bone

Cartilage

Flesh

Fig. 3-5

2 YEARS

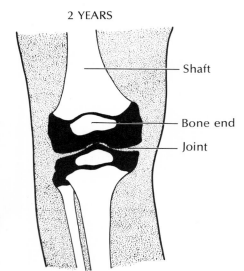

Shaft

Bone end

Joint

Fig. 3-6

5 YEARS

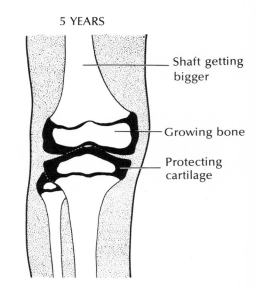

Shaft getting
bigger

Growing bone

Protecting
cartilage

Fig. 3-7

Fig. 3-4. Ossification of male knee at 3 months of age. (Traced from roentgenogram.)

Fig. 3-5. Ossification of male knee at 1 year of age. (Traced from roentgenogram.)

Fig. 3-6. Ossification of male knee at 2 years of age. (Traced from roentgenogram.)

Fig. 3-7. Ossification of male knee at 5 years of age. (Traced from roentgenogram.)

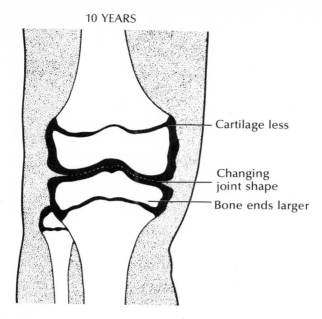

10 YEARS

Cartilage less

Changing
joint shape

Bone ends larger

Fig. 3-8. Ossification of male knee at 10 years of age. (Traced from roentgenogram.)

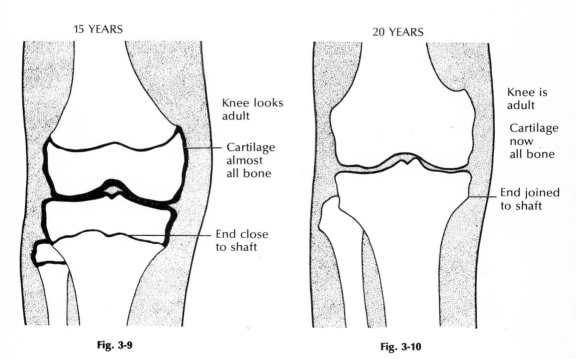

15 YEARS

Knee looks
adult

Cartilage
almost
all bone

End close
to shaft

Fig. 3-9

20 YEARS

Knee is
adult

Cartilage
now
all bone

End joined
to shaft

Fig. 3-10

Fig. 3-9. Ossification of male knee at 15 years of age. (Traced from roentgenogram.)
Fig. 3-10. Ossification of male knee at 20 years of age. (Traced from roentgenogram.)

33

seal cartilages contribute unequally to the total increase in length. The end contributing the greater or lesser share varies among the several bones but is constant for individual bones. The end in which a secondary center first appears is the last to unite with the shaft; therefore, this end grows for the longer period of time and contributes the most to the total length of the bone. In the event of injury or disease to an epiphysis the ultimate degree of limb shortening would depend upon which epiphysis was affected.

The maintenance of the appropriate shape and proportions of a bone is achieved by constant remodeling during the growing period. This is clearly illustrated in a long bone by the relative circumference of the shaft and the diameter of the medullary canal. As the osteoblasts (bone builders) add layers of bone under the periosteum, osteoclasts (bone destroyers) excavate the marrow canal proportionately. This concomitant activity of osteoblast and osteoclast throughout the growing skeleton is the essence of the remodeling process.

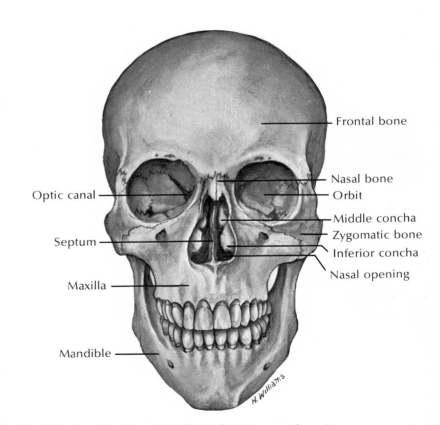

34   **Fig. 3-11.** Anterior view of skull. (Male, 25 years of age.)

The skull is composed of 21 bones closely joined together and one, the lower jaw or mandible, that is freely movable. To this may be added the three ossicles in each middle ear cavity.

The skull has certain very obvious features that are easy to identify and that should be learned before the separate bones are studied (Figs. 3-11 and 3-12). On the anterior aspect of the skull are the orbits, two large sockets lodging the eyeballs. Superior to them are the supraorbital ridges, and between and inferior to the orbits is the pear-shaped nasal opening subdivided by the nasal septum into two lateral halves. The scrolls of bone attached to either side wall of the nasal cavity are the conchae, or turbinates. The small, round, external ear opening (external auditory meatus) is in the lower part of the side of the skull. The zygomatic arch, or cheek bone, springs posteriorly from the side of the skull above and in front of the ear opening and is attached anteriorly to the face below the lateral edge of the orbit. The temporal fossa is the space superior to the zygomatic arch and posterior to the orbit. The mastoid process is the heavy projection of bone posterior and inferior to the external ear opening. On the undersurface of the skull is the large opening, the foramen magnum, through which

BONES OF THE SKULL

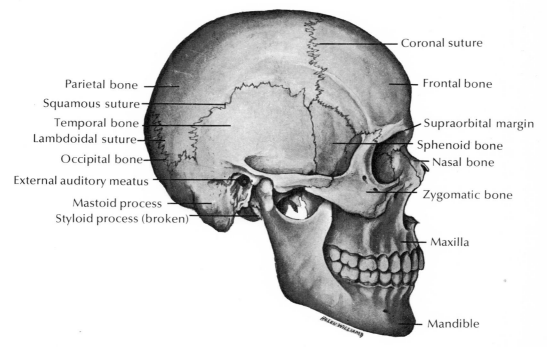

Fig. 3-12. Lateral view of skull. (Male, 25 years of age.)

35

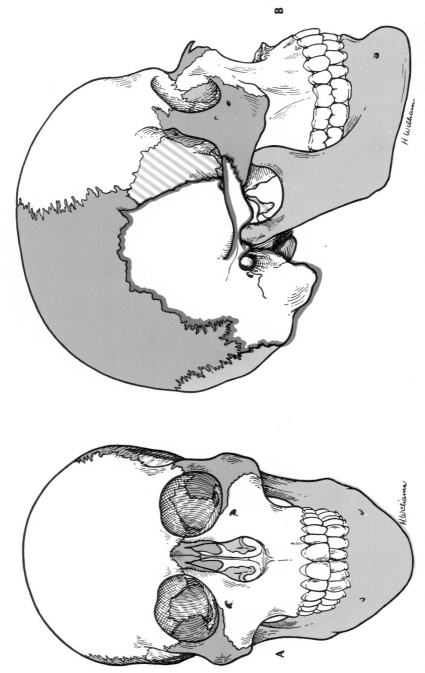

Fig. 3-13. A, Anterior view of skull (same skull as shown in Fig. 3-11). Solid blue, mandible, inferior concha; blue hatched, sphenoid; solid red, nasal, zygomatic ethmoid, and parietal bones; red outline, temporal; other bones uncolored. **B,** Lateral view of skull (same skull as shown in Fig. 3-12). Solid blue, mandible, occipital, and lacrimal bones; blue hatched, sphenoid; solid red, nasal, zygomatic, and parietal bones; red outline, temporal; other bones uncolored.

the spinal cord emerges. About 5 cm in front of that are the two choanae, or posterior openings of the nose. The hard palate, or roof of the mouth, forms the floor of the nose. The upper teeth are lodged in a rampart of bone known as the alveolar process, which forms a horseshoelike border for the hard palate. If the top of the skull is removed, the floor of the brain case is seen to consist of three large uneven areas called the anterior, middle, and posterior cranial fossae.

Frontal bone. The frontal bone is a saucer-shaped bone forming the forehead, the upper part of the orbit, the anterior portion of the anterior cranial fossa, and a part of the septum between the brain case and nasal cavity. There is a notch (or sometimes a foramen) in the supraorbital margin through which the supraorbital nerve passes. In the upper lateral part of the orbit there is a shallow depression for the lacrimal gland.

In the embryo the frontal bone is formed from two equal parts, with a suture in the midline that sometimes persists into adult life as the metopic suture.

In the substance of the frontal bone above the orbits are two large irregular cavities, the frontal sinuses, which communicate with the nasal cavity. These are further described in the discussion on air sinuses in Chapter 11.

Parietal bones. Each of the parietal bones is shaped rather like a square saucer and forms the upper portion of the side of the skull. On the inner surface there are well-marked grooves radiating upward from the inferior border of the bone for the middle meningeal blood vessels and there are shallow impressions produced by the gyri of the cerebrum.

Occipital bone. The occipital bone constitutes the back and a large part of the base of the skull. The part posterior to the foramen magnum is the squamous portion, which forms most of the posterior cranial fossa. The external occipital protuberance is a well-marked projection in the midline, halfway up the back of the bone. The superior nuchal line, an attachment site for muscles, extends laterally to either side of this projection.

The internal occipital protuberance is the central projection on the inner surface of the squamous portion. Extending upward from this landmark is the sulcus for the superior sagittal blood sinus, and extending to either side is a lateral sulcus for a transverse blood sinus. The occipital poles of the cerebral hemispheres lie in the fossae superior to these lateral sulci and the cerebellar hemispheres lie in the fossae inferiorly.

The lateral parts of the occipital bone lie on either side of the foramen magnum. The smooth, convex area on the inferior surface on

37

Text continued on p. 42.

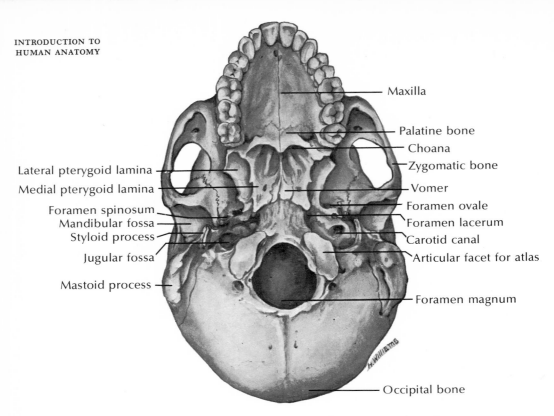

Maxilla

Palatine bone

Choana

Lateral pterygoid lamina

Zygomatic bone

Medial pterygoid lamina

Vomer

Foramen ovale

Foramen spinosum

Foramen lacerum

Mandibular fossa

Styloid process

Carotid canal

Jugular fossa

Articular facet for atlas

Mastoid process

Foramen magnum

Occipital bone

Fig. 3-14. Undersurface of skull. (Male, 25 years of age.)

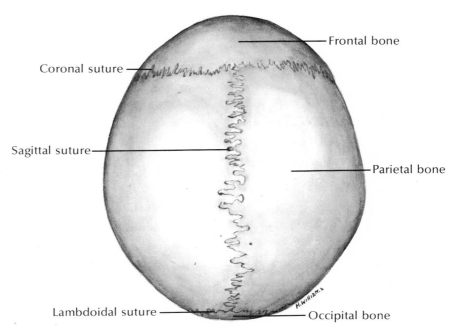

Frontal bone

Coronal suture

Sagittal suture

Parietal bone

Lambdoidal suture

Occipital bone

Fig. 3-15. Vault of skull. (Male, 25 years of age.)

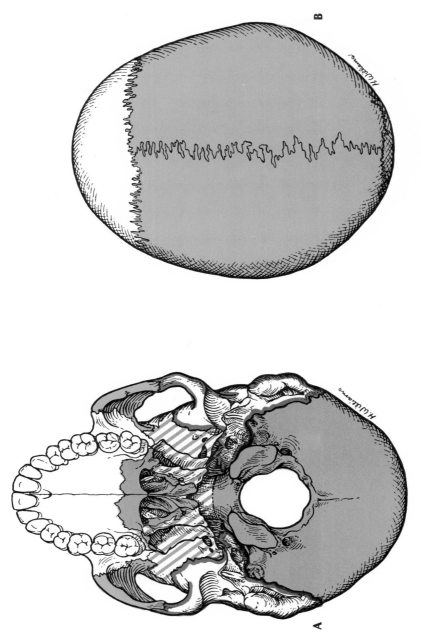

Fig. 3-16. A, Base of skull (same skull as shown in Fig. 3-14). Solid blue, occipital and palatine bones; blue hatched, sphenoid; solid red, vomer and zygomatic bones; red outline, temporal bone; maxilla uncolored. **B,** Vault of skull (same skull as shown in Fig. 3-15). Solid blue, occipital bone; solid red, parietal bones; frontal bone uncolored.

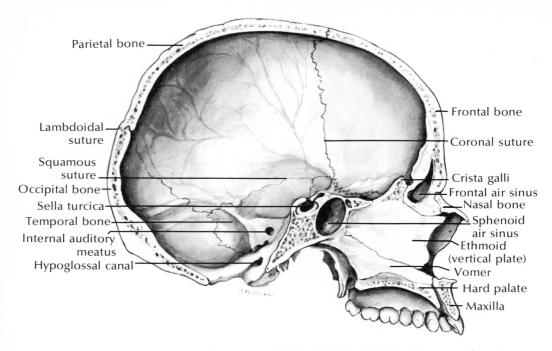

Parietal bone

Lambdoidal suture

Squamous suture

Occipital bone

Sella turcica

Temporal bone

Internal auditory meatus

Hypoglossal canal

Frontal bone

Coronal suture

Crista galli

Frontal air sinus

Nasal bone

Sphenoid air sinus

Ethmoid (vertical plate)

Vomer

Hard palate

Maxilla

Fig. 3-17. Sagittal section of left half of skull. (Male, 25 years of age.)

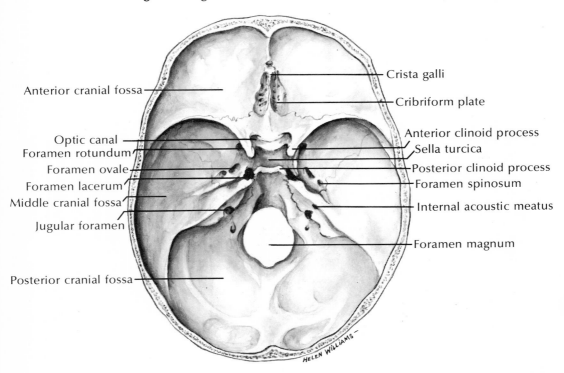

Anterior cranial fossa

Optic canal

Foramen rotundum

Foramen ovale

Foramen lacerum

Middle cranial fossa

Jugular foramen

Posterior cranial fossa

Crista galli

Cribriform plate

Anterior clinoid process

Sella turcica

Posterior clinoid process

Foramen spinosum

Internal acoustic meatus

Foramen magnum

HELEN WILLIAMS

Fig. 3-18. Floor of cranial cavity. Petrous portions of temporal bones asymmetrical. (Male, 25 years of age.)

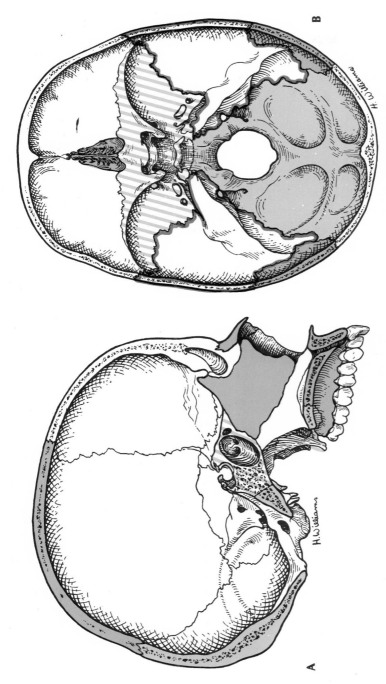

Fig. 3-19. A, Sagittal section of left half of skull (same skull as shown in Fig. 3-17). Solid blue, occipital and palatine bones; solid red, maxilla, parietal, ethmoid, and nasal bones; blue hatched, sphenoid; maxilla colored to distinguish it from vomer. **B,** Floor of cranial cavity (same skull as shown in Fig. 3-18). Solid blue, occipital bone; solid red, parietal and ethmoid bones; blue hatched, sphenoid; red outline, temporal; other bones uncolored.

41

each side is the occipital condyle for articulation with the first cervical vertebra or atlas. A channel through the bone above this articular surface transmits the twelfth cranial nerve on its way to the tongue and, therefore, is called the canal for the hypoglossal nerve. The terminal portion of the transverse sinus, the sigmoid sinus, grooves the deep surface of the lateral part of the occipital bone.

The basilar part of the occipital bone is the heavy bar extending anteriorly from the foramen magnum to the body of the sphenoid.

Temporal bones. The temporal bone forms a part of the lateral wall of the skull as well as of the base. The large, winglike, squamous portion forms the lateral wall of the middle cranial fossa. The mastoid portion forms the prominence that can be felt posterior to the ear. Within the substance of the mastoid are air cells connected with the middle ear cavity. The long, slender, bony spike extending inferiorly and anteriorly, medial to the mastoid process, is the styloid process. (This is frequently broken off in dry skulls.) To the styloid are attached several important muscles and ligaments of the neck. Just anterior to the root of the styloid is the round, smooth, mandibular fossa for the lodgment of the head of the mandible.

The inner surface of the mastoid is grooved by the distal or sigmoid portion of the transverse blood sinus. This portion of the blood sinus is separated from the mastoid air cells by a thin plate of bone, and infections occasionally extend from the mastoid air cells to the sinus, causing lateral sinus thrombosis.

The petrous portion of the temporal bone is an uneven, wedge-shaped projection lying mainly in the floor of the middle cranial fossa between the great wing of the sphenoid and the lateral border of the basilar part of the occipital bone. This wedge of bone also forms part of the posterior fossa of the skull. On this face of the petrous portion of the temporal bone can be seen the internal acoustic meatus, which transmits the eighth cranial nerve to the internal ear, and the seventh cranial nerve, which passes through the petrous portion to emerge at the stylomastoid foramen just posterior to the root of the styloid process. Within the petrous portion are the cavities of the middle and inner ear. On the undersurface there is a depression, the jugular fossa, for the dilated beginning of the internal jugular vein.

In the line of articulation between the petrous portion of the temporal bone and the basal portion of the occiput are two important openings. The anterior and more medial slitlike opening is the foramen lacerum. The jugular foramen is the more posterior and lateral opening through which pass the internal jugular vein and the ninth, tenth, and eleventh cranial nerves. Superiorly the jugular foramen leads into the posterior cranial fossa. The carotid canal is a channel within the petrous portion that transmits the internal carotid artery. This canal begins just anterior to the jugular foramen and takes a curved path through the bone to emerge above at the foramen lacerum. In the fissure between the anterior border of the petrous portion and the posterior edge of the great wing of the sphenoid there is an irregular opening that is the inner end of the bony part of the auditory tube (eustachian tube).

Sphenoid bone. The sphenoid bone is quite irregular in shape and somewhat resembles a butterfly with its two pairs of outspread wings (Fig. 3-20). It forms part of the floor of the anterior cranial fossa above the eyes and nose (small wings of sphenoid) and also part of the floor and lateral wall of the middle cranial fossa (great wings). The body of the sphenoid is shaped more or less like a cube, and its posterior portion extends backward in the midline into the posterior cranial fossa where it unites with the basilar part of the occipital. Within the substance of the central portion of the sphenoid are the sphenoid air sinuses. The pterygoid canal passes through the body of the sphenoid below and lateral to the air sinuses, each canal being about 1 cm from the midline and running horizontally posterior to anterior. The pit in the upper surface of the sphenoid bone superior to the air sinuses is the sella turcica for the lodgment of the hypophysis (pituitary gland).

The pterygoid processes of the sphenoid are downward projections from the body of the sphenoid flanking the posterior opening of the nose. The lower end of each process is subdivided into two thin, flat sheets of bone, the medial and lateral pterygoid plates or laminae.

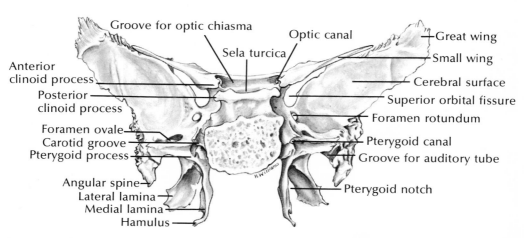

Fig. 3-20. Sphenoid bone, posterior view.

43

The lower end of the medial pterygoid plate ends in a hooklike process, the hamulus of the pterygoid.

The optic canal (foramen) is the round opening communicating with the orbit at the root of the lesser wing. Lateral to the optic canal is a long slit communicating with the orbit, known as the superior orbital fissure. The foramen rotundum is the opening at the base of the greater wing, and the foramen ovale pierces the lower portion of the greater wing.

The inferior orbital fissure is a cleft between those portions of the great wing of the sphenoid and the maxilla, which form the back of the orbit. The inferior orbital fissure is continuous posteriorly with a slit between the lateral pterygoid plate and the maxilla called the pterygomaxillary or pterygopalatine fissure.

Ethmoid bone. The ethmoid bone is very irregular in shape and difficult to define in a complete skull (Fig. 3-21). It lies anterior to the sphenoid between the eyes and forms part of the nasal roof where it is perforated by foramina for branches of the first cranial nerve. This sievelike plate, the lamina cribrosa or cribriform plate, helps to complete the floor of the anterior cranial fossa. The crista galli is the upward projection of the median perpendicular plate of the ethmoid between the two cribriform plates, and the upper part of the nasal septum is formed by the lower portion of the median plate. On each side of the median plate of the ethmoid bone is the lateral mass enclosing many small spaces, called the ethmoid air cells or ethmoid labyrinth, and bearing on its inner face the superior and middle nasal conchae, or turbinates, which are scroll-like leaves of bone projecting into the nose from its lateral wall. The medial wall of each orbit is formed by the outer face of the lateral mass of the ethmoid.

Nasal bones. Two small flat bones form the bridge of the nose.

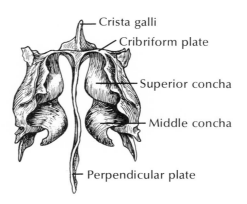

Crista galli
Cribriform plate
Superior concha
Middle concha
Perpendicular plate

Fig. 3-21. Ethmoid bone, posterior view. A semidiagrammatic drawing.

44

They articulate with each other in the midline and superiorly with the midportion of the frontal bone.

Lacrimal bones. Each lacrimal bone is a thin scalelike bone the size of a fingernail, lying in the medial wall of the orbit on the ethmoid bone and helping to form the side wall of the nasal cavity where it touches the maxilla and inferior nasal concha.

Maxillary bones. The maxillary bones constitute the anterior aspect of face and upper jaw, and each forms the floor of the corresponding orbit and lateral wall of the lower part of the nasal cavity. Within the central portion or body is a large air sinus called the maxillary sinus, which communicates with the nasal cavity.

The orbital surface is marked off from the facial surface by a ridge of bone that forms the lower and medial half of the orbital opening. Just below the lateral part of this ridge is the infraorbital foramen.

The zygomatic process is the lateral projection that articulates with the zygomatic bone and forms the anterior end of the zygomatic arch.

The alveolar process is the dental arch in which are set the upper (maxillary) teeth.

The palatine process is the horizontal shelf of bone within the dental arch that forms the anterior and lower part of the hard palate. The two palatine processes meet in the midline.

Inferior nasal conchae. Each inferior nasal concha is a shell-like scroll of bone covered with mucous membrane that projects medially as a rolled plate of thin bone into the nasal cavity.

Zygomatic bones. The zygomatic or malar bone forms the midportion of the zygomatic arch, and an upward projection completes the lateral wall of the orbit.

Palatine bones. The palatine bone forms the posterior portion of the hard palate and part of the lateral wall of the posterior nasal opening, or choana. The vertical portion forms part of the lateral wall of the nose and above, a little of the medial portion of the posterior part of the orbit.

Vomer. The vomer forms the posterior part of the nasal septum. In dried skulls, it is frequently broken into fragments.

Mandible. The mandible is the bone of the lower jaw. It consists of a horseshoe-shaped body, the upper or alveolar portion of which lodges the lower (mandibular) teeth, and a strong ramus extending superiorly and posteriorly from each free end of the horseshoe (Fig. 3-22). Each ramus bears a condyle that articulates with the undersurface of the temporal bone. There is a flat tongue of bone anterior to the condyle, called the coronoid process, to which the temporal muscle is attached.

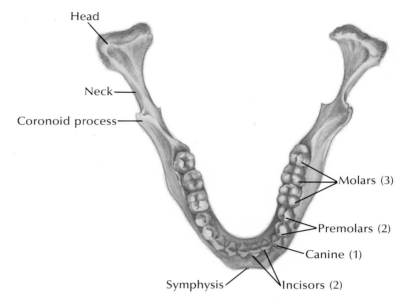

Head

Neck

Coronoid process

Molars (3)

Premolars (2)

Canine (1)

Symphysis

Incisors (2)

Fig. 3-22. Mandible, superior view. (Male, 25 years of age.)

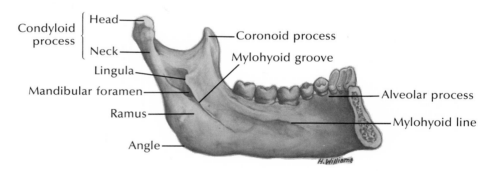

Condyloid process

Head

Coronoid process

Neck

Mylohyoid groove

Lingula

Mandibular foramen

Alveolar process

Ramus

Mylohyoid line

Angle

Fig. 3-23. Medial surface, left half of mandible. (Male, 40 years of age.)

Above the center of the inner surface of the ramus is the mandibular foramen through which the nerves and arteries for the lower teeth pass into the bone. Overhanging the foramen is a spine of bone, the lingula. The mylohyoid groove extends downward and forward from the foramen. The mylohyoid line is the marked horizontal ridge on the inner surface of the mandible, below the alveolar portion (Fig. 3-23).

In the newborn child the mandible is composed of two halves that meet in the midline to form the symphysis of the mandible. During infancy the two halves fuse.

Table 2. Skull bones

Name	Location	Distinguishing features	Articulations
Frontal	Front of skull and upper part of each orbit	Frontal part with air sinuses, tuberosities, and zygomatic processes; orbital part	Sphenoid; ethmoid; each parietal; nasal; zygomatic; maxilla; lacrimal
Parietal	Vault of skull	Grooves on inner surface for middle meningeal vessels	Frontal; temporal; sphenoid; occipital; other parietal
Occipital	Back of skull and posterior part of base	Squamous part with internal and external occipital protuberances and grooves for blood sinuses; lateral part with articular facets and hypoglossal canals; basal part with foramen magnum and jugular fossae	Sphenoid; atlas; each temporal and parietal
Temporal	Lateral part of vault and base of skull	Squamous part with zygomatic process and mandibular fossa; tympanic part with external auditory meatus, stylomastoid foramen, and styloid process; mastoid part with air cells and grooves for blood sinuses; petrous part with jugular fossa, carotid canal, and internal acoustic meatus	Parietal; occipital; zygomatic; sphenoid; mandible
Sphenoid	Anterior part of base of skull and deep part of face	Body with air cells, sella turcica, posterior clinoid processes, optic groove, rostrum, and pharyngeal canal; small wings with optic canal, anterior clinoid processes, and superior orbital fissure; great wings with foramen ovale, foramen rotundum, and foramen spinosum; pterygoid processes with pterygoid canals and medial and lateral pterygoid plates	Frontal; vomer; ethmoid; each parietal; temporal; zygomatic and palatine
Ethmoid	Anterior part of base of skull, medial part of each orbit, and upper part of nose	Perpendicular plate with crista galli; cribriform plates; lateral parts with air cells and superior and middle nasal conchae	Sphenoid; vomer; frontal; each nasal; maxilla; lacrimal; palatine and inferior nasal concha
Nasal	Bridge of nose		Frontal; ethmoid; maxilla; other nasal
Lacrimal	Medial wall of orbit		Frontal; ethmoid; maxilla; inferior nasal concha
Maxilla	Upper jaw, face, and lower part of orbit	Body with air sinus, lacrimal groove, infraorbital foramen, and greater palatine groove; frontal process; zygomatic process; alveolar process with upper teeth and incisive canal; palatine process	Frontal; nasal; ethmoid; zygomatic; lacrimal; inferior nasal concha; vomer; palatine; other maxilla
Inferior nasal concha	Lower lateral wall of nose		Palatine; maxilla; lacrimal; ethmoid
Zygomatic	Cheek	Temporal process; orbital process; frontosphenoidal process	Temporal; frontal; sphenoid; maxilla
Palatine	Part of hard palate, nasal cavity, and orbit	Horizontal plate; perpendicular part with pyramidal process and sphenopalatine notch	Sphenoid; maxilla; ethmoid; inferior nasal concha; vomer; other palatine
Vomer	Back of nasal septum		Ethmoid; sphenoid; each maxilla; palatine
Mandible	Lower jaw	Body with alveolar process and lower teeth, mylohyoid line and mental foramina; two rami each with coronoid process, condyloid process, head, neck, and mandibular foramen	Each temporal

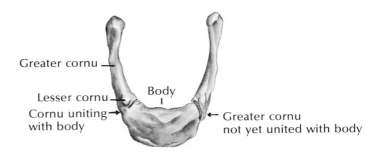

Greater cornu

Lesser cornu

Body

Cornu uniting
with body

Greater cornu
not yet united with body

Fig. 3-24. Hyoid bone, superior view. (Male, 40 years of age.)

Hyoid. The hyoid bone, though not a portion of the skull, can best be described here. It is a slender, horseshoe-shaped bone found below the mandible at the upper border of the larynx. It may be felt just above the anterior margin of the thyroid cartilage (Fig. 3-24).

The greater horns or cornua of the hyoid are the superior and posterior projections of bone from either extremity. The lesser horns are the two small, upward projections from the upper edge of the bone anterior to the greater horns.

Ear bones. Within the middle ear cavity of the petrous portion of each temporal bone are three tiny bones called malleus (hammer), incus (anvil), and stapes (stirrup), thus named from their respective shapes.

The arterial or nutrient foramina for the vessels that nourish bones have been omitted as well as many inconstant foramina for emissary veins. Emissary veins are short communicating vessels between the venous sinuses within the skull and the veins outside the skull.

VERTEBRAL COLUMN

The vertebral column typically has seven cervical, 12 thoracic, and five lumbar vertebrae, a sacrum composed of five vertebrae fused together in an adult, and a coccyx in which there are four fused vertebrae. The vertebrae, separated from each other by discs of fibrocartilage, are closely bound together by ligaments.

Since the body weight that must be borne increases progressively as one passes rostral to caudal, the vertebral bodies and discs are more massive in the lumbar region (Fig. 3-25).

The adult vertebral column has a forward curve in the cervical and lumbar regions and a backward curve in the thoracic and sacral regions, whereas at birth there is a single backward curve from neck to sacrum. The forward cervical curve appears at about 3 to 4 months of age when the baby learns to hold up or steady his head. The forward convexity in the lumbar region follows at about 3 years of age.

48

and blunt. It may be felt at the back of the base of the neck as the uppermost projection in the midline of that region.

Thoracic vertebrae. Thoracic vertebrae are characterized by having long spinous processes and articular facets for ribs (Fig. 3-29). The tip of each transverse process bears an articular surface for the tubercle of the rib corresponding to that vertebra. The head of the rib meets the body of the vertebra at its junction with the pedicle, so there are two articular areas on each vertebra for the corresponding rib. In the case of the upper ten ribs the head articulates not only with the body of the corresponding rib but also with the body of the vertebra above (Fig. 3-30).

The superior and inferior articular processes form joints with the corresponding processes of the vertebrae above and below. Spinous and transverse processes serve for attachment of the muscles and ligaments of the back.

Lumbar vertebrae. The lumbar vertebrae are larger than the thoracic. The superior and inferior articular processes are large. On the posterior and lateral part of each superior articular process there is a small mass called the mammillary process. The spinous processes are short, thick, and blunt. The transverse processes are thin and are not

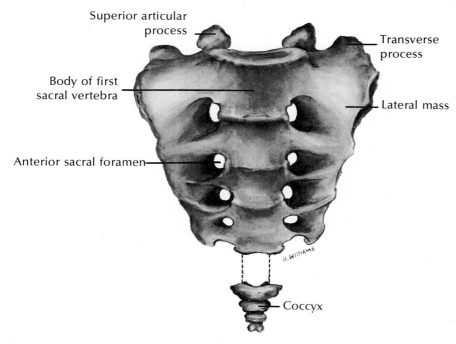

Superior articular process

Transverse process

Body of first sacral vertebra

Lateral mass

Anterior sacral foramen

H. Williams

Coccyx

Fig. 3-32. Sacrum and coccyx, anterior view. (Male, 26 years of age.)

53

perforated. There are no articular surfaces for ribs, but the transverse processes of the first lumbar vertebra are sometimes free and closely resemble short ribs (Fig. 3-31).

Sacrum. The sacrum in the adult consists of five fused sacral vertebrae (Fig. 3-32). Together with the two hip bones, it forms the bony pelvis. The smooth, concave, anterior or pelvic surface forms the hollow of the sacrum. The posterior or dorsal surface is rough and uneven for the attachment of the muscles and heavy ligaments of the back. The portion of the vertebral canal within the sacrum is called the sacral canal, and its lower aperture is the sacral hiatus. On each surface there are four pairs of intervertebral foramina for the exit of the upper four sacral nerves. On each side there is a large, sharply defined, ear-shaped area for articulation with the ilium (upper portion of the hip bone).

Coccyx. The coccyx is a small, rough, triangular bone forming the caudal most part of the spinal column and articulating with the inferior end of the sacrum. It is composed of four coccygeal vertebrae, which are fused in the adult (Fig. 3-33).

BONES OF THE THORAX

The bony thorax surrounds the heart and lungs. Participating in its composition are 12 pairs of ribs attached behind to the 12 thoracic vertebrae. Anteriorly the upper ten ribs are attached either directly

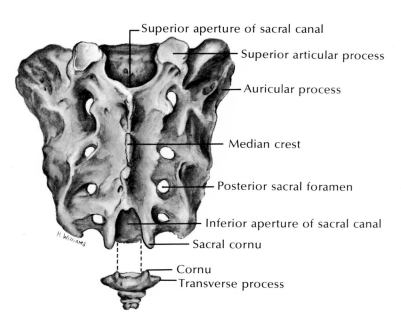

Fig. 3-33. Sacrum and coccyx, posterior view. (Male, 26 years of age.)

Superior aperture of sacral canal

Superior articular process

Auricular process

Median crest

Posterior sacral foramen

Inferior aperture of sacral canal

Sacral cornu

Cornu
Transverse process

or indirectly to the sternum or breast bone by means of costal cartilages.

Ribs. A typical rib is a long, slender, curved bone. Its head articulates with two thoracic vertebrae, namely, the one corresponding to it and the one just above it. The lowest two ribs, however, possess only one articular surface, namely, that for the corresponding vertebra. The first rib may have but one.

Beyond the head of the rib is a narrow portion called the neck, and just beyond this again, except in the lowest two ribs, is a knob called the tubercle, which has a smooth area articulating with a transverse process of the corresponding vertebra.

The first rib is short, sharply curved, and relatively broader than any of the others. The great vessels and lowest nerves for the arm pass over this rib, making distinct grooves on its upper surface (Fig. 3-34).

The second to seventh ribs are increasingly longer, whereas the succeeding ones diminish regularly in length. Each of the upper seven ribs is joined to the sternum by a separate costal cartilage. The costal cartilages of the eighth, ninth, and tenth ribs are joined respectively to the costal cartilage of the rib next above and so indirectly to

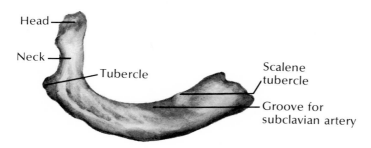

Fig. 3-34. First rib, right side, superior view. (Male, 31 years of age.)

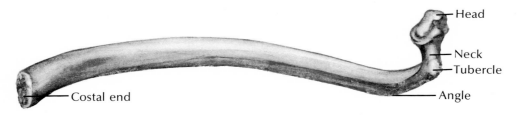

Fig. 3-35. Seventh rib, right side, deep aspect. Rib shown is two-fifths life size, whereas rib in Fig. 3-34 is drawn two-thirds life size. (Male, 31 years of age.)

55

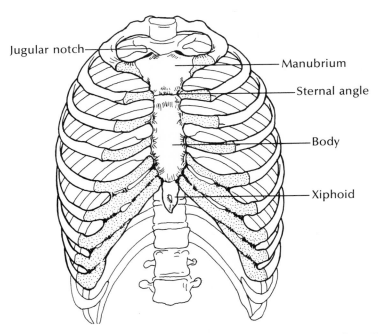

Fig. 3-36. Sternum, anterior view. Note junction of second costal cartilage with sternal angle.

the lower part of the sternum. The costal cartilages of the eleventh and twelfth ribs are not joined to the sternum, and these ribs are therefore sometimes called "floating ribs." The free tips of their costal cartilages are easily felt low down on the lateral wall of the thorax.

Sternum. The sternum or breast bone is shaped somewhat like a blunt dagger. It forms the chest wall in the midline anteriorly. Its upper end is broad and articulates on each side with the clavicle, or collar bone, and with the first rib. The sternum tapers toward the lower end, or xiphoid, which forms a small projection in the upper portion of the "pit of the stomach" between the costal margins.

The sternum consists of a superior portion (the manubrium), a middle portion (the body), and an inferior portion (the xiphoid). The concave superior border of the manubrium is called the jugular notch. The inferior border of the manubrium articulates with the superior border of the body at a slight angle, called the sternal angle. Quite often the sternal angle can be seen as a transverse ridge in a living subject. The sternal angle is an important bony landmark, since it normally also marks the level of the second costal cartilage (Fig. 3-36). The xiphoid is cartilaginous in early life but later ossifies and fuses with the body of the sternum.

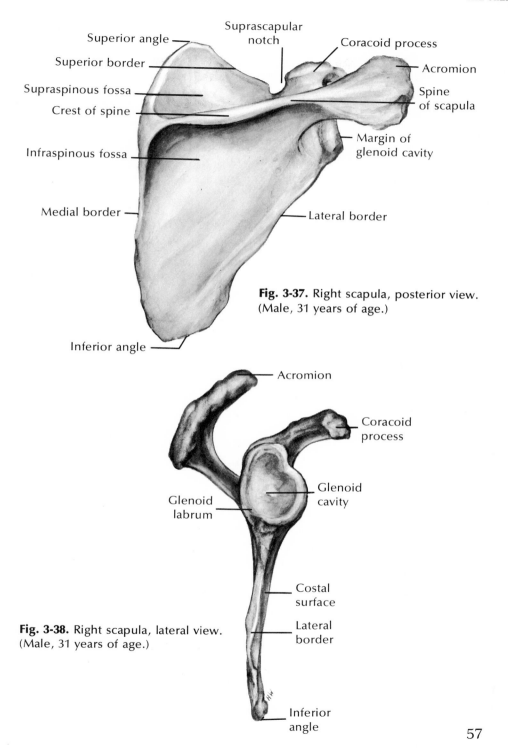

Superior angle

Suprascapular notch

Coracoid process

Superior border

Acromion

Supraspinous fossa

Spine of scapula

Crest of spine

Infraspinous fossa

Margin of glenoid cavity

Medial border

Lateral border

Fig. 3-37. Right scapula, posterior view. (Male, 31 years of age.)

Inferior angle

Acromion

Coracoid process

Glenoid labrum

Glenoid cavity

Costal surface

Lateral border

Fig. 3-38. Right scapula, lateral view. (Male, 31 years of age.)

Inferior angle

57

BONES OF UPPER EXTREMITY

In the upper extremity, or superior member, are the shoulder girdle, upper arm, forearm, wrist, and hand.

Scapula. The scapula, or shoulder blade, is largely covered by muscles. The main portion is a flat, triangular body. The lateral angle nearest the armpit bears a smooth, slightly depressed, oval area, the glenoid cavity, for articulation with the head of the humerus (Figs. 3-37 and 3-38).

The other two angles delimit the vertebral or medial border that parallels the vertebral column. The deep face of the scapula is concave and is known as the costal surface because it lies next to the ribs. In movements of the shoulder the scapula glides freely over the posterior chest wall. The superficial surface of the scapula presents a backwardly projecting spinous process terminating laterally in an expanded knob, called the acromion, which forms the tip of the shoulder. The acromion articulates anteriorly with the lateral end of the clavicle. The entire length of the spinous process is subcutaneous. On the superior border of the scapula there is a hooklike process, the coracoid, which curls forward beneath the clavicle.

Clavicle. The clavicle, or collar bone, is a long, curved, slender bone that lies in the root of the neck between the superior end of the sternum and the acromion. The medial end is rounded, articulates with the sternum, and is the only joint between the upper extremity and the trunk, for all the other attachments are made by means of muscles and tendons. The lateral end is broad and flat and articulates with the acromion (Fig. 3-39).

Humerus. The humerus is the bone of the upper arm (Figs. 3-40 and 3-41). Its proximal end has a thick, rounded knob on the medial side, called the head, which articulates with the glenoid cavity of the scapula. There are two rough projections lateral to the head, the greater and lesser tubercles, or tuberosities, with an intermediate groove, the intertubercular sulcus, for the tendon of the long head of the biceps brachii muscle. When the arm hangs freely by the side, the greater tubercle of the humerus projects just below the acromion of the scapula.

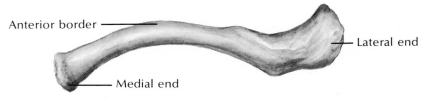

Anterior border
Lateral end
Medial end

Fig. 3-39. Right clavicle, posterosuperior view. (Male, 31 years of age.)

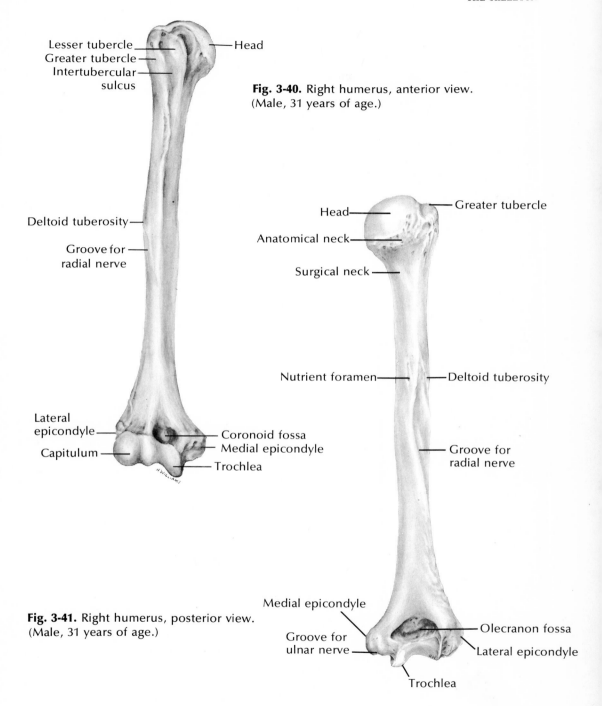

Lesser tubercle

Greater tubercle

Intertubercular
sulcus

Head

Fig. 3-40. Right humerus, anterior view.
(Male, 31 years of age.)

Deltoid tuberosity

Groove for
radial nerve

Head

Anatomical neck

Surgical neck

Greater tubercle

Nutrient foramen

Deltoid tuberosity

Lateral
epicondyle

Capitulum

Coronoid fossa

Medial epicondyle

Trochlea

Groove for
radial nerve

Fig. 3-41. Right humerus, posterior view.
(Male, 31 years of age.)

Medial epicondyle

Groove for
ulnar nerve

Olecranon fossa

Lateral epicondyle

Trochlea

59

On the lateral side of the shaft of the bone, about halfway between the two ends, there is a V-shaped, roughened area for attachment of the deltoid muscle, below which is a spiral groove for the radial nerve.

The central portion of the shaft is round, but the bone becomes flattened in the distal portion. The sharp border, thus formed on either side, ends in a roughened projection, the medial and the lateral epicondyles. The entire lower portion of the humerus is called the condyle, and its articular surface is divided into two parts. The lateral is a smooth, round knob, called the capitulum, which articulates with

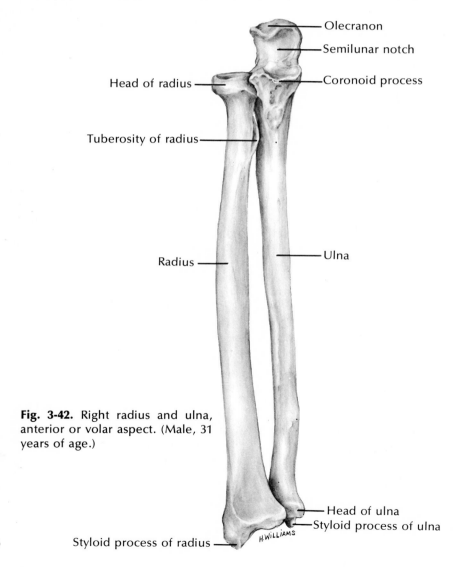

Olecranon

Semilunar notch

Head of radius

Coronoid process

Tuberosity of radius

Ulna

Radius

Head of ulna

Styloid process of ulna

Fig. 3-42. Right radius and ulna, anterior or volar aspect. (Male, 31 years of age.)

H.WILLIAMS

Styloid process of radius

the proximal end of the radius. The medial is a smooth, pulley-shaped surface, called the trochlea, which articulates with the proximal end of the ulna.

On the front of the lower end of the shaft of the humerus just above the articular area is the coronoid fossa, so called because it lodges the coronoid process of the ulna when the elbow is flexed. On the back of the distal end of the shaft of the humerus is the olecranon fossa, which lodges the olecranon process of the ulna when the elbow is extended.

Ulna. The ulna is the longer of the two bones in the forearm. It is

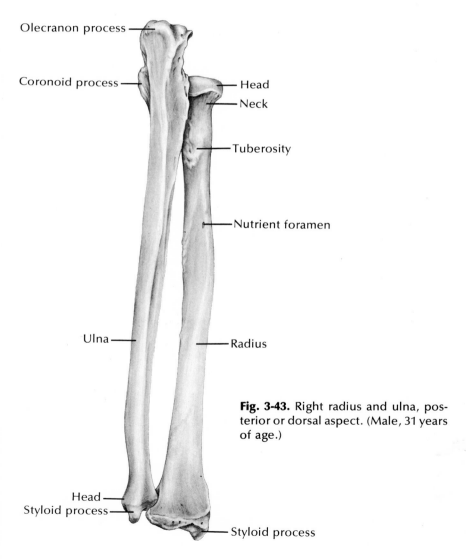

Olecranon process

Coronoid process

Head

Neck

Tuberosity

Nutrient foramen

Ulna

Radius

Head
Styloid process

Styloid process

Fig. 3-43. Right radius and ulna, posterior or dorsal aspect. (Male, 31 years of age.)

on the medial side and can easily be felt in its entire length by running the finger from the tip of the elbow down the posterior aspect of the forearm to the small projection on the back of the wrist on the little finger side.

The upper end of the ulna has two large, beaklike projections between which the trochlea of the humerus snugly fits in the semilunar or trochlear notch. The superiorly projecting process is the olecranon and the anteriorly projecting process is the coronoid. The distal end of the ulna, smaller than the proximal end, has a knobbed portion called the head, beside which is a conical projection known as the styloid process.

Radius. The shorter of the two bones of the forearm is called the radius. It lies on the lateral, or thumb, side and is for the most part well covered by muscles. At the proximal end is a circular disc, the head, which articulates with the capitulum of the humerus and also with the ulna. A short distance below the upper end there is a low,

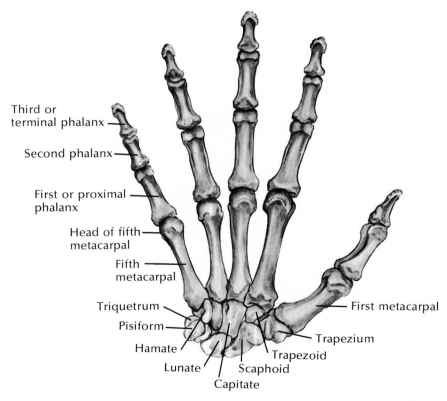

Third or
terminal phalanx —

Second phalanx —

First or proximal —
phalanx

Head of fifth —
metacarpal

Fifth —
metacarpal

Triquetrum —
Pisiform —
Hamate —
Lunate —
Capitate
Scaphoid
Trapezoid
Trapezium
First metacarpal

Fig. 3-44. Bones of right wrist and hand, volar aspect. (Male, 31 years of age.)

Table 4. Bones of upper extremity

Name	Location	Distinguishing features	Articulations
Scapula	Back of shoulder	Shoulder blade; head with neck and glenoid cavity; acromion; spine; coracoid process; supraspinous fossa; infraspinous fossa; subscapular fossa	Lateral end of clavicle; head of humerus
Clavicle	Junction of neck and thorax	Collar bone; medial and lateral ends	Medial end with sternum; lateral end with scapula
Humerus	Upper arm	Head; anatomical neck; surgical neck; lesser and greater tubercles; intertubercular sulcus; deltoid tuberosity; medial and lateral epicondyles; capitulum; trochlea; coronoid and olecranon fossae	Head with scapula; capitulum with radius; trochlea with ulna
Radius	Lateral part of forearm	Head; neck; tuberosity; styloid process; ulnar notch	Head with humerus and ulna; lower end with ulna and carpal bones
Ulna	Medial part of forearm	Olecranon; semilunar notch; coronoid process; radial notch; head; styloid process	Upper end with humerus and radius; lower end with radius
Carpus	Wrist	Eight bones arranged in two rows; proximal row-scaphoid, lunate, triquetrum, and pisiform; distal row-trapezium trapezoid, capitate, and hamate	Proximal row with lower end of radius; distal row with metacarpals; with each other; the pisiform with triquetrum only
Metacarpus	Hand	Five bones each with head, shaft, and base; numbered from one to five beginning on the thumb side	Bases with each other and with distal row of carpal bones; heads with corresponding finger bone
Phalanges	Fingers	Fourteen; two for thumb and three for each of the other fingers	Proximal with respective metacarpal; with each other

rough projection on the inner side (toward the ulna) called the tuberosity, to which is attached the tendon of the biceps brachii.

The distal end of the radius is much larger than the upper end and has a final tip on the thumb side called the styloid process. At its lower end the radius articulates with two bones of the wrist, the scaphoid and lunate. There is also an articulation with the head of the ulna.

Carpus. The eight bones in the carpus or wrist are arranged in two rows. In the proximal row are scaphoid, lunate, triquetrum, and pisiform; in the distal row are trapezium, trapezoid, capitate, and hamate. The projection at the anterior part of the wrist on the little finger side is produced by the pisiform bone. The other bones, being firmly held together by ligaments, cannot be separately distinguished through the skin.

Hand bones. In the palm there are five metacarpal bones; the four medial ones articulate at their bases with each other and are closely bound together by ligaments; the first metacarpal articulates at its base with the trapezium and is freely movable. The other metacarpals articulate proximally with other carpal bones, and the head of each metacarpal articulates distally with its proper finger bone. The heads of the metacarpals form the knuckles.

In the fingers there are 14 phalanges, two in the thumb and three in each of the fingers. In the flexor tendons of the thumb are found sesamoid bones near the metacarpophalangeal and interphalangeal joints, and there is occasionally a sesamoid bone near the metacarpophalangeal joint of the index and of the little finger.

BONES OF LOWER EXTREMITY

The bones of the lower extremity, or inferior member, include those of the hip, thigh, leg, ankle, and foot. The term "thigh" refers to that part between the hip and knee joints, and the term leg is sometimes used to designate that part between the knee and ankle joints.

The two hip bones are firmly held together with the sacrum by strong ligaments to form the pelvic girdle, a rigid ring of bone that supports the weight of the body on the two lower extremities.

Os coxae or os innominatum. Each hip bone has a broad, expanded blade, the ilium; a downwardly projecting posterior portion, the ischium; and a remaining part, the pubis, which completes the ring or obturator foramen. On the lateral side at the junction of these three is the acetabular cavity. Capping the ilium is the iliac crest, which ends anteriorly and posteriorly in bony bosses known respectively as the anterior and the posterior superior spines to distinguish these from other projections placed lower on the margins of the blade and designated anterior and posterior inferior spines. The ilium forms the upper portion of the acetabulum into which fits the head of the femur. The ischium forms the lower and posterior portion of the acetabulum and ends in a rough knob called the ischial tuberosity (tuber). The pubis forms the anterior lower portion of the acetabulum. The two pubic bones articulate with each other in the midline (symphysis pubis) at the anterior part of the pelvic girdle, and their inferior rami diverge to form the pubic arch (Figs. 3-45 and 3-46).

Femur. The femur is the thigh bone. It is the longest and heaviest bone of the body and, for the most part, is deeply embedded within the large thigh muscles (Figs. 3-47 and 3-48).

At the proximal end are the head, the neck, and the greater and lesser trochanters. The smooth and almost spherical head fits into the acetabulum, and the neck is the stout bar of bone that supports the head on the upper end of the shaft. The angle of the neck with

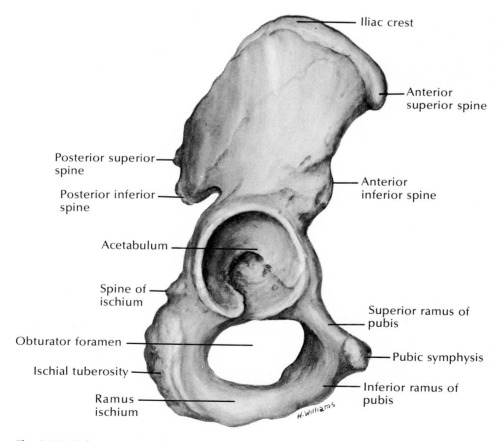

Fig. 3-45. Right os coxae. The bone has been turned to give a view directly into the acetabulum. (Male, 31 years of age.)

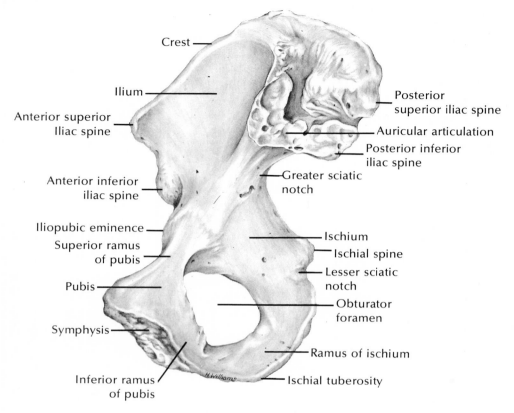

Crest

Ilium

Anterior superior
Iliac spine

Posterior
superior iliac spine

Auricular articulation

Posterior inferior
iliac spine

Anterior inferior
iliac spine

Greater sciatic
notch

Iliopubic eminence

Superior ramus
of pubis

Ischium

Ischial spine

Lesser sciatic
notch

Pubis

Symphysis

Obturator
foramen

Ramus of ischium

Inferior ramus
of pubis

Ischial tuberosity

Fig. 3-46. Right os coxae, medial view. (Male, 31 years of age.)

the shaft is characteristically greater than a right angle. The greater
trochanter is the massive projection on the lateral side of the shaft
at its junction with the neck, and the lesser trochanter is the smaller,
rounded boss of bone on the medial side of the shaft just below the
neck. The ridge for attachment of muscles in the midline of the back
of the shaft is called the linea aspera. The trochanteric fossa is a pit
on the inner side of the greater trochanter. The ridge on the back of
the upper end of the shaft joining the two trochanters is the intertrochanteric crest, and the quadrate tubercle is a small mound near
the center of the crest. The intertrochanteric line begins on the front
of the shaft just below the greater trochanter, runs medially and distally around the bone below the lesser trochanter, and blends with
the medial side of the linea aspera.

The distal end of the femur is modeled into the medial and lateral
66   condyles, between which there is a deep groove, the intercondylar

fossa, especially marked behind and below. The condyles bear articular surfaces for the upper end of the tibia and for the patella.

Patella. The patella, or kneecap, is a large sesamoid bone embedded in the tendon of the great extensor muscle of the thigh (Fig. 3-49). It is the bony prominence on the anterior aspect of the knee when the leg is extended, but it sinks into the intercondylar fossa during flexion at the knee joint.

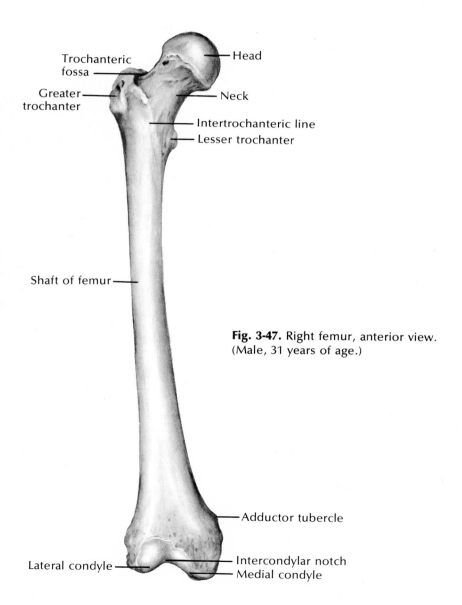

Trochanteric fossa

Greater trochanter

Head

Neck

Intertrochanteric line

Lesser trochanter

Shaft of femur

Fig. 3-47. Right femur, anterior view. (Male, 31 years of age.)

Adductor tubercle

Lateral condyle

Intercondylar notch
Medial condyle

67

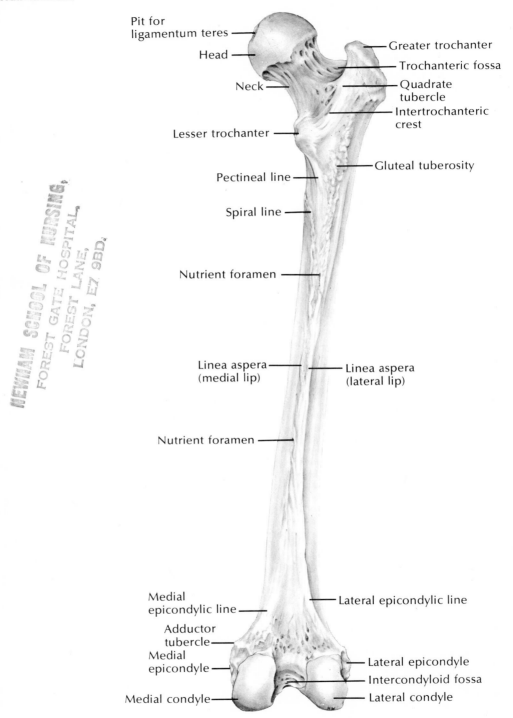

68 **Fig. 3-48.** Right femur, posterior view. (Male, 31 years of age.)

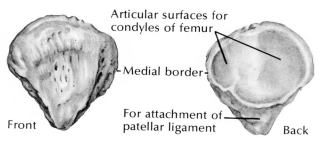

Articular surfaces for
condyles of femur

Medial border

For attachment of
patellar ligament

Front

Back

Fig. 3-49. Right patella. (Male, 31 years of age.)

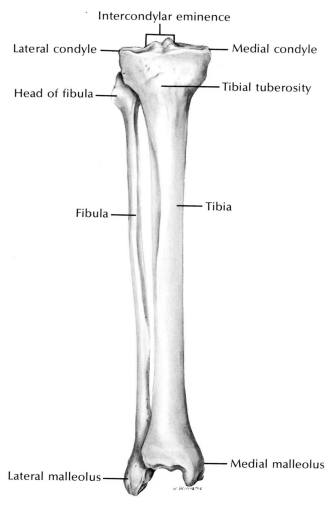

Intercondylar eminence

Lateral condyle

Medial condyle

Head of fibula

Tibial tuberosity

Fibula

Tibia

Lateral malleolus

Medial malleolus

Fig. 3-50. Right tibia and fibula, anterior view. (Male, 31 years of age.)

69

Tibia. The tibia, or shin bone, is the larger bone of the leg. The medial surface is entirely subcutaneous. The thickened proximal end supports the medial and lateral condyles with their articular surfaces for the lower end of the femur. Between these two smooth articular surfaces projects the intercondylar eminence. On the anterior aspect of the bone, about 2 cm below the proximal end, is the tibial tuber-

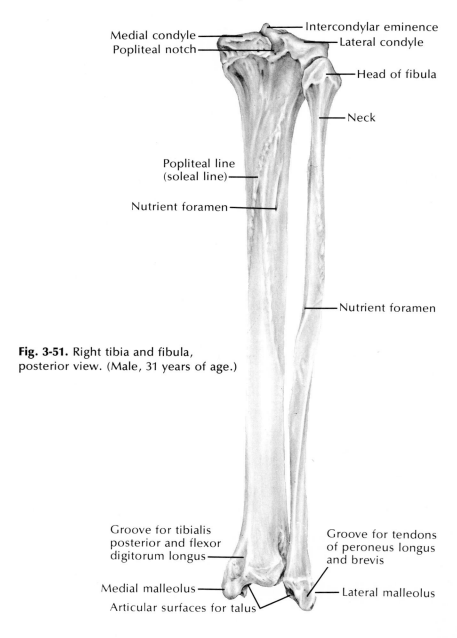

Medial condyle
Popliteal notch
Intercondylar eminence
Lateral condyle
Head of fibula
Neck
Popliteal line (soleal line)
Nutrient foramen
Nutrient foramen

Fig. 3-51. Right tibia and fibula, posterior view. (Male, 31 years of age.)

Groove for tibialis posterior and flexor digitorum longus
Groove for tendons of peroneus longus and brevis
Medial malleolus
Articular surfaces for talus
Lateral malleolus

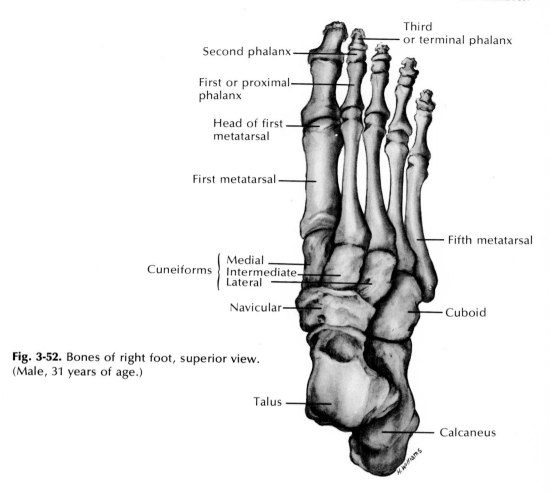

Third
or terminal phalanx

Second phalanx

First or proximal
phalanx

Head of first
metatarsal

First metatarsal

Fifth metatarsal

Cuneiforms { Medial
Intermediate
Lateral

Navicular

Cuboid

Talus

Calcaneus

H. Williams

Fig. 3-52. Bones of right foot, superior view.
(Male, 31 years of age.)

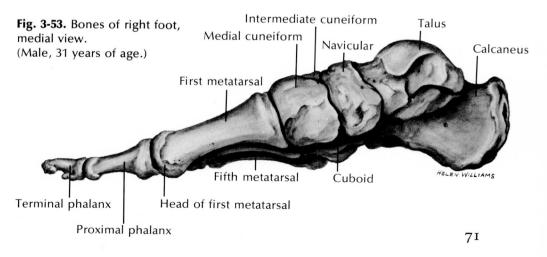

Fig. 3-53. Bones of right foot,
medial view.
(Male, 31 years of age.)

Intermediate cuneiform

Medial cuneiform

Navicular

Talus

Calcaneus

First metatarsal

Terminal phalanx

Proximal phalanx

Head of first metatarsal

Fifth metatarsal

Cuboid

HELEN WILLIAMS

71

osity, into which is inserted the tendon of the quadriceps, the great extensor muscle of the thigh. Immediately beneath the outer ridge of its lateral condyle, the tibia has an articular facet for the fibula. The line for the popliteus muscle is seen on the back of the shaft of the tibia, beginning just below the articular facet for the fibula and passing inferiorly and medially to the inner border of the bone. The distal end of the tibia has an inferior projection on its inner side, the medial malleolus, which forms the prominence on the medial side of the ankle. The lateral side of the lower end articulates with the fibula and the distal surface with the talus.

Fibula. The fibula is a slender bone on the lateral side of the leg. The knoblike upper end, or head, articulates with the lateral side of the lateral condyle of the tibia just beneath the lateral ridge. The fibula does not articulate with the femur nor the patella and does not help to form the knee joint. The fibula ends distally in the lateral malleolus, the prominence of the lateral side of the ankle.

Tarsus. The seven tarsal bones form the posterior half of the foot. Of these the talus is the bone that articulates with the tibia and fits between the malleoli of the tibia and fibula. Below the talus is the calcaneus, which is the largest of the tarsal bones and forms the heel. Anterior to these on the lateral side is the cuboid; on the medial side, the navicular; and in front of the navicular, the three cuneiform bones in a row. The calcaneus, navicular, and cuneiforms together with the three medial metatarsals and corresponding phalanges constitute the medial longitudinal arch of the foot. The calcaneus, cuboid, two lateral metatarsals, and corresponding phalanges form the lateral longitudinal arch.

Metatarsus. Anterior to the tarsus lie the five metatarsal bones. The bases of the inner three articulate with the three cuneiform bones and those of the outer two with the cuboid. The heads of the five metatarsal bones form the ball of the foot. The head of the innermost (first) metatarsal forms the main feature of the front end of the medial longitudinal arch, and the head of the outermost (fifth) metatarsal, the main feature of the front end of the lateral longitudinal arch. There is also a transverse arch produced by the manner of interarticulation of the anterior tarsal and of the five metatarsal bones.

Toe bones. Theoretically there should be 14 phalanges in the toes, two for the great toe and three for each of the others. Often the middle phalanx of the fifth toe and sometimes that of the fourth is absent or fused with the corresponding terminal phalanx.

Sesamoid bones are found in the tendons passing to the great toe and also in the tendons passing from the leg into the foot on either side of the ankle.

Table 5. Bones of lower extremity

Name	Location	Distinguishing features	Articulations
Os coxae (innominate)	Hip	Acetabulum; pubic arch; obturator foramen; greater and lesser sciatic notches; formed by union of ilium, pubis, and ischium	Sacrum, femur, and other pubis
		ilium with crest, anterior superior and inferior spines, posterior superior and inferior spines, auricular articulation	
		pubis with crest, tubercle, symphysis, superior and inferior rami	
		ischium with ramus and tuberosity	
Femur	Thigh	Head; neck; greater and lesser trochanters; trochanteric fossa and crest; intertrochanteric line; shaft with linea aspera; medial and lateral condyles and epicondyles; adductor tubercle; intercondylar fossa	Head with acetabulum; condyles with patella and tibia
Patella	Knee	Kneecap	Femur
Tibia	Medial bone of leg	Shin bone; medial and lateral condyles; intercondylar eminence; tuberosity; medial malleolus	Femur, fibula, and talus
Fibula	Lateral bone of leg	Splint bone; head; neck; lateral malleolus	Tibia and talus
Tarsus	Back of foot	Seven bones; talus, calcaneus, cuboid, navicular, medial, intermediate, and lateral cuneiforms	Talus with lower end of tibia and fibula; cuneiforms and cuboid with metatarsals; with each other
Metatarsus	Front of foot	Five bones each with head, shaft, and base; numbered from one to five beginning on the great toe side	With distal tarsals; with each other; with corresponding toe bone
Phalanges	Toes	Fourteen (some may be fused); two for great toe; three for each of the other toes	Proximal with respective metatarsal; with each other

**SEX DIFFERENCES
IN THE SKELETON**

As a general rule the bones of a man are heavier and larger than those of a woman. The articular ends are more massive in comparison to the size of the shaft, and the various ridges, tuberosites, and lines are proportional to the relative size of the muscles.

Specific sex features in the skeleton are largely limited to the bony pelvis. The pubic arch in the female is broad; in the male it is narrow. Although the bones of the pelvic girdle are smaller in a woman, the pelvic cavity is relatively capacious, and the greater sciatic notch between ilium and ischium on each side in the articulated pelvis is large (Figs. 3-54 to 3-57).

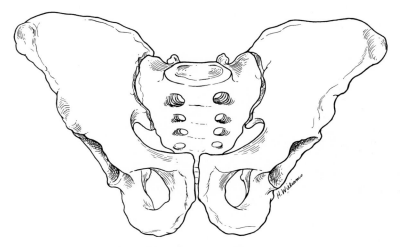

Fig. 3-54. Pelvis, anterior view. (Male, 44 years of age.)

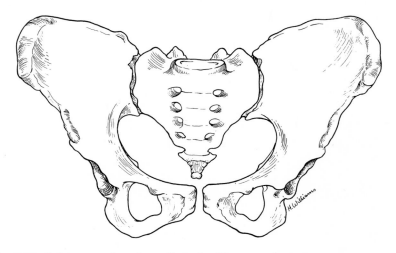

74 **Fig. 3-55.** Pelvis, anterior view. (Female, 23 years of age.)

Throughout the entire life of a person, changes are occurring in the skeleton. Because of the ossification of cartilaginous ends of bones, these changes are more obvious in childhood. After the adult features of the bones are completed, age changes are confined to the texture and to the margins of articular surfaces. The approximate age of a person at death can be estimated from an examination of the skeleton.

During infancy the skull grows rapidly because it houses the rapidly growing brain. The unossified areas are gradually replaced by bone, and by 18 months of age the fontanelles are closed.

At birth the brain case has a capacity of about 350 cc; this has

AGE CHANGES IN THE SKELETON

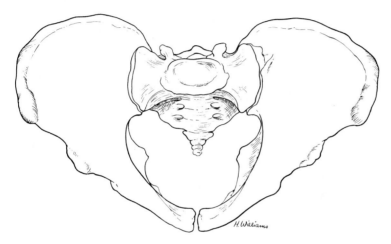

Fig. 3-56. Pelvis, superior view. (Male, 44 years of age.)

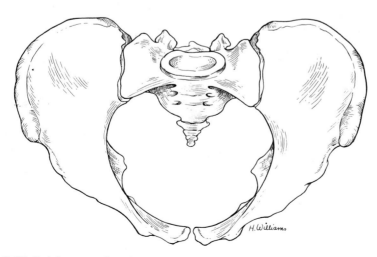

Fig. 3-57. Pelvis, superior view. (Female, 23 years of age.)

75

increased to 750 cc by the age of 1 year, and at 2 years of age it is 900 cc. The brain case reaches its approximate adult size of about 1,500 cc by the age of 6 years, and in well-grown children, it may be practically adult in size by 4½ years of age. Thereafter the increase in the size of the brain case is very small. The sutures or joints between the bones of the skull begin to fuse between the ages of 20 and 30 years. By the age of 60 years, almost all the sutures have united.

Since much of the brain case is still membranous at birth, during delivery the skull may be molded into various irregular shapes. These irregularities usually disappear during the first few months of life, and the head becomes fairly symmetrical. If an infant is too frequently left lying on its back or on one side, the side next to the pillow becomes flattened. This is one reason for altering the baby's position at frequent intervals.

After the fontanelles have ossified, the brain case becomes a closed box, and alterations of intracranial pressure are possible only by way of the circulation. Therefore any disease or injury that increases intracranial pressure soon gives rise to serious symptoms.

The bones forming the face grow steadily but relatively slowly until the late teens. This contrasts with the practical cessation of growth in the brain case in earlier childhood and is conditioned by the need for increasing the size of the respiratory passages and the jaws, which lodge the teeth.

The early growth of the brain case results in its relatively large size as contrasted with the small face. The facial region makes up about one eighth of the skull at birth, about one fourth at 5 years of age, and about one half in the adult. Part of the increase in size of the face during childhood is due to the development of air sinuses, rudiments of only the maxillary and mastoid sinuses being present at birth. This explains why small babies rarely have mastoiditis, although middle ear infections are common. The sphenoid, ethmoid, and frontal sinuses are present as shallow grooves in the nasal mucosa in infancy. The sphenoid sinus and ethmoid air cells usually appear as definite structures at about 6 years of age, and the frontal sinus, at about 7 years. The sinuses, particularly the frontal, increase rapidly in size at adolescence. These air spaces are extensions of the nasal chambers and permit increase in size without corresponding increase in weight. The mandible and maxilla continue to grow until the last teeth, the third molars or wisdom teeth, have erupted.

In a newborn infant the external auditory canal is short and the tympanic membrane is more obliquely placed than that in an adult. When the eardrum of a baby is examined, it is usually necessary to pull the ear down and back, whereas in an adult the ear is pulled up and back.

Definite changes appear in the proportions of the skeleton during childhood. The chest is barrel shaped during infancy, and the downward slope of the ribs is less pronounced than it is in later childhood and in adult life. During infancy the pelvis is relatively small, and organs that lie within the abdomen in a child sink into the pelvis as, with approaching adolescence, the pelvic cavity grows larger. The change in gait evident at about the age of 3 years results from a widening of the pelvic girdle and an increase in the relative length of the legs.

In an infant the head is large, the trunk is long, and the limbs are short. During childhood, limb growth is more rapid than the growth in trunk length. In the preadolescent years, arms and legs appear to be too long for the trunk. During the teenage years the legs stop growing before the trunk, and the final adult proportions are attained at about 18 years of age. These changes in bodily proportion are a part of the normal process of growing up.

In old age, bones tend to lose mineral salts, thus becoming lighter in weight and more easily broken. The margins, particularly of articular surfaces, become roughened and more pronounced and may interfere with freedom of movement. This piling up of bone about an articulation may be associated with arthritis and may actually produce ankylosis or pathologic union of the bones that form the joint.

REVIEW QUESTIONS

1. What are the functions of the skeleton?
2. What are the two main subdivisions of the skeleton?
3. What bones are included in each subdivision?
4. How may bones be classified? Give an example of each class.
5. List the bones of the skull. Which are paired and which unpaired?
6. What bones form the brain case?
7. What bones enter into the formation of the face?
8. Name five foramina in the base of the skull. What structures pass through each?
9. What bones form the orbit?
10. Describe a typical vertebra.
11. List the bones that form the vertebral column.
12. Describe the sacrum.
13. What bones are located in the upper extremity?
14. What bones are located in the lower extremity?
15. Name three ways in which the female pelvis differs from the male pelvis.
16. Describe briefly the differences between the skull of a newborn child and that of an adult.
17. How are the bones of an aged person different from those of a young adult?
18. Describe briefly the growth of a long bone such as the tibia.
19. With what bones does the clavicle articulate?
20. With what bones does the femur articulate?
21. List the bones of the carpus.
22. List the bones of the tarsus.
23. With what bones does the tibia articulate?

CHAPTER 4

ARTICULATIONS

A joint may be defined as a union of two or more rigid skeletal elements. This concept recognizes that joints exist not only between two or more bones but also between bone and cartilage or between two or more cartilages.

The primordium of the skeleton develops as condensations of mesenchyme. A layer of undifferentiated mesenchymal cells connects the perichondrium or periosteum of the primordium and encloses tissue known as interzonal mesenchyme. If this interzonal mesenchyme differentiates into a uniting layer, nonsynovial joints are formed. This union may be by fibrous tissue, cartilage, or bone. In other joints the interzonal mesenchyme develops a cavity and differentiates into the synovial membrane. The perichondrium or periosteum enclosing the joint cavity forms the joint capsule and most of its ligaments. Intra-articular accessory structures, such as articular discs, develop from the capsule or from adjacent cartilaginous primordia.

Nerve fibers and blood vessels are distributed to joints from adjacent nerve trunks and vascular channels. Generally, nerves supplying muscles that pass over joints also send branches into the capsule of the joint. In addition to conveying pain, sensory neurons convey "position sense" so that one can appreciate the position of the body parts without visualizing them.

When a tendon lies in contact with a bony surface or with another tendon the intervening connective tissue is converted into a well-defined sac with a mesothelial lining, identical to the synovial membrane of a joint cavity. These sacs are called *bursae*. They function as small water cushions to minimize the effects of pressure and fric-

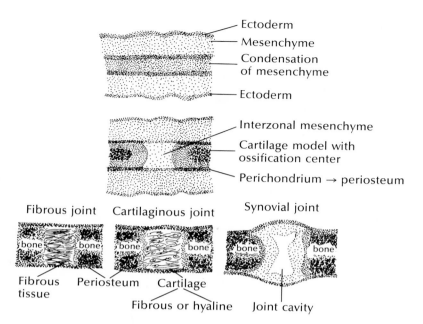

Ectoderm
Mesenchyme
Condensation
of mesenchyme
Ectoderm

Interzonal mesenchyme
Cartilage model with
ossification center
Perichondrium → periosteum

Fibrous joint   Cartilaginous joint   Synovial joint

bone   bone   bone   bone   bone   bone

Fibrous   Periosteum   Cartilage   Joint cavity
tissue
Fibrous or hyaline

Fig. 4-1. Schematic representation of the development of different types of joints. (Modified from Rosse, C., and Clawson, D.: Introduction to musculoskeletal system, New York, 1970, Harper & Row, Publishers.)

tion. Some also lie between the skin and bony prominences, as over the kneecap, and others are found as *tendon* or *vaginal sheaths* surrounding tendons as they pass through bony channels.

There are two general classifications of joints, synovial and non-synovial. A synovial joint is one in which the articulating elements are separated by a cavity that contains synovial fluid. In nonsynovial joints the skeletal elements are directly continuous with each other, and the type of intervening substance (fiber or cartilage) is used as the basis for subdivision.

Synovial joints are best subdivided on the basis of movement. Most skeletal movements are angular (circular) and occur in a plane around an axis. The plane in which a movement occurs is always at right angles to the axis around which it takes place. The axes of rotation, planes of movement, and types of movement possible are summarized in Table 6.

A joint that permits movement in only one plane is classified as uniaxial; one that permits movement in two planes is biaxial. If movement occurs in all three planes, it can occur also in any intermediate plane, and the joint is said to be multiaxial. Nonangular or plane sur-

CLASSIFICATION OF JOINTS

79

Table 6. The axes of rotation

Axis	Direction of axis	Plane of movement	Movements possible
Transverse	Horizontally from side to side	Sagittal	Flexion and extension
Anteroposterior	Horizontally from front to back	Frontal or coronal	Abduction and adduction
Vertical	Perpendicular to ground	Transverse or horizontal	Rotation

face movements may also occur, and such synovial joints are known as gliding joints.

I. Synovial joints

Synovial joints permit variable amounts of movement. There are a series of investing ligaments, a true joint cavity, and hyaline cartilage over the articulating surfaces. Synovial joints may be subdivided according to the type of movement allowed.

A. Gliding joints

Examples are the joints between carpal bones and between tarsal bones.

B. Uniaxial (pivot)

Movement is in the long axis of the bone. Examples are the joints between the dens of the axis and the atlas, and between the radius and ulna.

C. Uniaxial (hinge)

Example is the elbow joint.

D. Biaxial joints

Movements occur in two planes at right angles to each other. The condyloid joint at the wrist (between the radius and carpal bones) is biaxial.

E. Multiaxial (ball-and-socket)

Examples are shoulder and hip joints.

The movements possible in synovial joints are the following:

1. Sliding or gliding.
2. Medial and lateral rotation.
3. Flexion or decreasing the angle of a joint.
4. Extension or increasing the angle of a joint.
5. Abduction or drawing the part away from the midline.
6. Adduction or drawing toward the midline.
7. Circumduction, all three angular movements are combined in succession so that the limb revolves on a proximal point and the distal end describes a circle.

II. Nonsynovial joints
   A. Fibrous joint

In the fibrous joint there is no joint cavity, and there is close contact between the adjacent joint surfaces.

     1. Suture

Sutures are found only between bones of the skull, and union is effected by fibrous tissue. Sutures fuse with increasing age.

     2. Syndesmosis

In this type of joint the union is effected by dense connective tissue. The joints between the distal ends of the radius and ulna and between the tibia and fibula are examples.

     3. Gomphosis

The joint is between a tooth and its socket in an alveolar process.

   B. Cartilaginous joint

In the cartilaginous joint, union is effected by cartilage.

     1. Synchondrosis

Union is effected by hyaline cartilage. Such joints are found in growing bones, between the end of the shaft and the epiphysis. The joint disappears with fusion of the epiphysis after cessation of growth.

     2. Symphysis

Union is effected by fibrocartilage. There is a supporting capsule, and there may be a joint cavity. Symphyses occur in the midline of the body and include the joints between the bodies of the vertebrae, between the manubrium and the body of the sternum, and between the pubic bones.

Synovial joint. The tissues involved are (1) two or more rigid skeletal elements, (2) the joint capsule, (3) synovial membrane, (4) the synovial cavity and synovial fluid, (5) articular cartilage, and (6) ligaments.

Most often the skeletal elements are two or more bones, but these may be cartilage. The joint capsule is a fibrous tissue sleeve that encloses the joint and is continuous with the outer fibrous layer of the periosteum or perichondrium of the involved skeletal elements (Fig. 4-2). The synovial membrane is highly vascular connective tissue that lines the capsule and covers everything within the joint cavity except the articular surfaces. The synovia, produced by the synovial membrane, is a tissue fluid containing an appreciable amount of hyaluronic acid, which accounts for its viscosity and lubricating qualities. The articular cartilage covers the articulating surfaces and is usually of the hyaline variety. Joint ligaments are generally a band of collagenic

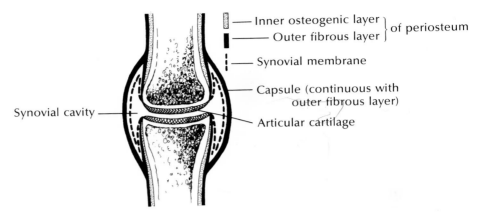

Inner osteogenic layer ⎫
Outer fibrous layer ⎭ of periosteum

Synovial membrane

Capsule (continuous with
outer fibrous layer)

Synovial cavity

Articular cartilage

Fig. 4-2. Typical synovial joint as seen in frontal section. Synovial cavity is enlarged to allow visualization of internal structures.

connective tissue placed so as to effectively limit certain motions of the joint, thus determining the direction of the movements and preventing excessive motion. In certain regions, ligaments contain an appreciable amount of elastic tissue, for example, ligamenta flava. This ligament completes the posterolateral walls of the vertebral canal and permits spreading of the vertebral laminae during movements of the vertebral column.

Temporomandibular joint. The temporomandibular, or mandibular, joint is the only movable joint between the skull bones. All the others are sutures and are immovable. The mandibular joint occurs between the concave cavity or mandibular fossa of the temporal bone and the head of the mandible. Interposed between the articular surfaces is a disc of fibrocartilage that separates the joint cavity into two parts. The capsular ligament has a thickening on the lateral side, the temporomandibular ligament, that helps to prevent displacement of the mandible. (Fig. 4-3). The stylomandibular ligament, a band of dense fascia running from the tip of the styloid process to the posterior edge of the angle of the mandible, is entirely separate from the joint but does give support to the mandible. The sphenomandibular ligament is another supporting band of fascia that runs from the spine of the sphenoid to the lingula on the inner surface of the ramus of the mandible (Fig. 4-4).

In the upper compartment of the joint the head of the mandible and the articular disc glide as one structure on the articular surface of the temporal bone, thus producing the movement of protraction and retraction of the lower jaw. In the lower compartment the head of the mandible rotates on the concave lower surface of the disc, thus

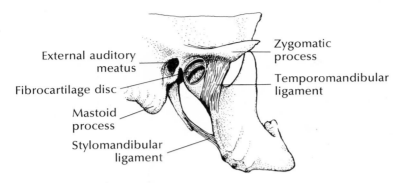

External auditory meatus

Zygomatic process

Fibrocartilage disc

Temporomandibular ligament

Mastoid process

Stylomandibular ligament

Fig. 4-3. Right temporomandibular joint, lateral view. Joint capsule has been opened to show articular disc.

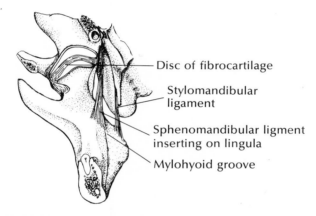

Disc of fibrocartilage

Stylomandibular ligament

Sphenomandibular ligment inserting on lingula

Mylohyoid groove

Fig. 4-4. Right temporomandibular joint, medial view.

permitting opening and closing of the mouth. This rotation occurs around a transverse axis running through the lingula of both rami of the mandible. The complicated grinding movements used in chewing food are produced by combinations of the simple movements just described.

Vertebral joints. The joints of the vertebral column, with the exception of the specialized joints between atlas and axis, are arranged on a common plan. The vertebral bodies, united by intervertebral fibrocartilaginous discs, form a series of nonsynovial cartilaginous joints. The intervertebral discs, because of their pliability, provide flexibility to the vertebral column and function as shock absorbers. The disc consists of a tough outer fibrocartilaginous ring, the annulus fibrosus, and an inner gelatinous mass, the nucleus pulposus. The discs are thickest in the lumbar region, where maximum vertical compression

83

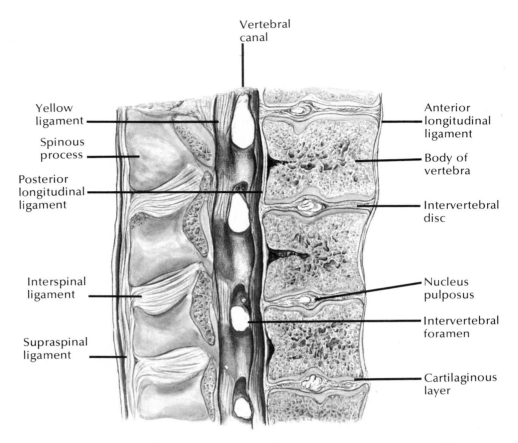

Vertebral
canal

Yellow
ligament

Spinous
process

Posterior
longitudinal
ligament

Interspinal
ligament

Supraspinal
ligament

Anterior
longitudinal
ligament

Body of
vertebra

Intervertebral
disc

Nucleus
pulposus

Intervertebral
foramen

Cartilaginous
layer

Fig. 4-5. Lumbar region of the vertebral column. Paramedian sagittal section to show four symphyses between the bodies of the vertebrae. (Drawing by Lili Ebstein-Loewenstein, courtesy Dr. R. Locchi.) (From DiDio, L. J. A.: Synopsis of anatomy, St. Louis, 1970, The C. V. Mosby Co.)

occurs. The amount of movement at a single joint is not great, but the range of movement in the entire series is considerable. Gliding movement also occurs at each of the synovial joints between articular processes of adjacent vertebrae.

Clothing the anterior and posterior aspects of the vertebral bodies are bands of connective tissue, the anterior and posterior longitudinal ligaments. These ligaments pass up the entire length of the column to insert into the occipital bone as the anterior atlantooccipital ligament and membrana tectoria, respectively (Fig. 4-6). The laminae of adjacent vertebrae are connected by sheets of yellow elastic connective tissue, the ligamenta flava, which is continued superiorly as the posterior atlantooccipital ligament. The tips of the spinous processes

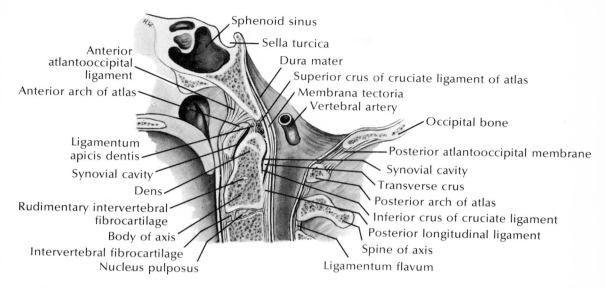

Fig. 4-6. Sagittal section of atlantoaxial joint and upper cervical joints.

are joined by supraspinous ligaments that, in the cervical regions, are especially well developed, forming the ligamentum nuchae. There are also fairly well-defined interspinous and intertransverse ligaments.

The movements of the vertebral column are described as flexion, extension, lateral flexion, and rotation.

Atlantooccipital joints. The two atlantooccipital joints, between the occipital condyles and the superior articular facets of the atlas, are uniaxial synovial joints placed on either side of the foramen magnum. The anterior and posterior atlantooccipital membranes, attached to the edge of the foramen magnum superiorly and the arch of the atlas inferiorly, strengthen the joints. Movement, occurring around a transverse axis, results in nodding or flexion and extension of the head.

Atlantoaxial joints. The atlantoaxial joints are a pair of synovial joints between the articular processes of the first and second cervical vertebrae (atlas and axis, respectively) and two median synovial joints formed by the articulation of the dens of the axis anteriorly with the anterior arch of the atlas and posteriorly with the transverse ligament (Fig. 4-6). The transverse ligament of the atlas is a stout band of connective tissue that passes posterior to the dens and attaches to the medial aspect of the lateral masses of the atlas. From the middle of the transverse ligament, longitudinal fibers pass superiorly to insert into the anterior edge of the foramen magnum and inferiorly to attach

85

to the posterior surface of the body of the axis. These longitudinal bands, together with the transverse ligament, form the cruciate ligament of the atlas. The axis is directly attached to the occipital bone by the apical and alar ligaments, which arise from the tip and either side of the dens, respectively.

Rotatory movements of the head occur between the atlas and axis. Movement is free; however, the alar ligaments limit rotation of the skull and atlas upon the axis, and the apical ligament tightens during extension.

Clavicular joints. A variable amount of movement occurs in the clavicular joints. At the medial end, limited movement can occur in any direction. When all the angular motions are performed in succession, the movement of circumduction occurs whereby the clavicle rotates at the sternal end and describes a circle at the acromial end carrying the scapula with it. This movement of the scapula and clavicle in unison is the most important action that occurs at the acromioclavicular joint, although the scapula also can rotate a certain amount around the anteroposterior axis of the joint.

Thoracic joints. The thoracic joints are those articulations involving the ribs. These articulations may be either costovertebral or costosternal.

COSTOVERTEBRAL. The joints of the heads of the ribs with the bodies of the vertebrae and of the tubercles of the ribs with the transverse process of the vertebrae are synovial joints, each one having a distinct capsular ligament.

COSTOSTERNAL. The anterior end of each of the first seven ribs is joined to the sternum by a bar of hyaline cartilage (Fig. 3-36). The union of the first costal cartilage with the manubrium is a synchondrosis. The remaining joints vary from the second, which is usually synovial, to the seventh, which is more often a symphysis. There may also be small cavities for the costal cartilages of the eighth and ninth ribs.

The joint between the manubrium and body of the sternum is similar to a symphysis, a type of cartilaginous joint. The connecting plate of fibrocartilage may be cavitated, and in approximately 10% of persons after reaching maturity, the fibrocartilaginous plate may be replaced by bone, a process known as synostosis.

Shoulder joint. The shoulder joint is a multiaxial synovial joint formed by the articulation of the head of the humerus with the glenoid cavity of the scapula. The strength of any joint depends upon three factors: (1) bony components, (2) ligaments, and (3) muscles. The rounded head of the humerus fits poorly with the shallow glenoid cavity, and although the glenoid labrum, a rim of fibrocartilage, deepens

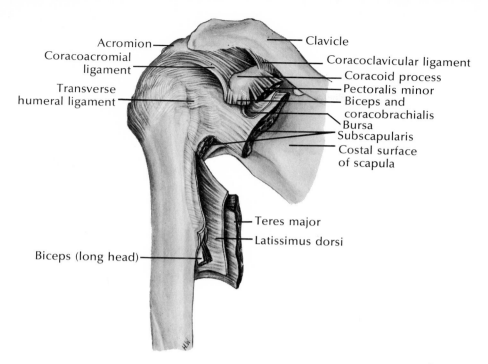

Fig. 4-7. Anterior aspect of right shoulder joint. This is a direct anterior view. (Male, 53 years of age.)

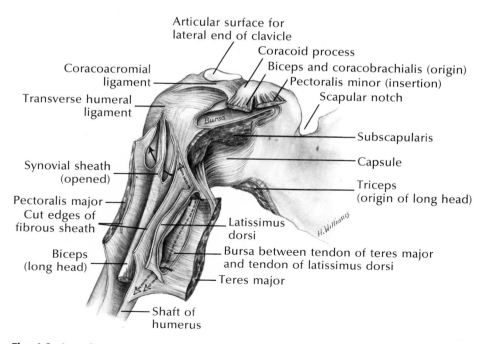

Fig. 4-8. Anterior aspect of right shoulder joint, showing the axilla and the relation of the muscle tendons to the joint. The clavicle has been removed, and the various bursae have been opened. (Male, 53 years of age.)

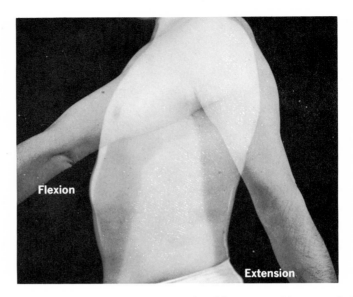

Fig. 4-9. Flexion and extension at the shoulder joint. (Photograph by Dr. D. R. L. Duncan.)

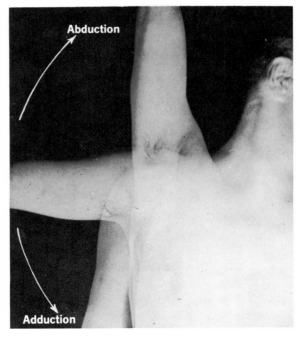

Fig. 4-10. Abduction and adduction at the shoulder joint. (Photograph by Dr. D. R. L. Duncan.)

the cavity, the shoulder joint remains extremely mobile and unstable. The capsular ligament, lax to allow free movement, is strengthened superiorly only by the coracohumeral and coracoacromial ligaments. Lacking substantial support from bony or ligamentous factors, the shoulder joint depends upon surrounding muscles to maintain its integrity. The tendons of four short muscles, the supraspinatus and infraspinatus, teres minor, and subscapularis, fuse with the capsule and strengthen the joint superiorly, posteriorly, and anteriorly, respectively. The tendon of the long head of the biceps brachii muscle also tends to hold the head of the humerus in the glenoid cavity. The inferior aspect of the capsule remains lax, and dislocation tends to occur in this direction.

There is a tubular extension of the synovial membrane of the joint inferiorly around the upper end of the tendon of the long head of the

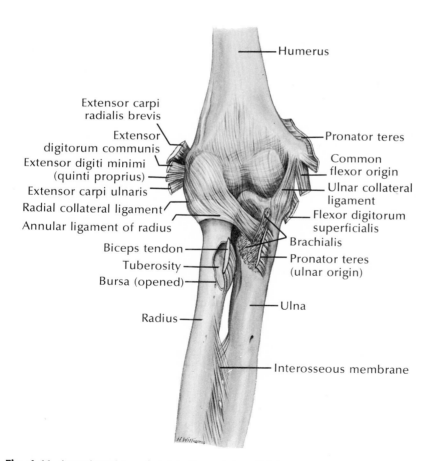

Fig. 4-11. Anterior view of right elbow joint. (Male, 53 years of age.)

biceps, and there is a bursa between the joint capsule and the tendon of the subcapularis muscle that communicates with the joint cavity. Several other bursae are in close proximity but do not communicate with the joint cavity. Beneath the deltoid muscle there is an extensive synovial sac called the subdeltoid or subacromial bursa. There is usually a bursa beneath the tendon of the infraspinatus and one between the tendons of insertion of the teres major and latissimus dorsi muscles; these bursae do not communicate with the joint cavity.

Elbow joint and radioulnar joint. The elbow joint is a uniaxial synovial joint between the humerus and the two bones of the forearm. The semilunar notch of the ulna articulates with the trochlea of the humerus; the head of the radius articulates with the capitulum. The capsule of the elbow joint also encloses the proximal radioulnar joint.

The joint capsule is thin and loose anteriorly and posteriorly to permit freedom of movement but is quite thick and strong on either side, forming the ulnar and radial collateral ligaments. The interosseous membrane between the radius and ulna is regarded as an accessory ligament of the radioulnar joints. The annular radial ligament is a thickened portion of the capsular ligament attached to the margins of the radial notch of the ulna and closely applied to the head and neck of the radius.

During flexion and extension of the elbow the proximal end of the ulna moves about the trochlea, and at the same time the head of the radius glides over the capitulum. The movements of supination and

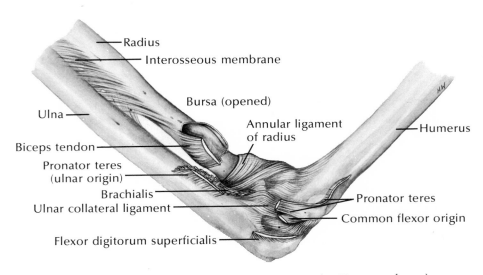

Radius
Interosseous membrane
Bursa (opened)
Ulna
Annular ligament of radius
Humerus
Biceps tendon
Pronator teres (ulnar origin)
Brachialis
Ulnar collateral ligament
Pronator teres
Common flexor origin
Flexor digitorum superficialis

90   **Fig. 4-12.** Medial view of right elbow joint. (Male, 53 years of age.)

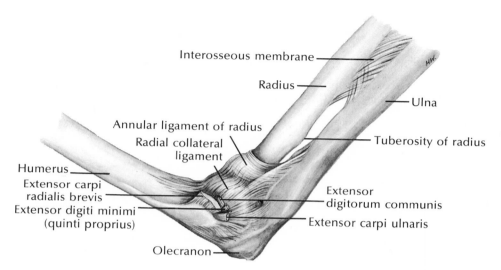

Fig. 4-13. Lateral view of right elbow joint. (Male, 53 years of age.)

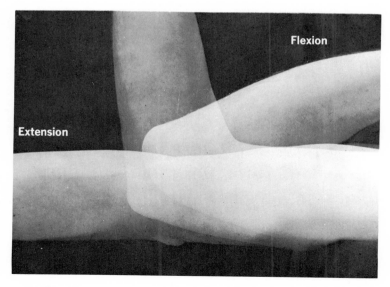

Fig. 4-14. Flexion and extension at elbow joint. (Photograph by Dr. D. R. L. Duncan.)

pronation of the palm result from movement of the radius upon the ulna. When the palm is turned upward (supination), the proximal end of the radius rotates about its own axis and the distal end moves about the head of the ulna to a position lateral to that bone. When the palm is turned downward (pronation), the radius moves in front of the head of the ulna, passing from the lateral side to occupy a position medial to the ulna. During supination and pronation the ulna does not move.

The distal radioulnar joint is separated from the wrist joint by a triangular articular disc of fibrocartilage, attached at its apex to the styloid process of the ulna and at its base to the radius. The joint cavity is separate from that of the wrist joint.

Wrist joint. The wrist joint is a biaxial synovial articulation between the distal end of the radius and the triangular articular disc proximally and the scaphoid, lunate, and triquetral bones distally. The tendons of the flexor and extensor muscles of the wrist and hand strengthen the joint, and the capsular ligament is further reinforced by flexor and extensor retinacula (volar and dorsal carpal ligaments).

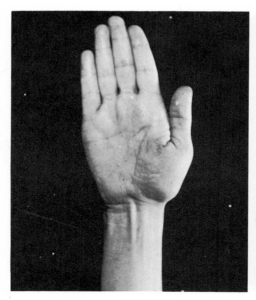 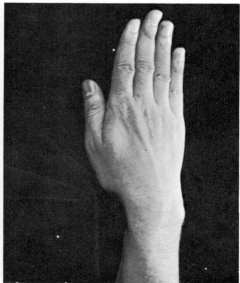

Fig. 4-15   **Fig. 4-16**

Fig. 4-15. Hand in position of supination. (Photograph by Dr. D. R. L. Duncan.)

Fig. 4-16. Hand in position of pronation. (Photograph by Dr. D. R. L. Duncan.)

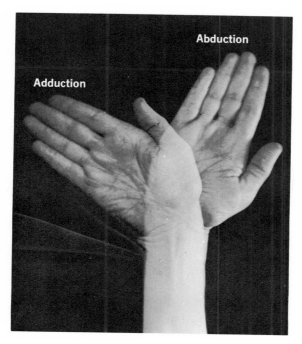

Fig. 4-17. Adduction (ulnar deviation) and abduction (radial deviation) with reference to the midplane of the body when the arms are in anatomical position. Considered in relation to the long axis of the forearm, both movements shown are abduction. (Photograph by Dr. D. R. L. Duncan.)

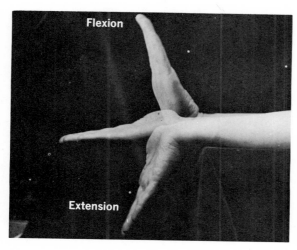

Fig. 4-18. Flexion and extension of the hand. The position of full extension is frequently termed hyperextension and the midposition, extension. (Photograph by Dr. D. R. L. Duncan.)

93

Movements of the wrist joint are in two planes, abduction-adduction in the frontal plane and flexion-extension in the sagittal plane.

Carpal joints. The carpal joints are all gliding synovial joints. The joint between the pisiform and triquetral bones is separate; the cavities between the other carpal bones communicate. There are numerous intercarpal ligaments on the volar and dorsal aspects of the wrist and also interosseous ligaments between most of the bones. The various bands are quite strong and hold the carpal bones firmly together. The joints are further reinforced by the flexor and extensor retinacula and by the long flexor and extensor tendons that pass over the wrist on their way to be attached on the finger bones. The range of movement between any two carpal bones is not great, but in combination, flexion, extension, abduction, and adduction can occur.

Hand joints. All of the joints in the hand are synovial. The joint between the base of the first metacarpal and the trapezium permits the thumb to be flexed and extended, abducted and adducted, and rotated and opposed. Much of the dexterity of the human hand is due to the great freedom of movement of this digit.

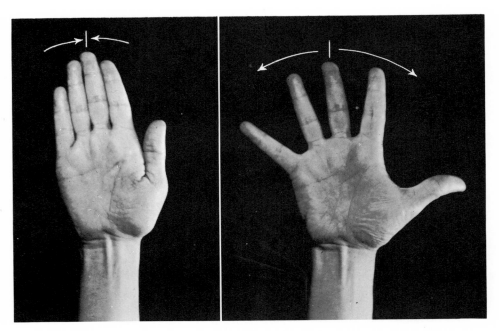

Fig. 4-19   **Fig. 4-20**

Fig. 4-19. Adduction of the fingers. (Photograph by Dr. D. R. L. Duncan.)

Fig. 4-20. Abduction of the fingers. (Photograph by Dr. D. R. L. Duncan.)

94

The remaining metacarpal and the metacarpophalangeal joints permit flexion and extension and a limited amount of abduction and adduction. It must be remembered that adduction of the fingers is a movement toward the midline of the middle digit or long finger, and abduction is movement away from the same line (Figs. 4-19 and 4-20). The interphalangeal joints are hinge joints, and their only movements are flexion and extension.

Sacroiliac joint. The sacroiliac joint is classified as a gliding synovial joint, but the joint cavity may become more or less obliterated after middle life. The sacrum fits like a wedge between the two iliac bones and is thus adapted to support the weight of the trunk; the joint is not primarily constructed for movement. The capsular ligament is

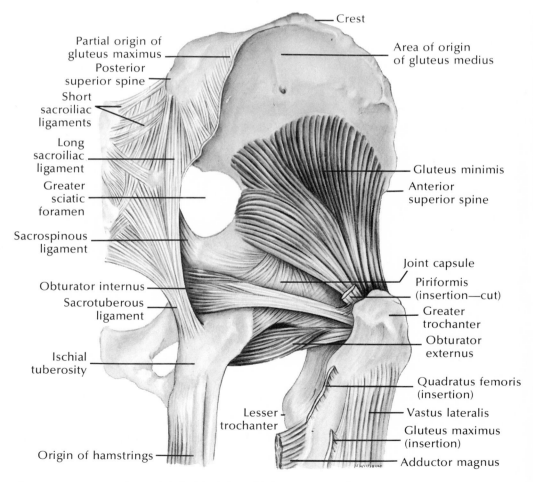

Fig. 4-21. Posterior view of right hip joint. (Male, 57 years of age.)   95

Table 7. Joints of upper extremity (all synovial)

Name	Type	Bones involved	Accessory ligaments
Sternoclavicular	Gliding	Sternum and medial end of clavicle	Costoclavicular; interclavicular
Acromioclavicular	Gliding	Lateral end of clavicle; acromion of scapula	Coracoclavicular
Shoulder	Multiaxial (ball-and-socket)	Glenoid cavity of scapula; head of humerus	Coracoacromial; coracohumeral; transverse humeral
Elbow			
Humeroradial	Gliding	Distal end of humerus; head of radius; proximal end of ulna	Radial collateral; ulnar collateral; annular radial; interosseous membrane of forearm
Humeroulnar	Uniaxial (hinge)		
Proximal radioulnar	Uniaxial (pivot)		
Distal radioulnar	Gliding	Distal end of radius and ulna	Interosseous membrane of forearm
Wrist	Biaxial	Distal end of radius and articular disc with scaphoid, lunate, and triquetrum	Volar carpal; dorsal carpal
Carpal	Gliding	Carpus; joint between pisiform and triquetrum is separate; the others communicate	Various interosseous; volar carpal; dorsal carpal
Metacarpal	Gliding	Bases of four medial metacarpals	Transverse
Carpometacarpal of thumb	Multiaxial	Base of first metacarpal with trapezium	Carpometacarpal
Carpometacarpal of fingers	Gliding	Bases of four medial metacarpals with distal row of carpals	Carpometacarpal
Metacarpophalangeal of thumb	Uniaxial (hinge)	Distal end of first metacarpal with base of proximal phalanx	Collateral
Metacarpophalangeal of fingers	Multiaxial (ball-and-socket)	Distal ends of metacarpals with bases of proximal phalanges	Collateral; transverse metacarpal
Phalangeal	Uniaxial (hinge)	Phalanges	Collateral

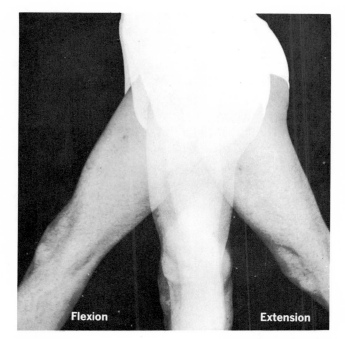

Fig. 4-22

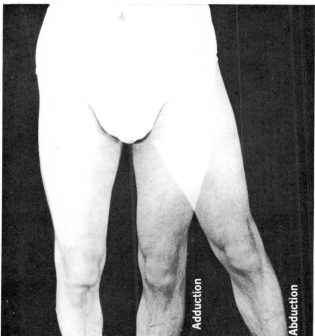

Fig. 4-23

Fig. 4-22. Flexion and extension of the hip joint. (Photograph by Dr. D. R. L. Duncan.)

Fig. 4-23. Abduction and adduction at the hip joint. (Photograph by Dr. D. R. L. Duncan.)

97

reinforced by a very strong interosseous sacroiliac ligament, by long and short posterior or dorsal sacroiliac ligaments, by the sacrotuberous ligament running from the sacrum to the ischial tuberosity, and by the sacrospinous ligament running from the sacrum to the spine of the ischium (Fig. 4-21).

Pubic symphysis. The pubic symphysis is a nonsynovial cartilaginous joint, but there is frequently a slitlike vertical cavity in the disc of fibrocartilage interposed between the two pubic bones. It is not lined with synovial membrane. The joint is strengthened on all sides by thickenings of fibrous tissue.

There is very little movement either in the sacroiliac joints or in the pubic symphysis, but during the later months of pregnancy the investing ligaments become somewhat softer, thus permitting more movement and occasionally causing much discomfort.

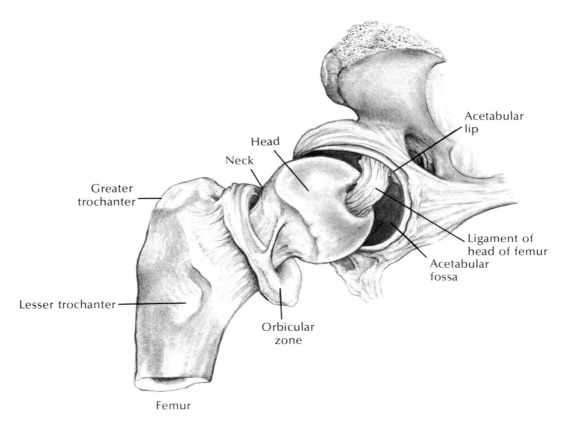

Fig. 4-24. Hip joint. Articular capsule has been opened. (Drawing by Lili Ebstein-Loewenstein, courtesy Dr. R. Locchi.) (From DiDio, L. J. A.: Synopsis of anatomy, St. Louis, 1970, The C. V. Mosby Co.)

Hip joint. The articulation between the head of the femur and the acetabulum of the hip bone is the best example in the human body of a multiaxial (ball-and-socket) synovial joint. It permits movements of flexion-extension, abduction-adduction, medial and lateral rotation, and circumduction (Figs. 4-22 and 4-23).

In contrast to those of the shoulder, the articular surfaces of the hip joint are very congruent. The acetabulum is deep, and a fibrocartilaginous rim, the acetabular labrum, as well as the transverse ligament literally grasp the head of the femur. The acetabulum is lined by a horseshoe-shaped cartilage that leaves a deficiency inferiorly called the acetabular notch. From the edge of the notch the ligamentum teres, or ligament of the head of the femur, runs within the capsule to a pit, fovea, in the central portion of the head of the femur (Fig. 4-24). Its function is not clearly understood, although a small

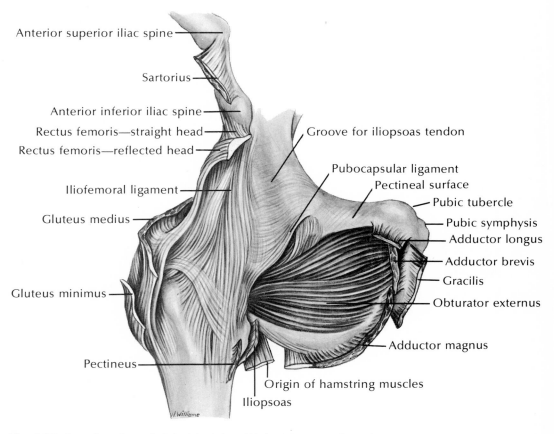

Anterior superior iliac spine
Sartorius
Anterior inferior iliac spine
Rectus femoris—straight head
Rectus femoris—reflected head
Iliofemoral ligament
Gluteus medius
Gluteus minimus
Pectineus
Iliopsoas
Origin of hamstring muscles

Groove for iliopsoas tendon
Pubocapsular ligament
Pectineal surface
Pubic tubercle
Pubic symphysis
Adductor longus
Adductor brevis
Gracilis
Obturator externus
Adductor magnus

Fig. 4-25. Anterior view of right hip joint. (Male, 62 years of age.)

artery, usually found within its substance, may supplement the blood supply to the head of the femur.

The articular capsule is a heavy fibrous sleeve that encloses not only the head but also the neck of the femur. The capsule is reinforced by three fairly well-defined thickenings: (1) the iliofemoral ligament, one of the strongest ligaments in the body, resembles an inverted Y and is attached superiorly to the ilium and inferiorly to the intertrochanteric line of the femur, (2) the pubofemoral, which passes from the pubic bone into the capsule, and (3) the ischiofemoral, which passes from the ischium into the capsule. All three ligaments, but in particular the iliofemoral, become taut upon extension, thereby increasing the stability of the hip joint in standing position without muscular effort. All three also limit medial rotation, and the pubofemoral prevents excessive abduction of the femur. There is occasionally a strong fibrous band, running from the tendon of origin of the reflected head of the rectus femoris muscle to the lateral side of the great trochanter, that may be regarded as an accessory ligament.

Knee joint. The knee joint, a modified hinge type of synovial joint between the distal end of the femur and the proximal end of the tibia, is the largest and most complex synovial articulation in the body. The main movements are flexion-extension, but there is also a slight degree of medial and lateral rotation possible between the tibia and femur. Both types of movement are complicated by linear movement of the joint surfaces on each other. When the macerated bones are moved one against the other, this joint appears to be very insecure, but in reality it is an unusually stable joint. Externally the joint capsule is strengthened by muscle tendons. Anteriorly the tendon of the quadriceps femoris muscle is fused with the capsule. The patella lies within this tendon, and the thickened central portion passing from the inferior edge of the patella to the tibial tuberosity is known as the patellar ligament. When the knee is completely extended, the back of the patella articulates with the lower end of the femur, but when the knee is completely flexed, the back of the patella occupies a deep grove between the two condyles. The patella never articulates with the tibia.

Posteriorly and on either side the articular capsule of the knee joint is further strengthened by tendons and tendinous expansions. On either side of the joint the tibial and fibular collateral ligaments, bands of dense connective tissue, become taut as full extension is reached.

Within the joint capsule are the anterior and posterior cruciate ligaments attached above to the sides of the intercondylar fossa of the femur and below to the intercondylar eminence of the tibia (Fig. 4-28). They are so named because they cross each other between

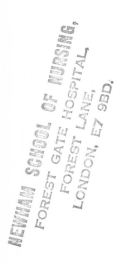

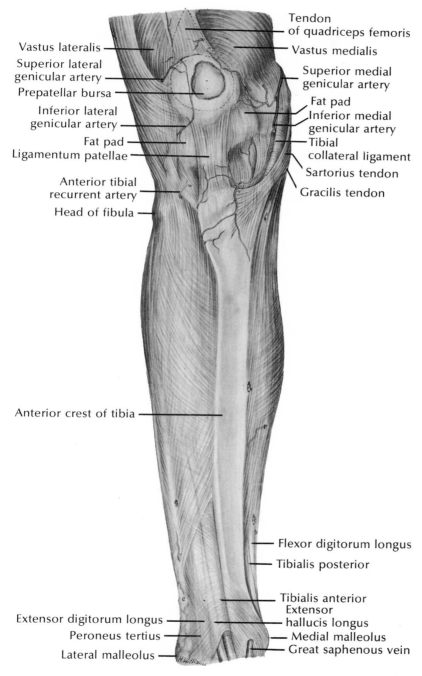

Vastus lateralis

Superior lateral genicular artery

Prepatellar bursa

Inferior lateral genicular artery

Fat pad

Ligamentum patellae

Anterior tibial recurrent artery

Head of fibula

Anterior crest of tibia

Tendon of quadriceps femoris

Vastus medialis

Superior medial genicular artery

Fat pad

Inferior medial genicular artery

Tibial collateral ligament

Sartorius tendon

Gracilis tendon

Flexor digitorum longus

Tibialis posterior

Tibialis anterior

Extensor hallucis longus

Medial malleolus

Great saphenous vein

Extensor digitorum longus

Peroneus tertius

Lateral malleolus

Fig. 4-26. Anterior view of right knee joint and deep fascia of leg. (Male, 62 years of age.)

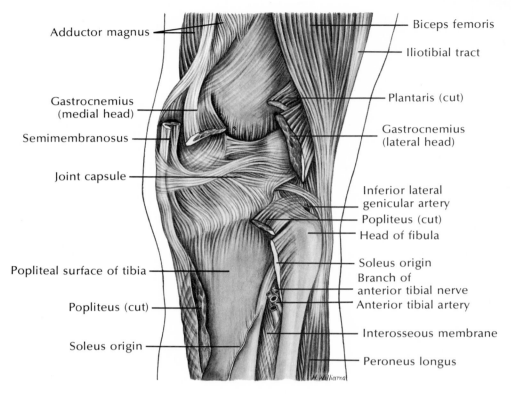

Fig. 4-27. Posterior view of right knee joint. (Male, 62 years of age.)

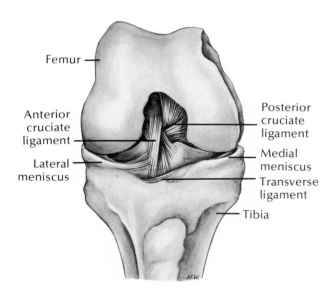

Fig. 4-28. Anterior view of right knee joint. The tibia is flexed on the femur, and the anterior portion of the capsule has been removed to show the cruciate ligaments and menisci. (Male, 57 years of age.)

their attachments. The anterior cruciate is more tense in extension, and the posterior, in flexion. Both prevent excessive anteroposterior movement. With anterior cruciate damage the tibia can be displaced forward; with posterior cruciate damage, posterior displacement is evident.

The semilunar menisci are two C-shaped fibrocartilaginous discs, one placed on the upper surface of each tibial condyle. Each cartilage is thick at its outer rim becoming thinner toward the center, thus producing a concave depression into which the respective femoral condyles fit. Both menisci are attached centrally to the intercondylar eminence of the tibia and peripherally to the fibrous capsule. The lateral meniscus also is attached to the femur by the meniscofemoral ligaments and receives slips from the popliteus muscle; therefore, its movements are guided by bony and muscular actions. The medial meniscus is more fixed due, in part, to its attachment to the tibial collateral ligament. Such attachment also explains why medial meniscus damage follows rupture of the tibial (medial) collateral ligament. There are numerous synovial bursae about the knee joint, and some of the deeper ones communicate with the joint cavity. Synovial tissue also invests the tendon of origin of the popliteus muscle.

Tibiofibular joints. The proximal tibiofibular joint is a gliding type of synovial joint between the head of the fibula and an articular facet on the undersurface of the lateral condyle of the tibia.

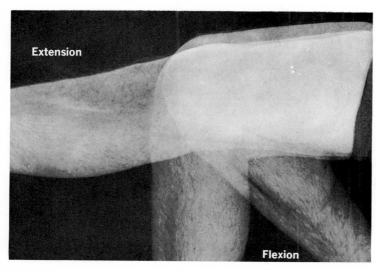

Fig. 4-29. Flexion and extension at the knee joint. (Photograph by Dr. D. R. L. Duncan.)

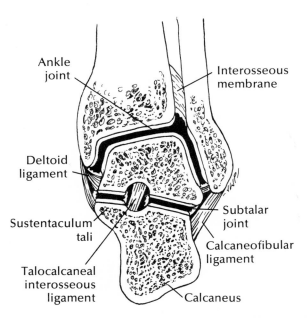

Fig. 4-30. Coronal section through the ankle showing the ankle joint, subtalar joint, and associated ligaments. (From Rosse, C., and Clawson, D.: Introduction to the musculoskeletal system, New York, 1970, Harper & Row, Publishers.)

The distal tibiofibular joint is a syndesmosis, and a very strong interosseous ligament joins the lower ends of the two bones. This ligament is the thickened distal portion of the interosseous membrane of the leg.

There is very little movement between the tibia and fibula, unlike the movement upon supination and pronation of the forearm.

Ankle joint. The distal ends of the tibia and fibula form a socket into which the upper portion of the talus fits, forming a uniaxial synovial joint, and the movements are dorsi-flexion and plantar flexion (Figs. 4-31 and 4-32).

The capsular ligament is reinforced by strong medial and lateral thickenings, and the long tendons of the foot muscles give additional support. The medial reinforcement is called the deltoid ligament and is attached to the medial malleolus and below to the talus, calcaneus, and navicular. The lateral ligament connects the lateral malleolus to the talus and calcaneus and is much weaker. A sprained ankle occurs when one of the collateral ligaments is stretched beyond its normal limit.

Foot joints. The foot is a weight-bearing structure, and the muscles, ligaments, and joints are arranged to support the weight of the

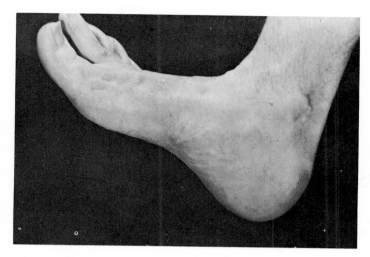

Fig. 4-31. Dorsiflexion at the ankle joint. (Photograph by Dr. D. R. L. Duncan.)

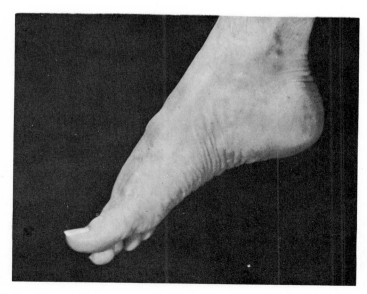

Fig. 4-32. Plantar flexion at the ankle joint. (Photograph by Dr. D. R. L. Duncan.)

body when standing and during locomotion. The joints between the tarsal bones are gliding synovial joints. Movement is limited but is rather free between talus and calcaneus and at the so-called transverse tarsal joint, between the talus and calcaneus posteriorly, and between the navicular and cuboid anteriorly. Actually there are two distinct joints, a medial one between talus and navicular and a lateral one between calcaneus and cuboid. Usually the joint cavity between each two tarsal bones is closed, and the various joints do not communicate with each other.

The joints of the bases of the metatarsals permit very little motion. The metatarsophalangeal joints permit flexion and extension of the toes and a limited amount of abduction and adduction. In the toes, movement toward the midline of the second toe is adduction, and movement in the opposite direction is abduction. The interphalangeal joints permit only flexion and extension.

Inversion of the foot turns the sole medially and eversion turns the sole laterally. This movement occurs largely at the talocalcaneal joint, but other foot joints are involved. Adduction of the foot turns the toes toward the midline of the body, and abduction turns the toes outward.

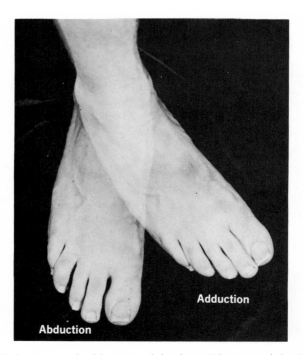

Fig. 4-33. Abduction and adduction of the foot. (Photograph by Dr. D. R. L. Duncan.)

The foot bones are held in position by capsular and interosseous ligaments, by powerful ligaments in the sole of the foot, and by the tendons of the long flexor muscles, all of which help in maintaining the stability of the foot.

Immediately deep to the skin on the plantar surface of the foot there is a sheet of dense connective tissue called the plantar aponeurosis (Fig. 4-36). Posteriorly, it is attached to the inferior surface of the cal-

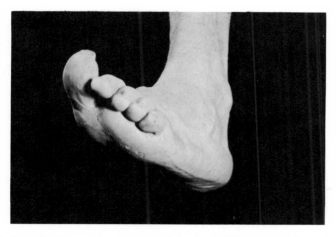

Fig. 4-34. Dorsiflexion and inversion of the foot. (Photograph by Dr. D. R. L. Duncan.)

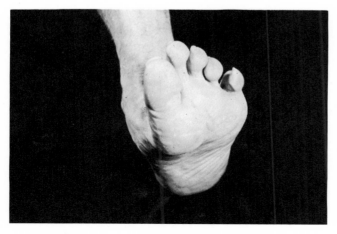

Fig. 4-35. Dorsiflexion and eversion fo the foot. (Photograph by Dr. D. R. L. Duncan.)

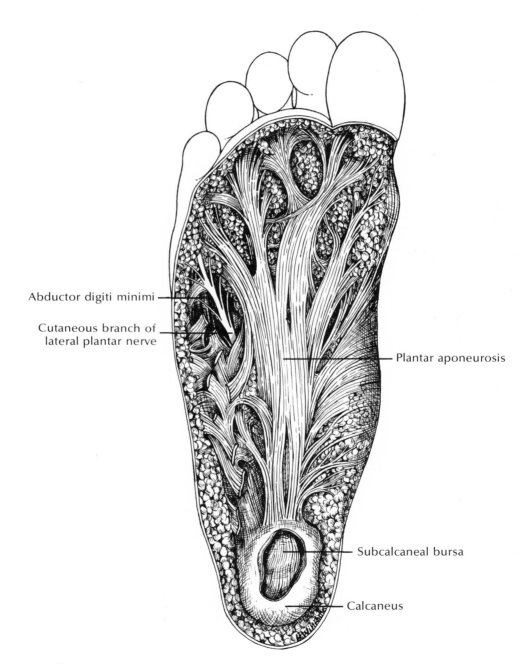

Abductor digiti minimi

Cutaneous branch of
lateral plantar nerve

Plantar aponeurosis

Subcalcaneal bursa

Calcaneus

Fig. 4-36. The plantar aponeurosis. (Male, 55 years of age.)

Table 8. Joints of lower extremity

Name	Type	Bones involved	Accessory ligaments
Sacroiliac	Gliding	Sacrum and ilium	Interosseous; long posterior sacroiliac; short posterior sacroiliac; sacrotuberous; sacrospinous
Pubic symphysis*	Cartilaginous	Pubes	Superior pubic and arcuate pubic ligament
Hip	Multiaxial (ball-and-socket)	Acetabulum with head of femur	Iliofemoral; pubofemoral; ischiofemoral; round
Knee	Biaxial (modified hinge)	Distal end of femur with patella and with proximal end of tibia	Patellar; tibial collateral; fibular collateral; anterior cruciate; posterior cruciate; medial meniscus; lateral meniscus; transverse
Proximal tibiofibular	Gliding	Head of fibula with lateral condyle of tibia	Interosseous membrane of leg
Distal tibiofibular*	Fibrous	Distal end of tibia and fibula	Interosseous membrane of leg
Ankle	Uniaxial (hinge)	Talus with distal end of tibia and fibula	Deltoid; anterior talofibular; posterior talofibular; calcaneofibular
Tarsal	Gliding	Tarsus	Interosseous; long plantar; short plantar; plantar; plantar calcaneonavicular; bifurcate
Tarsometatarsal	Gliding	Bases of metatarsals with distal tarsals	Interosseous; dorsal and plantar tarsometatarsal
Metatarsal	Gliding	Bases of metatarsals	Metatarsal
Metatarsophalangeal	Biaxial	Distal ends of metatarsals with bases of proximal phalanges	Plantar; collateral
Phalangeal	Uniaxial (hinge)	Phalanges	Plantar; collateral

* Indicates nonsynovial joints.

caneus; anteriorly the fibers fan out, and small branches pass to the metatarsophalangeal articulations and blend with the capsular ligaments. Other fibers pass from the deep surface of the aponeurosis between the small muscles of the foot and the long flexor tendons of the sole to attach to the deep fascia below the bones. The interosseous ligament between the talus and calcaneus is particularly strong, and it is very unusual to see a dislocation occurring between these two bones. The long plantar ligament is attached posteriorly to the inferior surface of the calcaneus and passes anteriorly to attach to the plantar surface of the cuboid and to the bases of the three lateral metatarsal bones. Deeper than this ligament is a short, broad, very strong band of fibers, running from calcaneus to cuboid, called the plantar calcaneocuboid or short plantar ligament. The plantar calcaneonavicular ligament, the spring ligament, is a very strong band of fibers extending from the anterior end of the calcaneus to the navicular and supporting the anterior end of the talus. It is an important factor in maintaining the medial longitudinal arch of the foot. The bifurcate ligament is a U-shaped fibrous band attached posteriorly to the calcaneus; anteriorly, one arm goes to the lateral side of the navicular, and the other arm, to the cuboid (see Fig. 5-42).

SUMMARY OF LIMB JOINTS

The upper and lower extremities have the same skeletal system pattern. There is one large long bone in the upper part of each, two long bones in the forearm and in the leg, a group of irregular bones in the carpus and in the tarsus, and five rays in the hand and in the forefoot. The joints in each extremity are similar but are modified for different functions. The upper extremity is structured to enable us to place the hand in almost any position and to perform many varied and complex actions. The lower extremity is structured to enable us to maintain balance in the erect position and to walk upright.

The shoulder and hip joints are ball-and-socket joints, but they display marked anatomical modifications. In the shoulder joint the glenoid cavity is shallow, and the articular surface of the head of the humerus is proportionally large. The capsular ligament is loose. Therefore, the head of the humerus has very free movement, and dislocations are frequent. Stability has been sacrificed for mobility. In the hip joint the acetabulum is deep, and the head of the femur fits snugly into the cavity. The head of the femur is rarely dislocated. The capsular ligament has thick, strong reinforcing bands. Mobility has been sacrificed for stability.

The elbow and knee joints are hinge joints. The knee joint is large and is reinforced by semilunar cartilages, muscles, and special ligaments. The radius moves freely about the ulna in supination and pronation. There is almost no movement between the tibia and fibula.

The wrist joint permits flexion and extension and some medial (ulnar) and lateral (radial) deviation. The ankle joint permits limited dorsal and plantar flexion. In the non-weight-bearing foot there is some inversion and eversion of the foot, but in the weight-bearing foot there is practically none.

The thumb has a great range of complex movements, but the great toe is almost immovable.

Trauma to a joint can cause damage to any or all of the structures of the joint (articular cartilage, synovial membrane, capsule, or supporting ligaments). When the ligaments are strained beyond their normal capacity, they may tear. These tears are called sprains. In severe tears the joint may become dislocated, in which case the articular surfaces are no longer congruent.

JOINT TRAUMA OR DISEASE

Arthritis, derived from the Greek *arthron* (joint) and *itis* (inflammation), is a term used to indicate inflammatory joint disease. The primary site of inflammation in arthritis is the synovial membrane.

Degenerative joint disease is characterized by a localized degeneration of articular cartilage. This condition, also called osteoarthritis, is not a true arthritis, since inflammation is not a primary event.

REVIEW QUESTIONS

1. Define a joint.
2. Define synovial joint versus nonsynovial joint.
3. Describe axis of rotation and plane of movement.
4. List five types of synovial joints and give an example of each.
5. List five types of nonsynovial joints and give an example of each.
6. Describe the development of a joint.
7. List the distinguishing features of a synovial joint.
8. What movements occur in the temporomandibular joint?
9. At what joints do nodding movements of the head occur? Where do rotatory movements of the head occur?
10. Describe briefly the bones and movements involved in supination and pronation of the hand.
11. What are the important ligaments that strengthen the capsular ligament of the hip joint?
12. Name four structures that increase the stability of the knee joint?
13. With what other bones does the femur articulate?
14. Define sprain.

CHAPTER 5

MUSCLES

Movements of the body are produced by muscular action. Muscles that are under the control of the will are referred to as voluntary or skeletal muscles. In the description of the individual muscles, one or two principal actions will be given, but since no movement is brought about by the action of a single muscle, many other muscles will be contracting simultaneously to a greater or lesser degree. For example, a person wishing to raise his arm laterally (abduction) does so primarily by contraction of the deltoid muscle, called the prime mover. Muscles that directly oppose this movement, pectoralis major, teres major, and latissimus dorsi, are called antagonists. The movement of abduction is brought about by coordination of prime mover contraction with simultaneous relaxation of the antagonists. At the same time the head of the humerus must be held in the rather ill-fitting glenoid cavity, and the capsule must be pulled out of the way of the humerus. Both actions are performed by the supraspinatus muscle, which also contracts throughout abduction, thereby acting as a synergist. To allow the deltoid and supraspinatus to abduct the upper limb, it is necessary to stabilize, or fix, the entire shoulder girdle, an action performed by the trapezius, serratus anterior, pectoralis minor, and rhomboids.

A further example of muscle interaction occurs during flexion and extension of the elbow, during which the biceps brachii and triceps act as antagonists. However, during supination of the forearm and hand, as would occur when one is using a screwdriver, the biceps is the prime mover. To cancel out unwanted components of biceps action and to stabilize the elbow joint, the triceps contracts, thereby acting as a synergist during supination.

A muscle has two areas of attachment: that nearer the center of the body is usually described as the origin, and that more peripherally situated is generally termed the insertion. Usually the origin is from a relatively immovable structure, and the insertion is into a relatively movable structure. In this text the conventional origin and insertion of the various muscles have been described. In many activities the area that is conventionally called the origin really becomes the functional insertion, and the insertion becomes the origin. For example, the pectoralis major muscle is described as originating from the chest wall and as being inserted into the humerus. This is true in a freely swinging arm, but in the exercise of chinning on a horizontal bar the arms are fixed on the bar, and the body is drawn upward. Therefore, the area of attachment on the humerus becomes the functional origin, and the attachment on the chest wall, the functional insertion. Bones carry the majority of muscular attachments, but there are some muscles affixed to the costal cartilages and some to the cartilages of the larynx and air passages. Muscles have attachments also to the fibrous tissue surrounding them and to the prolongations of their sheaths. Finally, there are small muscles in the actual substance of the skin as well as in the subcutaneous tissue beneath it. The fleshy portion of a muscle is occasionally attached directly to the bone, but the attachment is usually made by means of fibrous tissue, tendon, or aponeurosis. A tendon is a narrow ribbonlike band of dense connective tissue; an aponeurosis is a broad flat tendon.

The constituent fibers of a muscle are parallel to the long axis of the muscle when extent of contraction rather than power is the main requirement. Where power is needed, muscle fibers are short, are ar-

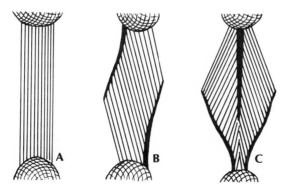

Fig. 5-1. Fiber arrangement in muscle. **A,** Fibers parallel to the long axis. **B,** Pennate arrangement of muscle fibers. **C,** Bipennate arrangement of muscle fibers. (After Murk Jansen.)

ranged in a pennate fashion, and are attached to tendons or fibrous bands penetrating the substance of the muscle (Fig. 5-1).

Each muscle is supplied with at least one nerve that transmits impulses from the central nervous system, causing the muscle to contract. A single motor nerve fiber innervates a number of muscle fibers, and it has been found that muscles performing very delicate movements have a smaller number of muscle fibers per nerve fiber than do the muscles used in gross movements. It has been reported that in the extrinsic muscles that move the eyeball there are from 6 to 12 muscle fibers for each nerve fiber, but that in the semitendinosus, a large muscle of the thigh, there are about 50 muscle fibers per nerve fiber. A motor nerve fiber with the muscle fibers it innervates is called a motor unit. Sensory impulses are carried by nerves from the muscle to the central nervous system, giving information on the degree and strength of contraction.

During infancy, muscles have a small amount of connective tissue, and frequently the muscle fibers attach directly to bone without any intervening tendon or aponeurosis. With increasing age the amount of connective tissue and of elastic fibers increases. This is the only definite age change that occurs in muscles, and there is some evidence that the lessened strength of later years is due to changes within the central nervous system or to vascular changes rather than to changes in the muscles themselves. Muscles have no definite or fixed rate of growth but grow in accordance with the structures to which they are attached and with their use. The eye and ear muscles grow very little, whereas the large muscles of the lower extremity increase greatly.

**MUSCLES OF
EXPRESSION**

The many small muscles beneath the skin of the scalp and face, particularly about the eyes and mouth, alter facial expression, a very important means of communication (Fig. 5-2). All the muscles described in this discussion are innervated by branches of the seventh cranial, or facial nerve. When this nerve is paralyzed, there is marked distortion. On the affected side the face becomes masklike, the lower eyelid falls away from the eyeball, and the lower lip hangs loosely due to paralysis of the muscles, a condition known as Bell's palsy.

The orbicularis oculi muscle is an oval sphincter lying in the subcutaneous tissue of the eyelids and of the forehead. It keeps the lids closely applied to the eyeball, closes the eye, and draws down the eyebrow. the corrugator supercilii muscle lies between the eyebrows and when contracted, as in frowning, produces vertical folds in the skin of the forehead.

The orbicularis oris lies within the lips and is the sphincter of the

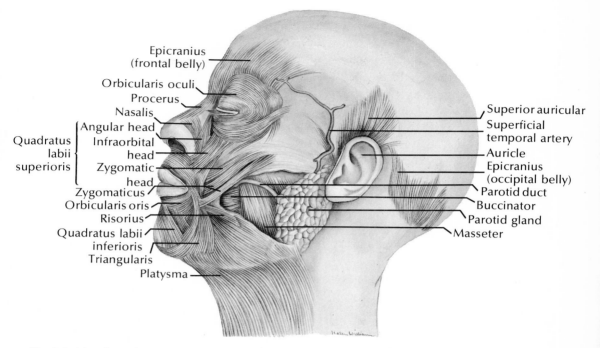

Fig. 5-2. Muscles of expression. View of the left side of the face. The lateral portion of the capsule of the parotid gland has been removed. (Dissection by Dr. Frank Vecchio.) (Male, 40 years of age.)

mouth. The other muscles associated with the lips have been variously named and subdivided. Only the more important and more constant ones will be mentioned. The levators of the upper lip and of the angle of the mouth arise from the zygomatic bone and maxilla and are inserted into the upper lip. They prevent drooping of the upper lip and corner of the mouth. The depressors of the lower lip and of the angle of the mouth arise from the mandible and pass superiorly to be inserted into the lower lip. They pull the lower lip and corner of the mouth down.

The buccinator muscle arises form the side of the maxilla superiorly, from the inner surface of the mandible inferiorly, and from the pterygomandibular raphe, which is a dense band of the deep fascia of the pharynx. The buccinator thus constitutes the essential muscular coat of the cheek and is inserted into the corner of the mouth. The buccinator aids in chewing movements by keeping the cheek more firmly in contact with the teeth, thus preventing food from being pocketed between teeth and cheek.

The platysma muscle arises from the deep surface of the skin in the upper chest wall and passes within the subcutaneous tissue of the neck to be attached to the lower lip and corner of the mouth. The platysma acts particularly on the skin of the lower lip and neck. The risorius is a small muscle extending laterally from the corner of the mouth. It is more or less intermingled with the platysma, as are all of the muscles that converge to this point.

The epicranius muscle has four bellies, two anterior bellies in the deep fascia of the forehead and two posterior bellies in the fascia over the back of the head, and a strong intervening fibrous sheet, the galea aponeurotica, stretched tightly over the dome of the skull. Contraction of the anterior bellies pulls the scalp anteriorly, raises the eyebrows, and wrinkles the forehead. Contraction of the posterior bellies pulls the scalp posteriorly.

The scalp by itself forms a thick cushioning layer that protects the underlying brain from all but the most severe and direct trauma. It is composed of five layers, which from exterior to interior are as follows:

Skin—with layer of hair
Cutaneous—with vessels and nerves
Aponeurosis—dense connective tissue
Loose space—emissary veins and small arteries
Pericranium—outer periosteum of the skull

The three outer layers of the scalp, with associated musculature, are intimately fused and move as a unit. The subcutaneous layer, containing many blood vessels and nerves, is rather dense and inelastic due to fibrous bands that unite the skin to the underlying galea aponeurotica. In scalp lacerations the fibrous bands tend to hold the wound and any divided vessels open, thereby creating often alarming hemorrhages. The three outer layers are separated from the periosteum of the skull by a loose connective tissue space that in addition to allowing movement upon the pericranium also allows the spread of fluid or infection, because of which it is often called the "danger space." Furthermore, the subaponeurotic space is also traversed by small arteries and by the important emissary veins that connect the superficial veins of the scalp with the intracranial venous sinuses (Fig. 6-5). Infections, failing to find ready exit from the subaponeurotic space, can spread along these emissary veins and enter the dural sinuses.

ANTERIOR MUSCLES OF THE NECK

The hyoid muscles, both suprahyoids and infrahyoids, also called the strap muscles because of their shape, are included in this group (Figs. 5-3 and 11-6). Since these muscles are part of the extrinsic

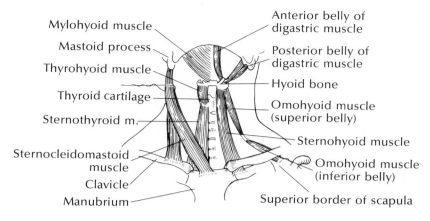

Mylohyoid muscle

Mastoid process

Thyrohyoid muscle

Thyroid cartilage

Sternothyroid m.

Sternocleidomastoid muscle

Clavicle

Manubrium

Anterior belly of digastric muscle

Posterior belly of digastric muscle

Hyoid bone

Omohyoid muscle (superior belly)

Sternohyoid muscle

Omohyoid muscle (inferior belly)

Superior border of scapula

Fig. 5-3. Anterior muscles of the neck.

musculature of the larynx, they are described in Chapter 11. The sternocleidomastoid muscle also must be discussed here. This muscle arises from the anterior surface of the manubrium of the sternum and from the medial portion of the clavicle and is inserted into the mastoid portion of the temporal bone. Both sternocleidomastoid muscles acting together extend the head on the atlas and flex the cervical spine against resistance. One muscle acting alone rotates the head to the opposite side and elevates the chin. The muscle receives its nerve supply from the spinal accessory nerve as well as from the second and third cervical nerves. Since the spinal accessory nerve is a purely motor nerve, it is postulated that sensory fibers from the sternocleidomastoid pass back to the central nervous system by the dorsal root ganglia of the cervical nerves.

The upper extremity in man is specialized for grasping. Its very powerful muscles, which give it strength, are arranged in the shoulder, upper arm, and forearm; the many smaller muscles used for precision are situated in the hand.

Muscles of pectoral region. The pectoralis major arises from clavicle, sternum, and adjacent costal cartilages and from the sheath of the superficial muscle of the abdominal wall (Fig. 5-4). From this broad origin the fibers converge to their insertion into the superior and anterior aspect of the humerus. The muscle draws the arm across the chest in such actions as chopping wood and is a powerful adductor. The clavicular portion has a nerve supply and a lymphatic drainage system separate from those of the other part of the muscle and from the breast. In radical amputation of the breast the costosternal

MUSCLES OF UPPER EXTREMITY

117

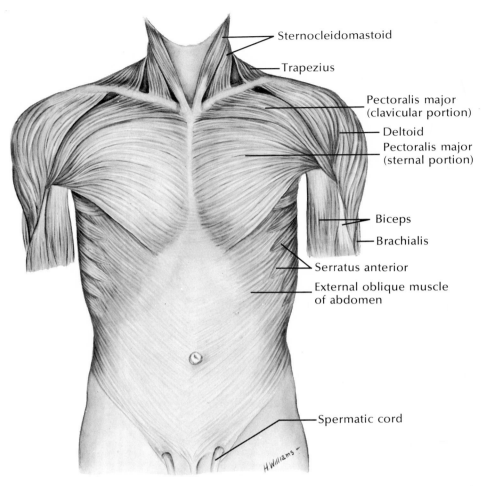

Fig. 5-4. Muscles of anterior surface of the trunk. (Male, 65 years of age.)

portion of the pectoralis major is removed along with the pectoralis minor, but the clavicular part of the muscle, which is inserted relatively low on the humerus, is occasionally left. Since the lower fibers of the pectoralis major are attached high up on the humerus, there is an overlapping of the tendon of insertion, the lower fibers lying behind the upper or clavicular fibers. This overlapping produces the rounded contour of the anterior axillary border.

The pectoralis minor arises from the second, third, and fourth ribs and is inserted into the coracoid process of the scapula. It assists in depressing and protracting the shoulder. It has the same nerve supply as the pectoralis major (the medial and lateral anterior thoracic nerves, also known as medial and lateral pectoral nerves). The pectoralis minor is removed in radical breast amputations.

The serratus anterior arises from the lateral chest wall from the second to the eighth or ninth rib and is inserted into the vertebral margin of the scapula on the costal surface. The portion arising from each rib is a distinct muscle belly that gives a serrated or saw-tooth appearance to the line of origin, hence the name. The serratus anterior draws the scapula anteriorly over the thoracic wall. The long thoracic nerve is its nerve supply.

Muscles of back attached to scapula. The trapezius is a large triangular muscle arising from the occipital bone, from the ligamentum nuchae, and from the spines of the vertebrae from the seventh cervical to the twelfth thoracic, inclusive. The ligamentum nuchae, by its attachment to the spines of the cervical vertebrae, separates from each other the two muscular columns of the back of the neck. The trapezius is inserted into the lateral third of the clavicle and the spine of the scapula. It is used in bracing and raising the shoulders and in rotating the scapula. It is innervated by the accessory nerve.

The latissimus dorsi is a large muscle arising from the spines of the lower six thoracic vertebrae, from a short layer of fascia in the loin known as the lumbodorsal fascia, from the iliac crest, and occasionally also from the lower angle of the scapula. It is inserted into the humerus medial to the pectoralis major. The thick lateral margin of the muscle forms the posterior wall of the axilla. This muscle is a very powerful adductor and extensor of the arm and is the main muscle used in sweeping the arm inferiorly and posteriorly during swimming. It is supplied by the thoracodorsal nerve.

The levator scapulae, rhomboideus major, and rhomboideus minor are three flat muscles beneath the trapezius that arise from the transverse processes of cervical and upper thoracic vertebrae and are inserted on the vertebral margin of the scapula. The levator and rhomboids retract and elevate the scapula and help to steady that bone during movements of the arm. The rhomboids are innervated by the dorsal scapular nerve, and the levator scapulae, by twigs from the third and fourth cervical nerves.

Muscles of shoulder. The deltoid is a large and powerful muscle arising from the lateral end of the clavicle and from the acromion and spine of the scapula and is inserted into the deltoid tuberosity, a prominence midway down the lateral surface of the humerus. It is innervated by the axillary (circumflex) nerve and is the chief abductor of the humerus (Fig. 5-7).

The supraspinatus arises from the superficial surface of the scapula above the spine and passes over the shoulder joint to be inserted on 119 the top of the greater tubercle of the humerus. The infraspinatus arises from the superficial surface of the scapula below the spine and passes posterior to the shoulder joint to be inserted on the greater tubercle below the supraspinatus. The supraspinatus and infraspinatus muscles are supplied by the suprascapular nerve. The teres minor arises from the upper portion of the axillary (lateral) margin of the scapula and passes posterior to the humerus to be inserted on the greater tubercle of the humerus below the infraspinatus. It is supplied by the axillary (circumflex) nerve. The teres major arises from the

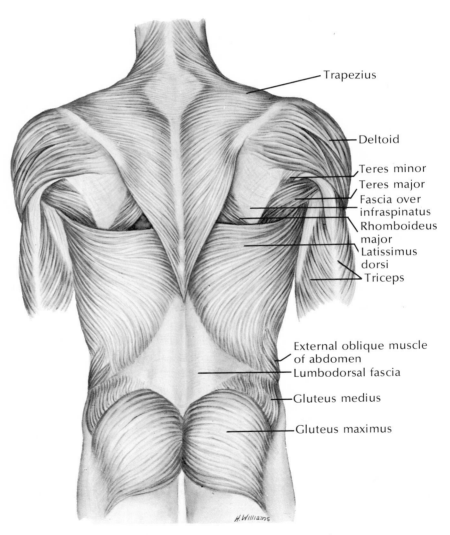

Trapezius

Deltoid

Teres minor
Teres major
Fascia over
infraspinatus
Rhomboideus
major
Latissimus
dorsi
Triceps

External oblique muscle
of abdomen
Lumbodorsal fascia

Gluteus medius

Gluteus maximus

H. Williams

120   **Fig. 5-5.** Superficial muscles of back. (Male, 65 years of age.)

axillary border of the scapula below the teres minor and passes anteriorly to be inserted on the humerus medial to the latissimus dorsi.
It is supplied by the lower subscapular nerve. The subscapularis muscle arises from the deep (costal) surface of the scapula and is inserted
into the lesser tubercle of the humerus. It is supplied by both subscapular nerves. The supraspinatus is an abductor of the arm, and the
others are adductors; the infraspinatus and teres minor rotate the

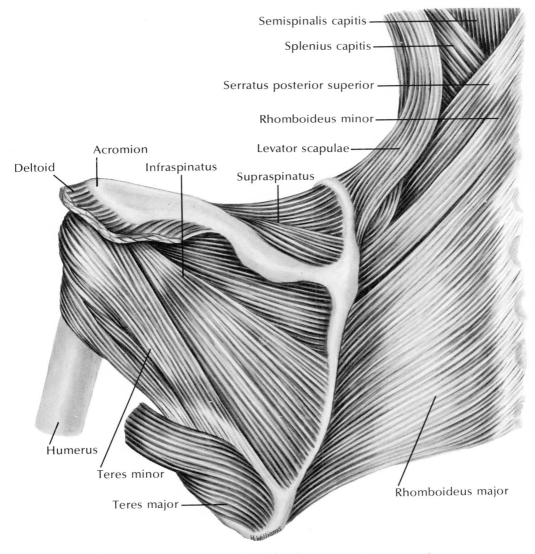

Fig. 5-6. Deep muscles attached to scapula; deltoid and trapezius removed.
(Male, 62 years of age.)

121

humerus laterally, and the teres major and subscapularis rotate the humerus medially. As the tendons of the supraspinatus, infraspinatus, teres minor, and subscapularis muscles pass across the shoulder joint, they are fused with the capsular ligament of that joint. This rein-

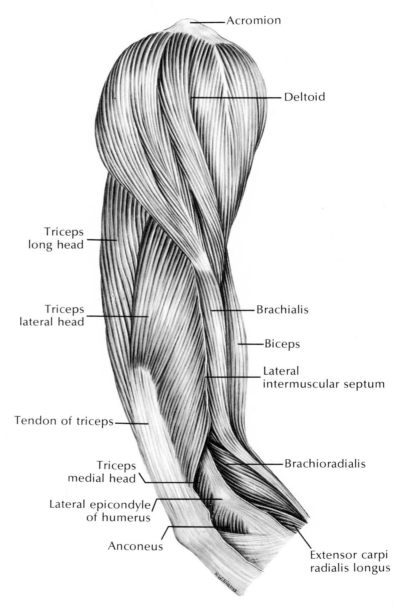

— Acromion

— Deltoid

Triceps
long head

Triceps
lateral head

Brachialis

Biceps

Lateral
intermuscular septum

Tendon of triceps

Triceps
medial head

Brachioradialis

Lateral epicondyle
of humerus

Anconeus

Extensor carpi
radialis longus

122   **Fig. 5-7.** Muscles of upper arm, lateral view. (Male, 62 years of age.)

forcement of the capsule is known as the musculotendinous or rotator cuff of the shoulder joint.

It is convenient to remember that the four great superficial muscles of the chest and shoulder, pectoralis major, trapezius, deltoid, and latissimus dorsi, are all triangular in outline. The fibers of each converge from a widespread origin to a small insertion. Small portions of each muscle are capable of functioning separately; for example, the posterior fibers of the deltoid, which arise from the spine of the scapula, extend and laterally rotate the arm. The anterior fibers, which arise from the clavicle, flex and medially rotate the arm, but when the muscle acts as a whole, it becomes an abductor of the humerus.

The action of many individual muscles can be demonstrated easily in a living human being, and movements at the shoulder joint illustrate this fact. The abducting action of the deltoid muscle can be palpated in anyone. The assisting action of the supraspinatus muscle is difficult to demonstrate. The opposite movement of adduction of the arm is brought about by two very powerful muscles, the pectoralis major anteriorly and the latissimus dorsi posteriorly.

PROTRACTION OF SHOULDER GIRDLE. Protraction or the drawing forward of the shoulder girdle is effected primarily by the serratus anterior pulling the scapula forward on the rib cage and by the pectoralis major pulling the humerus across the chest wall. The two muscles act simultaneously in the movement of reaching forward, and if the serratus is paralyzed, a typical "winging" outward of the medial border of the scapula is seen.

ABDUCTION OF THE SHOULDER. The deltoid and supraspinatus are the major abductors of the shoulder; however, with lateral rotation of the humerus, the long head of the biceps brachii will aid in abduction. The effectiveness of the deltoid and supraspinatus is largely dependent upon the synergistic action of the trapezius and serratus anterior. If these muscles are damaged, contraction of the abductors will cause medial rotation of the scapula with depression of the shoulder joint. Such depression would cause shortening and loss of effectiveness of the deltoid and supraspinatus. Either the deltoid or supraspinatus acting alone will abduct the upper limb although strength of abduction is obviously reduced.

FLEXION OF THE SHOULDER. Various muscles take part in flexing the shoulder: deltoid—axillary nerve, pectoralis major—medial and lateral pectoral nerves, and coracobrachialis and biceps brachii—musculocutaneous nerve. Because of the rather widespread nerve supply to these muscles, it is unlikely that flexion will be completely lost unless catastrophic damage occurs to the muscles of the shoulder or to the brachial plexus from which the nerve supply originates.

123

STABILIZATION OF SHOULDER JOINT. The muscles of the upper extremity that have just been described may be grouped differently to further emphasize certain of their combined actions. The shoulder joint is a very freely movable joint, and the various muscles of the region are arranged to give maximal stability without sacrifice of motility. There is a group of muscles extending from the trunk to the shoulder girdle; these include the trapezius, pectoralis minor, rhomboids, levator scapulae, and serratus anterior. These muscles bind the shoulder girdle closely and firmly to the trunk. Next there is a group of muscles extending from the shoulder girdle (mainly scapula) to the upper end of the humerus; these include the supraspinatus, infraspinatus, teres major and minor, and deltoid. These muscles hold the head of the humerus firmly against the glenoid cavity of the scapula. Finally there is a group of muscles extending from the trunk to the upper humerus; these are the latissimus dorsi and most of the pectoralis major. They aid in stabilizing the entire shoulder region in movements of forearm and hand.

Muscles of upper arm. On the front of the upper arm are the following muscles: (1) the coracobrachialis, which arises from the coracoid process of the scapula and is inserted into the medial border of the humerus, (2) the biceps brachii, which arises by two heads, one from the coracoid and the other from the tubercle overhanging the glenoid cavity of the scapula, and is inserted into the tuberosity of the radius and deep fascia of the forearm by an aponeurosis (lacertus fibrosus), and (3) the brachialis, which arises from the lowest portion of the anterior aspect of the humerus and is inserted into the coronoid process of the ulna. All are supplied by the musculocutaneous nerve. The biceps is the most superficial of the three and causes the bulge of the lower part of the front of the arm when the elbow is powerfully flexed.

The biceps is a supinator and flexor of the supinated forearm. The brachialis is the particular flexor of the forearm in the pronated position. The brachioradialis (a muscle of the forearm innervated by the radial nerve) is also a flexor of the forearm in the semisupinated, semipronated position. Flexion of the elbow is therefore possible after paralysis of the musculocutaneous nerve.

The triceps is the only important muscle of the posterior aspect of the upper arm. It arises from a prominence immediately below the glenoid cavity of the scapula, from the back of the humerus above and below the radial groove, and is inserted into the olecranon process of the ulna. This muscle is the extensor of the elbow joint and is innervated by the radial nerve.

124   The tendon of the long head of the biceps brachii muscle passing

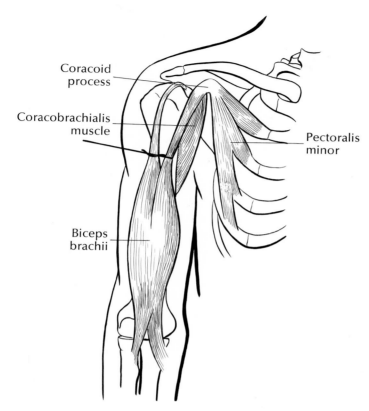

Coracoid process

Coracobrachialis muscle

Pectoralis minor

Biceps brachii

Fig. 5-8. Anterior view of muscles of upper arm and shoulder.

over the head of the humerus and the straight head of the triceps brachii lying beneath the head of the humerus also aid in maintaining the stability of the shoulder joint (Figs. 5-7 and 5-8).

After injuries to the radial nerve as it passes around the shaft of the humerus, active extension of the forearm is possible because the long head of the triceps is innervated by the nerve immediately beyond its emergence from the brachial plexus. After fractures of the olecranon the triceps pulls the proximal fragment upward, and this pull must be overcome to bring about reduction and must be counteracted during healing.

A point of importance is that all the muscles on the posterior or dorsal aspect of the arm, forearm, and hand are innervated by the radial nerve. Another important factor that has clinical implications is the nerve supply to muscles producing flexion of the elbow joint. Although the major elbow flexors are innervated by the musculocutaneous nerve, flexion against light resistance can be effected by the

125

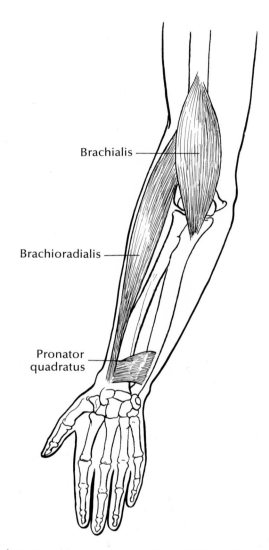

Fig. 5-9. Attachments of brachialis, brachioradialis, and pronator quadratus muscles.

brachioradialis and pronator teres muscles innervated by the radial and median nerves, respectively.

Muscles of forearm. The superficial muscles, namely, the flexor carpi radialis, palmaris longus, flexor carpi ulnaris, flexor digitorum superficialis (sublimis), and pronator teres, all arise by a common tendon of origin from the medial epicondyle; the flexor carpi ulnaris, flexor digitorum superficialis, and pronator teres have additional

126

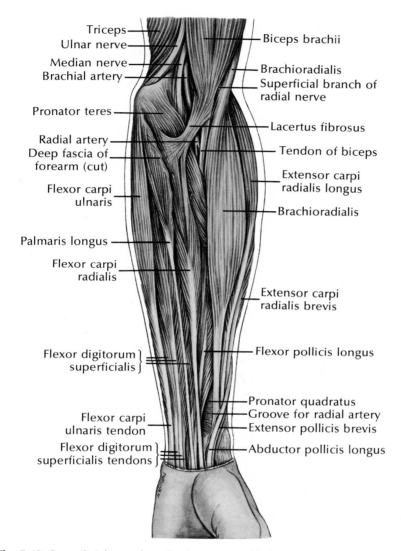

Triceps
Ulnar nerve
Median nerve
Brachial artery
Pronator teres
Radial artery
Deep fascia of forearm (cut)
Flexor carpi ulnaris
Palmaris longus
Flexor carpi radialis
Flexor digitorum superficialis
Flexor carpi ulnaris tendon
Flexor digitorum superficialis tendons

Biceps brachii
Brachioradialis
Superficial branch of radial nerve
Lacertus fibrosus
Tendon of biceps
Extensor carpi radialis longus
Brachioradialis
Extensor carpi radialis brevis
Flexor pollicis longus
Pronator quadratus
Groove for radial artery
Extensor pollicis brevis
Abductor pollicis longus

Fig. 5-10. Superficial muscles of volar aspect of left forearm. (Male, 68 years of age.)

origins from the ulna. After fracture of the medial epicondyle these muscles pull the fragment downward.

The flexor carpi radialis is inserted into the base of the second and third metacarpal bones, the flexor carpi ulnaris into the pisiform and base of the fifth metacarpal, and the palmaris longus into the apex of the palmar aponeurosis. These three muscles flex the wrist joint and aid in steadying that joint during movements of the fingers. The radial

127

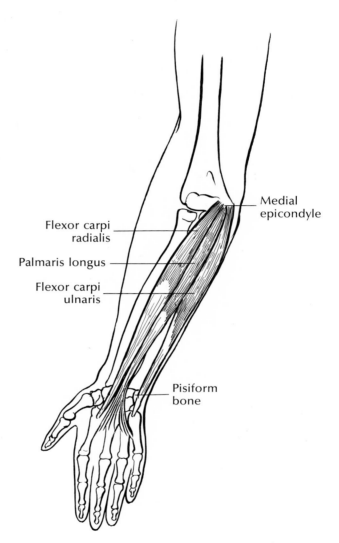

Fig. 5-11. Attachments of superficial muscles on anterior aspect of forearm.

flexor abducts the hand (lateral deviation), and the ulnar flexor adducts the hand (medial deviation). The pronator teres is inserted into the midportion of the shaft of the radius on the lateral side.

The flexor digitorum profundus and pronator quadratus have origins from the volar (front) aspect of the ulna. The flexor pollicis longus arises from the volar aspect of the radius. The flexors profundus and pollicis also have origins from the interosseous membrane. These three muscles lie deeper than the superficial group.

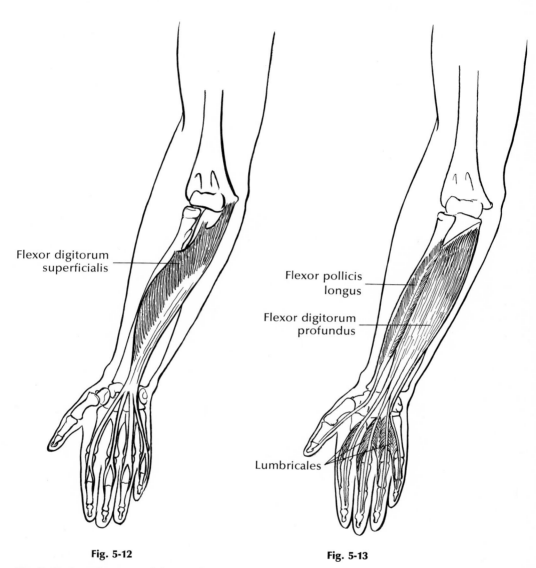

Fig. 5-12   **Fig. 5-13**

Fig. 5-12. Attachments of flexor digitorum superficialis.
Fig. 5-13. Deep muscles on anterior aspect of forearm.

The tendons of the long flexors of the fingers pass beneath the flexor retinaculum (transverse carpal ligament) into the palm and out along the fingers. The tendons of the flexor digitorum superficialis are inserted into the base of the middle phalanges of the four medial digits, and the tendons of the flexor digitorum profundus are inserted into the base of the terminal phalanges of the same fingers. The flexor

129

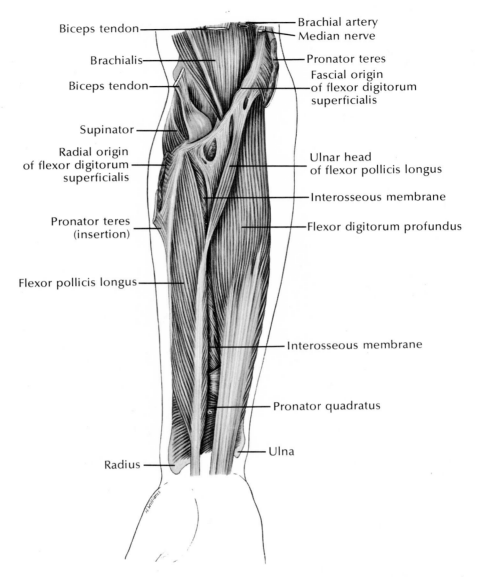

Biceps tendon

Brachialis

Biceps tendon

Supinator

Radial origin
of flexor digitorum
superficialis

Pronator teres
(insertion)

Flexor pollicis longus

Radius

Brachial artery
Median nerve

Pronator teres

Fascial origin
of flexor digitorum
superficialis

Ulnar head
of flexor pollicis longus

Interosseous membrane

Flexor digitorum profundus

Interosseous membrane

Pronator quadratus

Ulna

Fig. 5-14. Deep muscles of volar aspect of right forearm. (Male, 57 years of age.)

pollicis longus is inserted into the base of the terminal phalanx of the thumb. The pronator quadratus is inserted into the lower one-fourth of the anterior surface of the radius.

In the forearm the flexor carpi ulnaris and the ulnar portion of the flexor profundus are innervated by the ulnar nerve; all other muscles

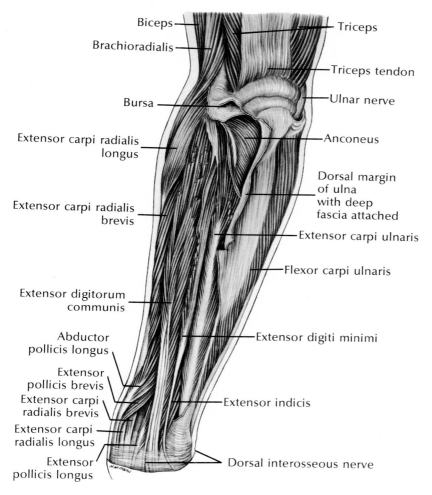

Biceps

Brachioradialis

Bursa

Extensor carpi radialis longus

Extensor carpi radialis brevis

Extensor digitorum communis

Abductor pollicis longus

Extensor pollicis brevis

Extensor carpi radialis brevis

Extensor carpi radialis longus

Extensor pollicis longus

Triceps

Triceps tendon

Ulnar nerve

Anconeus

Dorsal margin of ulna with deep fascia attached

Extensor carpi ulnaris

Flexor carpi ulnaris

Extensor digiti minimi

Extensor indicis

Dorsal interosseous nerve

Fig. 5-15. Superficial muscles of dorsal aspect of left forearm. (Male, 68 years of age.)

on the volar aspect of the forearm are innervated by branches of the median nerve.

On the dorsal aspect of the forearm there is a superficial group of muscles, namely, the brachioradialis, anconeus, extensors carpi radialis longus and brevis, extensor digitorum communis, extensor digiti minimi (proprius) and extensor carpi ulnaris. These arise from the lateral epicondyle of the humerus. There is likewise a deep group, namely, the supinator, extensors pollicis longus and brevis, abductor pollicis longus, and extensor indicis (proprius). These arise from the dorsal aspect of the bones of the forearm and interosseous mem-

131

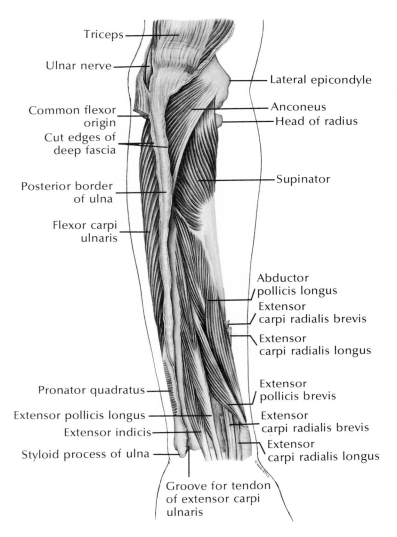

Triceps

Ulnar nerve

Common flexor origin

Cut edges of deep fascia

Posterior border of ulna

Flexor carpi ulnaris

Lateral epicondyle

Anconeus

Head of radius

Supinator

Abductor pollicis longus

Extensor carpi radialis brevis

Extensor carpi radialis longus

Extensor pollicis brevis

Pronator quadratus

Extensor pollicis longus

Extensor indicis

Styloid process of ulna

Extensor carpi radialis brevis

Extensor carpi radialis longus

Groove for tendon of extensor carpi ulnaris

Fig. 5-16. Deep muscles of dorsal aspect of right forearm. (Male, 57 years of age.)

brane—the supinator, extensor pollicis longus, and extensor indicis from the ulna; the extensor pollicis brevis from the radius; and the abductor pollicis longus from both bones. All are supplied by branches of the radial nerve. After fracture of the lateral epicondyle the extensor muscles pull the fragment downward.

The brachioradialis is inserted into the distal end of the radius on the lateral side. The anconeus is inserted into the ulna in common with the triceps muscle and may be regarded as an extra part of that muscle. The extensor carpi radialis longus is inserted into the base of the second metacarpal bone on the dorsal surface, and the extensor carpi radialis brevis is inserted similarly into the third metacarpal. The extensor carpi ulnaris is inserted into the base of the fifth metacarpal. The muscles just mentioned produce extension of the wrist joint. The radial extensors assist in movement of the hand to the thumb side (radial deviation), whereas the ulnar extensor assists in movement to the side of the little finger (ulnar deviation). The extensors of the fingers all become tendinous before reaching the wrist joint and pass beneath the extensor retinaculum on the back of the hand to be inserted into the dorsum of the various fingers by tendinous expansions. The supinator wraps around the lateral side of the upper portion of the radius and is inserted into the anterior aspect of that bone. The abductor pollicis longus is inserted into the lateral side of the base of the first metacarpal.

In thinking of the large number of complicated muscles of the forearm, one will find it helpful to remember a few general facts. The superficial flexor muscles arise from the region of the medial epicondyle of the humerus, and the muscle bundles pass downward into the forearm; at or near the wrist they become tendinous and are inserted into the various bones of the hand. These muscles are reinforced by deeper muscles that arise from the volar aspect of radius, ulna, and interosseous membrane. The flexor carpi ulnaris and part of the flexor digitorum profundus are supplied by the ulnar nerve, all the others by the median nerve.

The superficial extensor muscles arise from the region of the lateral epicondyle; their muscle bundles pass down the back of the forearm to become tendinous at the wrist and are inserted into hand and finger bones. They are also reinforced by deeper muscles arising from the dorsal aspect of the bones and interosseous membrane of the forearm. All are innervated by the radial nerve.

A very helpful way to associate the 12 muscles of the dorsal aspect of the forearm is to divide them into four functional groups of three each. There are three muscles, the anconeus, supinator, and brachioradialis, that are inserted into the bones of the forearm and act on the elbow joint. There are three muscles, the extensor carpi ulnaris and extensors carpi radialis longus and brevis, that are inserted into the metacarpal bones and are primarily extensors of the wrist joint. There are three muscles, the abductor pollicis longus and extensors pollicis longus and brevis, that go to the thumb. There are three muscles, the extensors digitorum communis, indicis, and digiti minimi, that are inserted into the fingers and act primarily as extensors of the metacarpophalangeal joints.

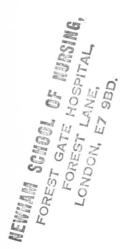
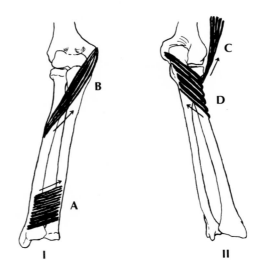

Fig. 5-17. Pronation and supination. **I,** Principal muscles used in pronating the forearm; *A,* pronator quadratus muscle; *B,* pronator teres muscle. **II,** Principal muscles used in supinating the forearm; *C,* biceps brachii muscle; *D,* supinator muscle.

The flexor muscles flex the wrist and fingers; associated with them are the pronators. The extensors extend the wrist and fingers; associated with them are the supinators.

The muscles of the upper arm and the forearm have been described separately because of their natural anatomical grouping. However, in many movements of the upper extremity, muscles from each of these two large groups act together. This is especially true in the very important movement of supination of the forearm (Fig. 5-17). The supinating action of the biceps brachii muscle can be demonstrated by palpating the muscle belly of the muscle while supinating the hand. The action of the supinator muscle itself cannot be felt. It is also difficult to palpate the muscles that bring about the opposite movement of pronation.

On the anterior surface of the wrist the flexor retinaculum (transverse carpal ligament) is a strong band of connective tissue attached on either side to carpal bones. Beneath this ligament the flexor tendons of the forearm pass into the palm. On the dorsal surface of the wrist the extensor retinaculum (dorsal carpal ligament) forms a strong band under which the extensor tendons pass on to the back of the hand (Figs. 5-18 and 5-19).

Palmar aponeurosis. The palmar aponeurosis is a dense sheet of fibrous connective tissue placed in the palm deep to a superficial fatty

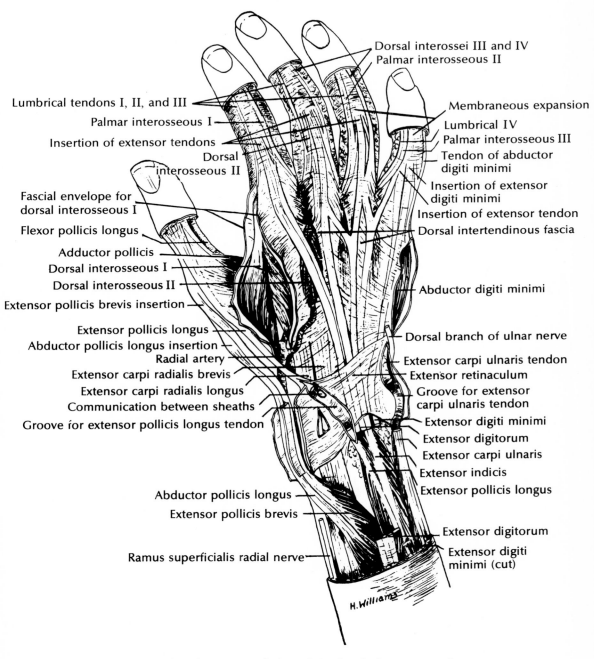

Dorsal interossei III and IV
Palmar interosseous II

Lumbrical tendons I, II, and III

Palmar interosseous I

Insertion of extensor tendons

Dorsal interosseous II

Membraneous expansion

Lumbrical IV

Palmar interosseous III

Tendon of abductor digiti minimi

Insertion of extensor digiti minimi

Insertion of extensor tendon

Dorsal intertendinous fascia

Fascial envelope for dorsal interosseous I

Flexor pollicis longus

Adductor pollicis

Dorsal interosseous I

Dorsal interosseous II

Extensor pollicis brevis insertion

Abductor digiti minimi

Extensor pollicis longus

Abductor pollicis longus insertion

Radial artery

Extensor carpi radialis brevis

Extensor carpi radialis longus

Communication between sheaths

Groove for extensor pollicis longus tendon

Dorsal branch of ulnar nerve

Extensor carpi ulnaris tendon

Extensor retinaculum

Groove for extensor carpi ulnaris tendon

Extensor digiti minimi

Extensor digitorum

Extensor carpi ulnaris

Extensor indicis

Extensor pollicis longus

Abductor pollicis longus

Extensor pollicis brevis

Ramus superficialis radial nerve

Extensor digitorum

Extensor digiti minimi (cut)

H. Williams

Fig. 5-18. Dorsum of the hand. (From Brickel, A. C. J.: Surgical treatment of hand and forearm infections, St. Louis, The C. V. Mosby Co.) (Male, 50 years of age.)

135

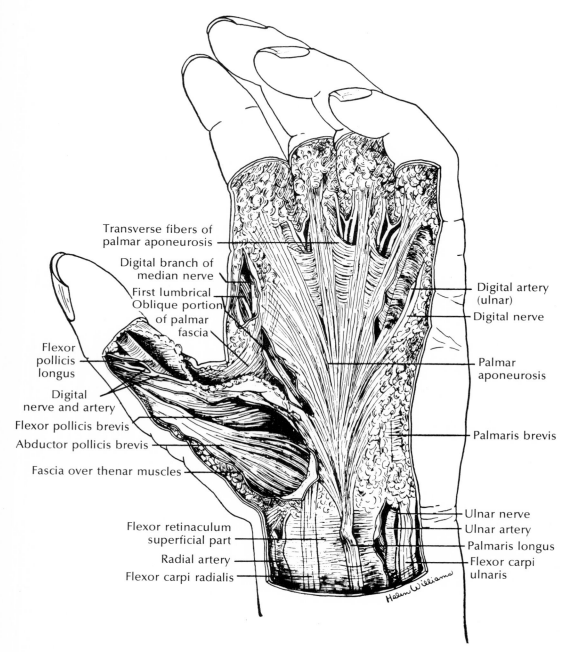

Transverse fibers of
palmar aponeurosis

Digital branch of
median nerve

First lumbrical
Oblique portion
of palmar
fascia

Flexor
pollicis
longus

Digital
nerve and artery

Flexor pollicis brevis

Abductor pollicis brevis

Fascia over thenar muscles

Flexor retinaculum
superficial part

Radial artery

Flexor carpi radialis

Digital artery
(ulnar)

Digital nerve

Palmar
aponeurosis

Palmaris brevis

Ulnar nerve

Ulnar artery

Palmaris longus

Flexor carpi
ulnaris

Helen Williams

Fig. 5-19. The palmar fascia. (From Brickel, A. C. J.: Surgical treatment of
hand and forearm infections, St. Louis, The C. V. Mosby Co.) (Male, 42
years of age.)

layer of connective tissue and superficial to the tendons of the long flexor muscles and the lumbrical and interosseous muscles. This aponeurosis is triangular in shape, with the apex toward the wrist and the base at the base of the fingers. The apex is continuous with the lower end of the tendon of the palmaris longus muscle and with some of the fibers of deep fascia of the wrist. At its base the fibers of the aponeurosis fan out, and slips pass to each of the four medial metacarpophalangeal joints and blend with the capsules of these joints.

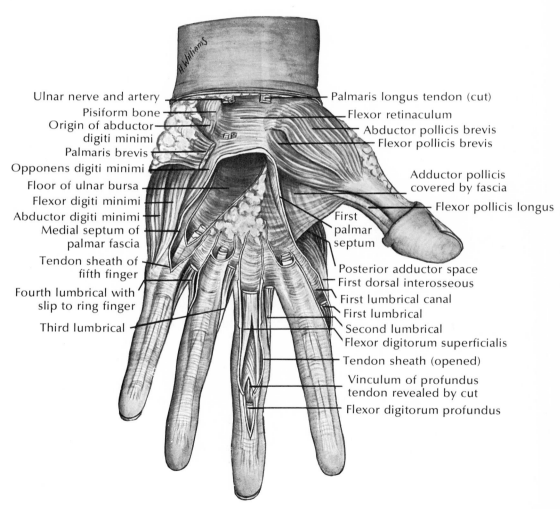

Fig. 5-20. Muscles of thenar and hypothenar eminences. (From Brickel, A. C. J.: Surgical treatment of hand and forearm infections, St. Louis, The C. V. Mosby Co.) (Male, 65 years of age.)

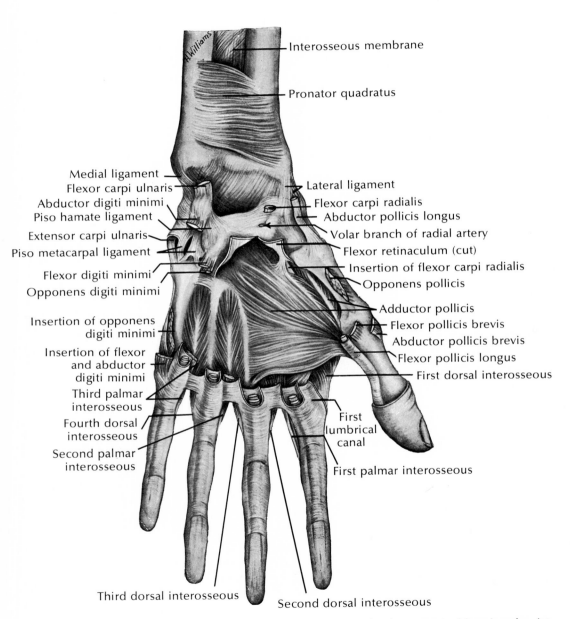

Interosseous membrane

Pronator quadratus

Medial ligament
Flexor carpi ulnaris
Abductor digiti minimi
Piso hamate ligament
Extensor carpi ulnaris
Piso metacarpal ligament
Flexor digiti minimi
Opponens digiti minimi

Lateral ligament
Flexor carpi radialis
Abductor pollicis longus
Volar branch of radial artery
Flexor retinaculum (cut)
Insertion of flexor carpi radialis
Opponens pollicis

Insertion of opponens
digiti minimi
Insertion of flexor
and abductor
digiti minimi
Third palmar
interosseous
Fourth dorsal
interosseous
Second palmar
interosseous

Adductor pollicis
Flexor pollicis brevis
Abductor pollicis brevis
Flexor pollicis longus
First dorsal interosseous

First
lumbrical
canal

First palmar interosseous

Third dorsal interosseous   Second dorsal interosseous

Fig. 5-21. Deep muscles and ligaments of volar aspect of hand and wrist.
(From Brickel, A. C. J.: Surgical treatment of hand and forearm infections,
St. Louis, The C. V. Mosby Co.) (Male, 50 years of age.)

There are septa that pass from the undersurface of the aponeurosis deeply into the palm, fusing with the fascia about the interosseous muscles. The palmar aponeurosis adds greatly to the strength of the hand.

Muscles of hand. There are 19 small muscles in the hand. Those for the thumb form the thenar eminence and include the abductor pollicis brevis, the opponens pollicis, the flexor pollicis brevis, and the adductor pollicis. There are also four muscles in the hypothenar eminence, the palmaris brevis, the abductor digiti minimi, the opponens digiti minimi, and the flexor digiti minimi brevis. There are four lumbrical muscles that arise in the palm from the tendons of the flexor digitorum profundus muscle and are inserted into the capsules of the metacarpophalangeal articulations of the four fingers.

In the spaces between the metacarpal bones are the three palmar and four dorsal interosseous muscles. Each palmar interosseous muscle arises by a single head from a metacarpal bone, and each dorsal

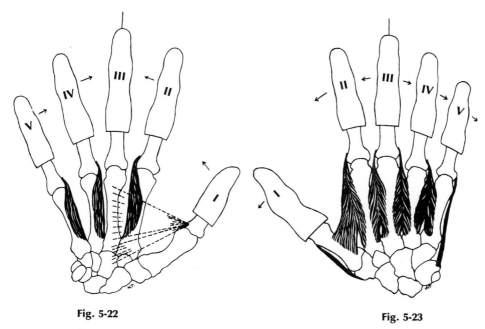

Fig. 5-22   **Fig. 5-23**

Fig. 5-22. Diagram showing action of the intrinsic muscles of the hand that adduct the fingers and thumb. The three palmar interosseous muscles are indicated by the heavy lines. The adductor pollicis is indicated by dotted outline. All are supplied by the ulnar nerve.

Fig. 5-23. Diagram showing action of the intrinsic muscles of the hand that abduct the fingers and thumb. All are supplied by the ulnar nerve except the abductor pollicis brevis, which is supplied by the median nerve.

arises by two heads, one from each bone bounding an intermetacarpal space. Each interosseous muscle is inserted into the posterior aspect of the base of a finger.

The abductor pollicis brevis, the opponens pollicis, the flexor pollicis brevis, and the two lateral lumbricals are supplied by branches of the median nerve. All the other muscles of the hand are supplied from branches of the ulnar nerve.

Certain distinctive functions of the muscles of the hand should and can be understood by referring to Figs. 5-22 to 5-25. The long extensors extend the wrist, the joints of the thumb, and the metacarpophalangeal joints of the fingers. The lumbricals flex the fingers at the metacarpophalangeal joints and extend them at the interphalangeal joints. The dorsal interossei abduct the fingers from the midline of the middle digit, and the palmar interossei adduct to the midline of the middle digits. Furthermore, both dorsal and palmar interossei flex the fingers at the metacarpophalangeal joints and extend the fingers at the interphalangeal joints. The long flexors flex the wrist and the metacarpophalangeal and interphalangeal joints.

Extensor expansion. As the long extensors enter the fingers,

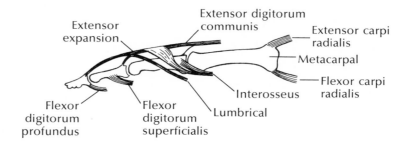

Fig. 5-24. Attachment of muscles of a finger, lateral view.

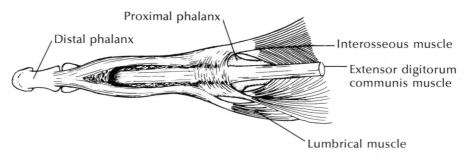

140   **Fig. 5-25.** Extensor expansion, dorsal view.

their tendons flatten out with the lateral portion inserting into the base of the proximal phalanges and the medial portion continuing to the middle phalanges. Joining the extensor tendons and forming a complex aponeurotic, "extensor expansion" are the tendons of the interossei and lumbrical muscles. Although the long extensors pass to the middle phalanges, their major function is as the sole extensors of the metacarpophalangeal joints. The lateral portions of the expansion, composed almost entirely of the interossei and lumbricals, continue and insert into the distal phalanges. It is this portion of the "expansion" that, passing dorsal to the interphalangeal joints, causes extension at these joints (Figs. 5-24 and 5-25). Ulnar nerve damage and the resulting hand deformity (claw hand) can also be explained by reference to Fig. 5-24. The ulnar nerve innervates the interossei and the ulnar half of the lumbricals, the actions of which are to flex the metacarpophalangeal joints and extend the interphalangeal joints. If these functions are lost, the opposite movements occur, namely, extension of the metacarpophalangeal joints by the unopposed action of the long extensors and flexion of the interphalangeal joints by the unopposed action of the long flexors of the fingers.

Eight muscles are inserted into the bones of the thumb. The long flexor, the long abductor, and the long and short extensors arise in the forearm; they are long, large muscles and are used in powerful actions such as gripping. The short flexor, the short abductor, the opponens, and the adductor are short muscles situated entirely within the lateral part of the hand; they are used in delicate movements. All the thumb muscles are named from a principle action, but all are used in combination, and all movements of the thumb are complex.

The lower extremity in man is specialized for use in standing erect and walking on two legs. These important functions involve approximately one half the total muscle mass of the body.

MUSCLES OF LOWER EXTREMITY

Muscles on anterior aspect of thigh. These muscles lie deep to the fascia lata and are separated on the medial side from the adductor group by the medial intermuscular septum and from the hamstring group laterally by the lateral intermuscular septum.

The sartorius, the longest muscle in the body, arises from the anterior superior iliac spine and passes distally and medially across the front of the thigh to be inserted high up on the medial surface of the tibial shaft. This is literally the tailor's muscle, and the position a tailor assumes when seated on the floor illustrates the functions of the muscle, that is, to flex the hip and knee joints, and to turn the thigh outward.

The quadriceps femoris forms the great bulk of the anterior aspect of the thigh and has four separate parts. The rectus femoris arises from the anterior inferior iliac spine and from the ilium above the acetabulum. The three vasti muscles (vastus medialis, vastus lateralis, and vastus intermedius) arise from the femur and ensheathe the lower two thirds of the bone except for its linea aspera and condyles. The four parts of the quadriceps are usually described as being inserted into the patella, but the patella is really a sesamoid bone developed within the central portion of the tendon by which the compound muscle is attached to the tuberosity of the tibia. There are expansions of insertion by aponeurotic fibers into the upper part of both condyles of the tibia. The central tendon and its expansions, also known as retinacula, replace to some extent the proper capsule of the knee joint. The articularis genus muscle consists of a few fibers that arise from the lower part of the front of the femur and are inserted into the capsule of the knee joint.

The quadriceps is a very powerful extensor of the knee and is brought into function in such movements as rising from a sitting position, kicking a football, and swimming. The articularis genus pulls the upper part of the joint capsule upward during extension and, thus, prevents pinching of the synovial membrane between the joint surfaces.

The fascia lata, a deep fascia of the thigh, is a relatively inelastic connective tissue sheath that envelops the entire thigh and is particularly well developed laterally. Superiorly the fascia lata attains attachment to the length of the iliac crest, sacrum, ischial tuberosity, ischial and pubic rami, and inguinal ligament. Inferiorly the fascia attaches to the bones of the leg, tibia and fibula and to the patella and then blends with the deep fascia of the leg.

Structures entering or leaving the lower extremity pass under the inguinal ligament. The area inferior to this ligament can be divided into two compartments, a lateral neuromuscular containing the iliopsoas muscle and femoral nerve and a medial vascular containing the femoral artery, vein, and an empty space, the so-called femoral canal. The nerves and vessels have a constant relationship that, from lateral to medial, can be remembered as N.A.V.E., Nerve, Artery, Vein, and Empty space. Femoral hernias descend through the femoral canal, and the importance of the topographical relationships is evident, since if an incision is necessary to enlarge the opening of the canal, the cut cannot be made laterally because the femoral vein and artery would be endangered (see Fig. 5-46).

The iliopsoas is a compound muscle, the iliac portion arising from the medial surface of the iliac blade and the psoas major arising from the anterior surface of the lowest thoracic and the upper four lumbar

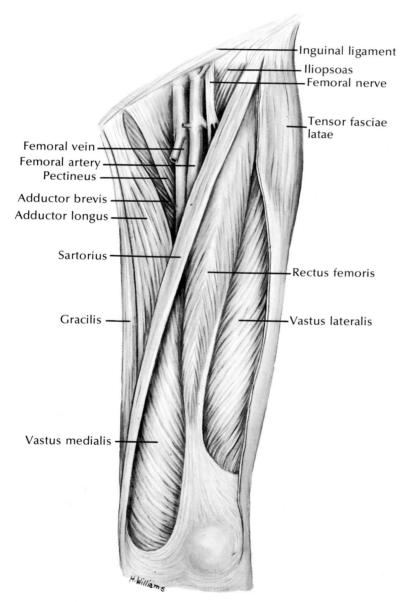

Fig. 5-26. Superficial muscles of left thigh, anterior view. The knee has been laterally rotated to show the adductor muscles. (Male, 64 years of age.) 143

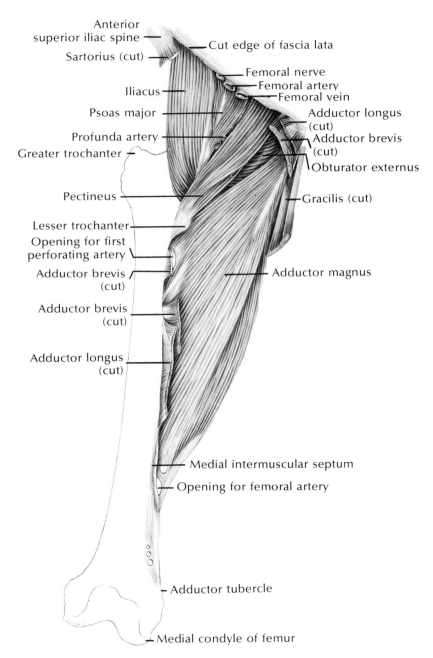

Anterior
superior iliac spine

Sartorius (cut)

Cut edge of fascia lata

Femoral nerve
Femoral artery
Femoral vein

Iliacus

Psoas major

Adductor longus
(cut)

Profunda artery

Adductor brevis
(cut)

Greater trochanter

Obturator externus

Pectineus

Gracilis (cut)

Lesser trochanter

Opening for first
perforating artery

Adductor brevis
(cut)

Adductor magnus

Adductor brevis
(cut)

Adductor longus
(cut)

Medial intermuscular septum

Opening for femoral artery

Adductor tubercle

Medial condyle of femur

Fig. 5-27. Deep muscles of medial side of right thigh. (Male, 57 years of age.)

144

vertebrae and intervening fibrocartilaginous discs. The iliac and psoas portions unite and pass beneath the inguinal ligament lateral to the femoral nerve to be inserted into the lesser trochanter. A large bursa is present beneath this muscle as it passes over the pubis and hip joint. The iliopsoas is the main flexor of the hip joint, and when the femur is fixed, it acts as a flexor of the trunk. As a flexor of the trunk, it is assisted by the portion of the rectus femoris that arises from the ilium. Occasionally a portion of the psoas muscle is partially separated and has a tendon inserted into the hip bone at the junction of the ilium and superior ramus of the pubis. When present, it is called the psoas minor muscle (Fig. 5-45).

The pectineus muscle arises from the upper surface of the superior pubic ramus and is inserted into the dorsum of the femur just below and behind the lesser trochanter. This muscle is an adductor and flexor of the hip joint.

The sartorius, quadriceps, iliacus, and pectineus muscles are supplied by branches of the femoral nerve. The psoas muscle is supplied directly from the lumbar nerves.

Muscles on medial aspect of thigh. These muscles include the gracilis, the three adductors, and the obturator externus.

The gracilis is a long, flat muscle that arises from the pubis just below the symphysis and is inserted by a strong tendon into the proximal end of the tibia behind the sartorius and in front of the semitendinosus.

The adductor longus arises from the body of the pubis just lateral to the symphysis and is inserted into the middle two fourths of the medial lip of the linea aspera. The adductor brevis arises from the inferior ramus and body of the pubis lateral to the gracilis and is inserted into the femur below the pectineus and into the upper end of the linea aspera behind the adductor longus. The adductor magnus is the largest of the adductors. It arises from the lower part of the inferior ramus of the pubis, from the ramus of the ischium, and from the tuberosity of the ischium. It is inserted into the posterior surface of the femur along the entire length of the linea aspera and into the adductor tubercle. The portion that arises from the ischial tuberosity and is inserted into the adductor tubercle is really not an adductor but a part of the hamstring group.

The obturator externus arises from the lateral surface of the obturator membrane and adjacent portion of the hip bone. The fibers pass posterior to the hip joint, and the tendon is inserted into the trochanteric fossa of the femur.

The name of this group of muscles indicates their main function, adduction at the hip joint; in addition, the obturator externus is a   145 lateral rotator of the femur, and the gracilis flexes the knee joint.

The adductors, gracilis, and the obturator externus are supplied by the obturator nerve, except the hamstring portion of the adductor magnus, which is supplied by the sciatic nerve.

The femoral triangle is a large triangular space bounded above by the inguinal ligament, laterally by the sartorius, and medially by the adductor longus. The more important structures in this area are the first part of the femoral artery and accompanying vein, the femoral nerve, numerous lymph nodes, and the terminal portion of the long

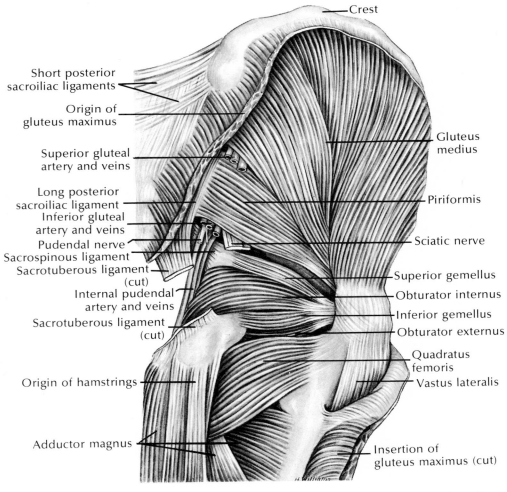

Fig. 5-28. Deep muscles of right buttock. (Male, 33 years of age.)

saphenous vein. Below, the femoral vessels pass beneath the sartorius muscle into a tunnel known as the adductor or Hunter's canal.

Muscles of buttock. This group of muscles includes the three glutei, the tensor fasciae latae, and a group of small muscles known as lateral rotators, including the obturator internus, the piriformis, quadratus femoris, and the two gemelli (Fig. 5-28).

The gluteus maximus arises from the posterior portion of the iliac blade, the dorsal surface of the sacrum and coccyx, the sacrotuberous ligament, and the lumbodorsal fascia. It is inserted into the dorsum of the iliotibial tract and also into the gluteal tuberosity of the femur. Through the iliotibial tract it has an indirect attachment to the tibia. This muscle has coarser fibers than any other muscle of the body. It is a very powerful extensor of the hip joint.

The tensor fasciae latae arises from the lateral anterior portion of the iliac crest and is inserted into the anterior portion of the iliotibial tract; it acts mainly as a flexor of the hip joint. The iliotibial tract is a wide, strong band of longitudinal fibers of the deep fascia attached above to the iliac crest and below to the lateral condyle of the tibia and capsule of the knee joint. In its upper portion it is split into two sheets that enclose the tensor fasciae latae muscle; below that muscle the two sheets fuse. Functionally the tract is the aponeurosis of the tensor fasciae latae and of the gluteus maximus.

The gluteus medius and minimus arise from the lateral surface of the iliac blade beneath the gluteus maximus and are inserted into the greater trochanter. These muscles are abductors of the femur and aid in stabilizing the pelvis on the femora during walking. The gluteus minimus is a medial rotator of the femur.

The gluteus maximus is supplied by the inferior gluteal nerve, and the tensor fasciae latae and the gluteus medius and minimus by the superior gluteal nerve.

The obturator internus arises from the medial surface of the obturator membrane and the adjoining bone. Its fibers converge to the lesser sciatic foramen, and the tendon passes behind the hip joint to be inserted into the medial side of the greater trochanter above the fossa. This muscle is a lateral rotator of the femur.

The superior gemellus muscle arises from the spine of the ischium; the inferior gemellus arises from the ischial tuberosity. The tendon of each gemellus muscle blends with that of the obturator internus and is inserted in common with that muscle. The quadratus femoris arises from the lateral margin of the ischial tuberosity and is inserted into the upper portion of the shaft of the femur. The piriformis arises from the anterior surface of the second, third, and fourth sacral vertebrae and passes through the greater sciatic foramen to be inserted in-   147 to a pit on the medial aspect of the greater trochanter. All are lateral rotators.

Hamstring muscles. The hamstring muscles are the biceps femoris, the semitendinosus, semimembranosus, and ischial portion of the adductor magnus. They are primarily flexors of the knee joint, and when the knee is fixed, they aid in extension of the hip joint.

The biceps femoris has a long head that arises in common with the semitendinosus from the medial portion of the ischial tuberosity and an additional origin or short head from the lateral lip of the linea aspera. The biceps is inserted into the head of the fibula and lateral condyle of the tibia. The semitendinosus arises with the long head of the biceps and is inserted into the upper end of the tibia behind the sartorius and below the gracilis. The semimembranosus arises from the lateral facet of the ischial tuberosity and is inserted into a groove on the back of the medial condyle of the tibia and into the deep fascia about the medial and posterior portions of the knee joint. The muscles of this group are innervated by the nerve to the hamstrings, a portion of the sciatic nerve.

The muscles of the thigh may be divided into three large groups: (1) an anterior knee extensor group innervated by the femoral nerve, (2) a medial hip adductor group innervated by the obturator nerve, and (3) a posterior knee flexor group innervated by a portion of the sciatic nerve. Each group has complex origins from the femur and from the pelvic girdle; therefore, each group is capable of moving the hip joint as well as the knee joint. Movements of abduction, medial rotation, and lateral rotation of the thigh are produced by a number of deeply placed muscles.

Muscles on anterior aspect of leg. These muscles lie anterior to the interosseous septum and between the lateral surface of the tibia and the anterior peroneal septum. They are the tibialis anterior, extensor digitorum longus, peroneus tertius, and extensor hallucis longus. All of these are supplied by the deep peroneal nerve, and all are dorsiflexors of the foot. In addition, the tibialis anterior acts as an invertor of the foot, and the peroneus tertius acts as an evertor.

The tibialis anterior arises from the upper lateral portion of the tibia and lateral intermuscular septum and is inserted into the medial aspect of the medial cuneiform and base of the first metatarsal. It is the most medial tendon in front of the ankle joint. The extensor digitorum longus arises from the lateral condyle of the tibia and the upper portion of the fibula and is inserted into the second, third, fourth, and fifth toes by tendons that are plainly visible on the dorsum of the foot. The peroneus tertius arises from the lower part of the fibula and is inserted into the dorsal aspect of the base of the fifth metatarsal. This muscle is not separated at its origin from the extensor digitorum longus. The extensor hallucis longus arises from the fibula deeper than the other muscles. At the ankle, its tendon becomes superficial and runs laterally to that of the tibialis anterior to its insertion into the base of the terminal phalanx of the first toe.

Muscles on lateral aspect of leg. The peroneus longus arises from the lateral condyle of the tibia and from the head and upper part of the lateral surface of the fibula. Its tendon passes posterior to the lateral malleolus, crosses the sole, and is inserted into the medial

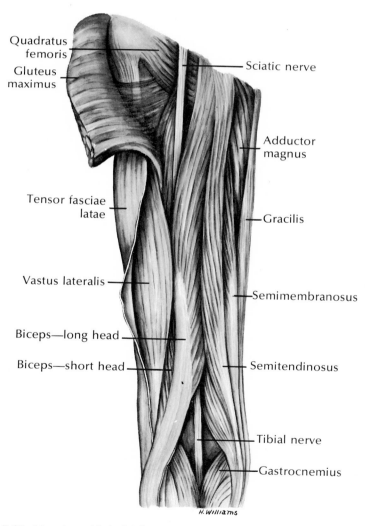

Fig. 5-29. Muscles of left thigh, posterior view. (Male, 64 years of age.)   149

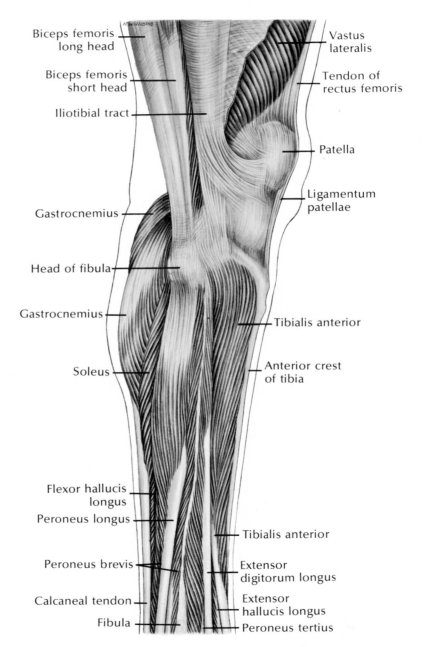

Biceps femoris long head

Biceps femoris short head

Iliotibial tract

Gastrocnemius

Head of fibula

Gastrocnemius

Soleus

Flexor hallucis longus

Peroneus longus

Peroneus brevis

Calcaneal tendon

Fibula

Vastus lateralis

Tendon of rectus femoris

Patella

Ligamentum patellae

Tibialis anterior

Anterior crest of tibia

Tibialis anterior

Extensor digitorum longus

Extensor hallucis longus

Peroneus tertius

Fig. 5-30. Muscles of lateral aspect of right leg. This dissection shows the close relationship of the muscle tendons around the knee to the joint capsule. (Male, 62 years of age.)

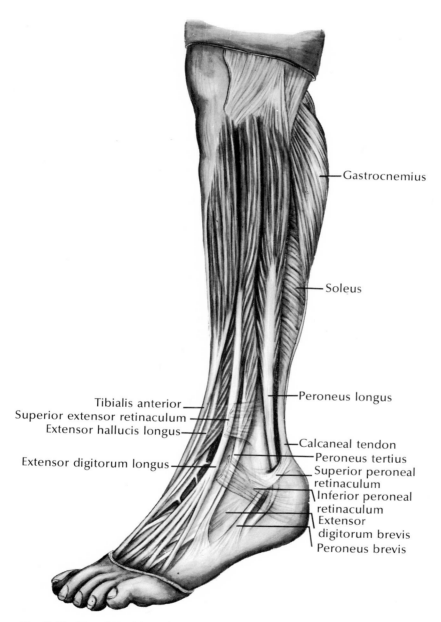

Gastrocnemius

Soleus

Tibialis anterior
Superior extensor retinaculum
Extensor hallucis longus

Extensor digitorum longus

Peroneus longus

Calcaneal tendon
Peroneus tertius
Superior peroneal
retinaculum
Inferior peroneal
retinaculum
Extensor
digitorum brevis
Peroneus brevis

Fig. 5-31. Muscles of lateral aspect of left leg. (Male, 64 years of age.)

cuneiform and base of the first metatarsal. The peroneus brevis arises from the lower part of the lateral surface of the fibula, passes behind the lateral malleolus, and is inserted into the tuberosity of the fifth metatarsal. The peroneus longus and brevis are supplied by the superficial peroneal nerve. They are plantar flexors of the ankle joint and evertors of the foot (Figs. 5-29 to 5-31).

Muscles on posterior aspect of leg. The muscles of the superficial group are the soleus, gastrocnemius, and plantaris, all inserted into the calcaneus and all acting as plantar flexors of the foot. The gastrocnemius arises from the dorsum of the condyles of the femur and from the posterior surface of the capsule of the knee joint. The soleus arises from the posterior surface of the fibula and tibia and arches over the popliteal vessels. Both of these muscles join in a common tendon of insertion, the calcaneal tendon or tendon of Achilles, into the back of the calcaneus. The plantaris is unimportant, arising from the back of the lateral condyle of the femur deeper than the gastrocnemius. By means of a long slender tendon it is inserted into the calcaneal tendon or directly into the calcaneus (Figs. 5-32 and 5-33).

The deep muscles of the back of the leg are the popliteus, flexor digitorum longus, flexor hallucis longus, and tibialis posterior. The popliteus arises from the lateral side of the lateral epicondyle of the femur, passes behind the knee joint, and is inserted into the upper medial posterior surface of the tibia. The flexor digitorum longus arises from the back of the tibia, passes behind the medial malleolus beneath the flexor retinaculum, and is inserted into the base of the terminal phalanges of the second, third, fourth, and fifth toes. The flexor hallucis longus arises from the posterior surface of the fibula and passes into the sole deeper than the tendon of the flexor digitorum longus to be inserted into the base of the terminal phalanx of the great toe. The tibialis posterior arises from the back of the tibia and fibula and the back of the interosseous membrane. The tendon passes behind the medial malleolus and spreads out in the sole of the foot to an insertion into the second, third, and fourth metatarsals and into all the tarsals except the talus; its greatest insertion is into the navicular. All of the muscles of the back of the leg are supplied from branches of the tibial nerve.

The popliteus aids in flexion of the knee joint. The remaining deep muscles of the back of the leg are plantar flexors at the ankle joint and flexors of the toes. The tibialis posterior, working with the tibialis anterior, inverts the foot. The deep fascia overlying the muscle tendons at the ankle has certain definite thickenings that strengthen the ankle joint and hold tendons in place. On the lateral side of the ankle are the superior and inferior peroneal retinacula passing from the lat-

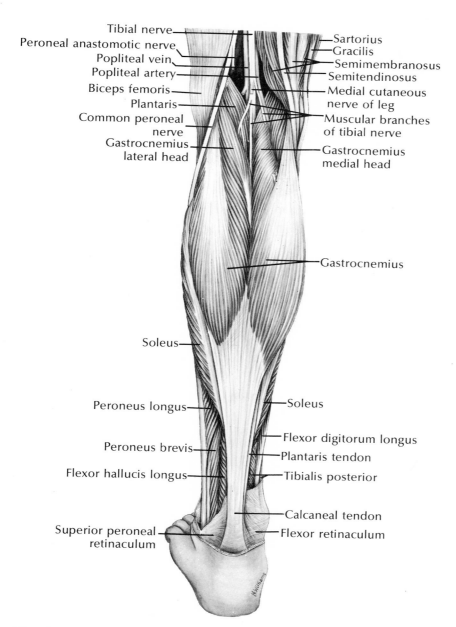

Fig. 5-32. Superficial muscles of left leg, posterior view. (Male, 62 years of age.)

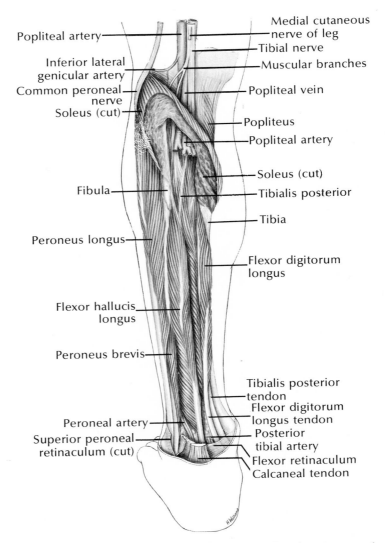

Popliteal artery

Inferior lateral genicular artery

Common peroneal nerve

Soleus (cut)

Fibula

Peroneus longus

Flexor hallucis longus

Peroneus brevis

Peroneal artery

Superior peroneal retinaculum (cut)

Medial cutaneous nerve of leg

Tibial nerve

Muscular branches

Popliteal vein

Popliteus

Popliteal artery

Soleus (cut)

Tibialis posterior

Tibia

Flexor digitorum longus

Tibialis posterior tendon

Flexor digitorum longus tendon

Posterior tibial artery

Flexor retinaculum

Calcaneal tendon

Fig. 5-33. Deep muscles of left leg, posterior view. (Male, 62 years of age.)

eral malleolus to the calcaneus and binding down the tendons of the peroneal muscles. In front is the superior extensor retinaculum (transverse ligament of the ankle), stretching between the two malleoli, and lower down is the inferior extensor retinaculum (cruciate ligament of the ankle). These two retinacula overlie the tendons of the muscles that dorsiflex the foot. On the medial side of the ankle is the flexor retinaculum (laciniate ligament) attached to the medial malleolus and

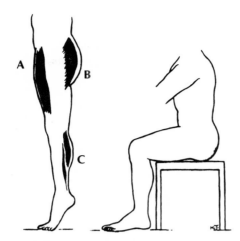

Fig. 5-34. Diagram of the great extensor muscles of the lower extremity. *A,* The quadriceps femoris muscle; *B,* the gluteus maximus muscle; *C,* the gastrocnemius and soleus muscles.

the calcaneus and stretched over the tendons of the long flexor muscles of the foot (the plantar flexors).

In studying the lower extremity it is helpful to remember how frequently the number three is associated with the structures. There are three main nerves: the obturator, the femoral, and the sciatic. The sciatic, in turn, has three main branches: the nerve to the hamstrings, the tibial nerve, and the peroneal nerve.

The muscles of the thigh are divided into three groups: the knee extensors, the adductors, of which there are three main ones, and the knee flexors or hamstrings, of which there are three. The muscles of the leg attached to tarsal bones are divided into three groups: the tibialis anterior and posterior on the inner side, the three peroneal muscles on the outer side, and the three muscles attached to the calcaneus behind, soleus, gastrocnemius, and plantaris. Three muscles that arise from points on the hip bone, the sartorius, gracilis, and semitendinosus, are inserted together into the tibia. There are also three gluteal muscles. At the ankle the tendons of three muscles pass beneath the extensor retinaculum, and the tendons of three muscles pass behind the medial malleolus beneath the flexor retinaculum.

At the beginning of this discussion it was stated that one half of the muscle bulk of the body in man is located in the lower extremities. The muscles that are especially large are the gluteus maximus, the quadriceps femoris, the gastrocnemius, and the soleus. For man to assume and maintain an erect posture these muscles must be very powerful. He uses them particularly to push the body weight upward

155

when arising from a seated position, to climb stairs, and to stand on tiptoe.

Muscles of foot. There are 18 small muscles in the plantar aspect of the foot: the quadratus plantae (flexor accessorius), four lumbricals, abductor hallucis, flexor digitorum brevis, abductor digiti minimi, flexor hallucis brevis, adductor hallucis, flexor digiti minimi brevis, four dorsal interossei, and three plantar interossei.

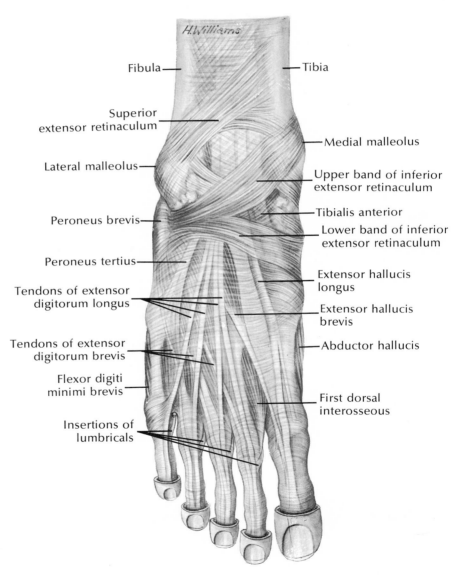

Fibula

Tibia

Superior
extensor retinaculum

Medial malleolus

Lateral malleolus

Upper band of inferior
extensor retinaculum

Tibialis anterior

Peroneus brevis

Lower band of inferior
extensor retinaculum

Peroneus tertius

Extensor hallucis
longus

Tendons of extensor
digitorum longus

Extensor hallucis
brevis

Tendons of extensor
digitorum brevis

Abductor hallucis

Flexor digiti
minimi brevis

First dorsal
interosseous

Insertions of
lumbricals

Fig. 5-35. Dorsal aspect of right foot. (Male, 51 years of age.)

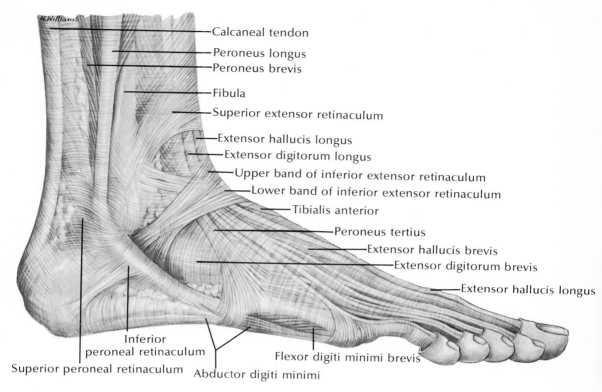

Calcaneal tendon
Peroneus longus
Peroneus brevis
Fibula
Superior extensor retinaculum
Extensor hallucis longus
Extensor digitorum longus
Upper band of inferior extensor retinaculum
Lower band of inferior extensor retinaculum
Tibialis anterior
Peroneus tertius
Extensor hallucis brevis
Extensor digitorum brevis
Extensor hallucis longus
Inferior peroneal retinaculum
Superior peroneal retinaculum
Abductor digiti minimi
Flexor digiti minimi brevis

Fig. 5-36. Lateral aspect of right foot. (Male, 51 years of age.)

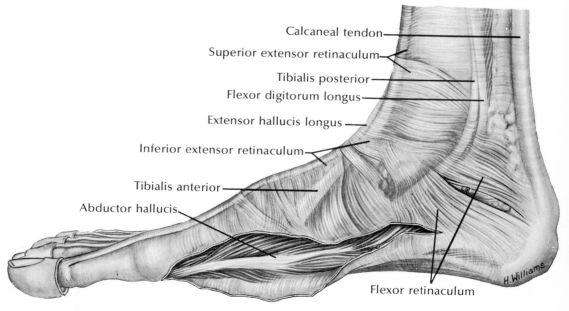

Calcaneal tendon
Superior extensor retinaculum
Tibialis posterior
Flexor digitorum longus
Extensor hallucis longus
Inferior extensor retinaculum
Tibialis anterior
Abductor hallucis
Flexor retinaculum

Fig. 5-37. Medial aspect of right foot. (Male, 51 years of age.)

157

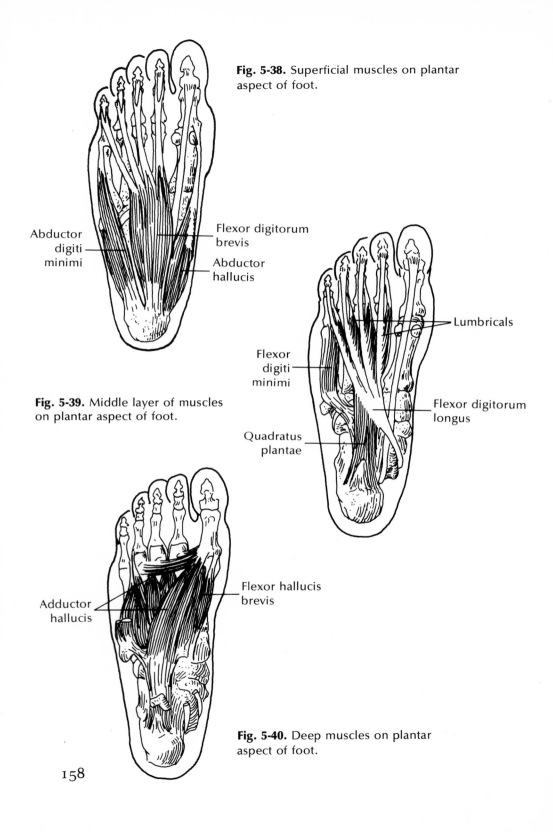

Fig. 5-38. Superficial muscles on plantar aspect of foot.

Abductor digiti minimi

Flexor digitorum brevis

Abductor hallucis

Fig. 5-39. Middle layer of muscles on plantar aspect of foot.

Lumbricals

Flexor digiti minimi

Flexor digitorum longus

Quadratus plantae

Adductor hallucis

Flexor hallucis brevis

Fig. 5-40. Deep muscles on plantar aspect of foot.

158

There is much less freedom of motion in the foot than in the hand, but the actions of the muscles are similar to those of the corresponding muscles in the hand. In the foot the midline anatomically is the middle of the second toe. The quadratus plantae is an accessory flexor arising from the undersurface of the calcaneus and strengthening the action of the long flexors of the toes; the flexor digitorum brevis has an action

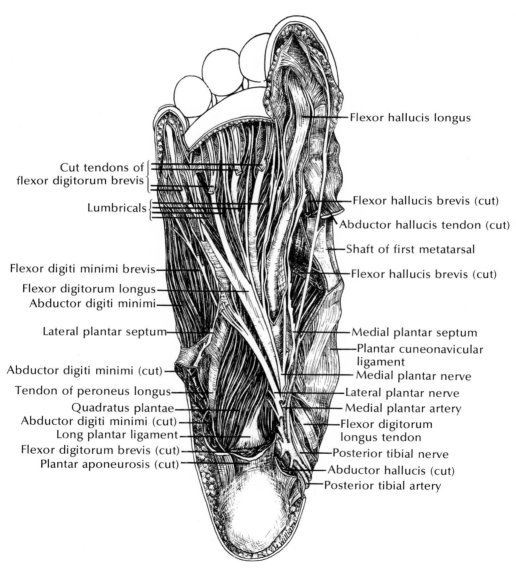

Cut tendons of flexor digitorum brevis

Lumbricals

Flexor digiti minimi brevis

Flexor digitorum longus

Abductor digiti minimi

Lateral plantar septum

Abductor digiti minimi (cut)

Tendon of peroneus longus

Quadratus plantae

Abductor digiti minimi (cut)

Long plantar ligament

Flexor digitorum brevis (cut)

Plantar aponeurosis (cut)

Flexor hallucis longus

Flexor hallucis brevis (cut)

Abductor hallucis tendon (cut)

Shaft of first metatarsal

Flexor hallucis brevis (cut)

Medial plantar septum

Plantar cuneonavicular ligament

Medial plantar nerve

Lateral plantar nerve

Medial plantar artery

Flexor digitorum longus tendon

Posterior tibial nerve

Abductor hallucis (cut)

Posterior tibial artery

Fig. 5-41. Plantar aspect of left foot. (Male, 55 years of age.)

159

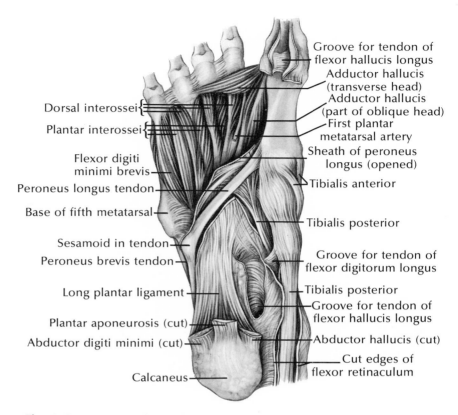

Dorsal interossei

Plantar interossei

Flexor digiti
minimi brevis

Peroneus longus tendon

Base of fifth metatarsal

Sesamoid in tendon

Peroneus brevis tendon

Long plantar ligament

Plantar aponeurosis (cut)

Abductor digiti minimi (cut)

Calcaneus

Groove for tendon of
flexor hallucis longus
Adductor hallucis
(transverse head)
Adductor hallucis
(part of oblique head)
First plantar
metatarsal artery
Sheath of peroneus
longus (opened)
Tibialis anterior

Tibialis posterior

Groove for tendon of
flexor digitorum longus

Tibialis posterior
Groove for tendon of
flexor hallucis longus
Abductor hallucis (cut)
Cut edges of
flexor retinaculum

Fig. 5-42. Deep muscles and ligaments of plantar aspect of right foot. (Female, 45 years of age.)

similar to that of the flexor digitorum superficialis of the hand. The abductor hallucis strengthens the medial longitudinal arch of the foot, and the abductor digiti minimi does the same for the lateral longitudinal arch.

The first lumbrical, the abductor hallucis, the flexor digitorum brevis, and the flexor hallucis brevis are supplied by the medial plantar branch of the tibial nerve. The remaining small muscles of the sole of the foot are supplied by branches of the lateral plantar nerve from the tibial nerve.

On the dorsum of the foot the extensor digitorum brevis muscle arises from the upper surface of the calcaneus and is inserted by four tendons into the four medial toes. The most medial muscle bundle and tendon is sometimes called the extensor hallucis brevis. The nerve supply comes from a branch of the peroneal nerve.

Functions of lower limb muscles in standing and walking. In an

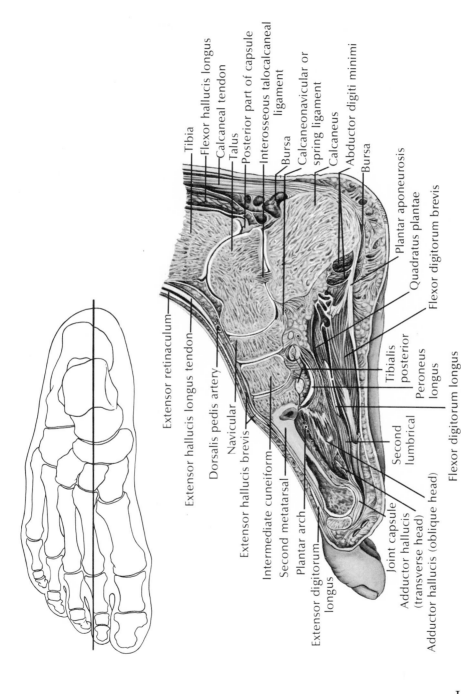

Tibia
Flexor hallucis longus
Calcaneal tendon
Talus
Posterior part of capsule
Interosseous talocalcaneal ligament
Bursa
Calcaneonavicular or spring ligament
Calcaneus
Abductor digiti minimi
Bursa

Plantar aponeurosis
Quadratus plantae
Flexor digitorum brevis

Extensor retinaculum
Extensor hallucis longus tendon
Dorsalis pedis artery
Navicular
Extensor hallucis brevis
Intermediate cuneiform
Second metatarsal
Plantar arch
Extensor digitorum longus
Joint capsule
Adductor hallucis (transverse head)
Adductor hallucis (oblique head)
Flexor digitorum longus

Tibialis posterior
Peroneus longus
Second lumbrical

Fig. 5-43. Longitudinal section through right foot. The small diagram shows the plane of the section. The drawing is of the medial surface of the lateral portion of the foot.

active standing position the gravity line of the body usually falls slightly in front of the hip joint, slightly behind the knee joint, and several centimeters in front of the ankle joint. The tendency for the weight of the body to cause flexion in these joints is opposed by the pull of the extensor muscles of the hip, knee, and ankle joint. This pull is not a constant one; rather there is alternate yielding and shortening that causes the body to sway forward and backward over the base of support. Lateral balance, when both feet are on the ground, is due to the interplay of the hip joint abductors and the peroneal muscles on the lateral aspect of the right and left legs. When the weight is supported on only one foot, the leg is stabilized on the foot by the interplay of the medial and lateral groups of lower leg muscles.

Walking involves weight-bearing and a backward-downward thrust of the propelling leg, a forward swing of the free leg, and a checking of momentum as the advanced leg strikes the floor. The propelling phase calls for contraction of the extensors of the hip, knee, and ankle joint and of the abductors of the hip joint. During this phase the force of gravity causes the body to fall forward and slightly medialward. Meanwhile, the forward swing of the free leg, started by the hip joint flexors and the force of gravity, has been completed. Then the hip, knee, and ankle joint extensors and the peroneal muscles again become active in checking momentum. The hip joint abductors on the side of the advanced foot become active when the rear foot leaves the ground.

MUSCLES OF ABDOMINAL WALL

The muscles in the abdominal wall are the external oblique, internal oblique, transverse, rectus, pyramidalis, and quadratus lumborum. Together they complete that portion of the abdominal wall not formed by bone (Fig. 5-44).

The external oblique muscle is a broad, thin sheet arising from the external surface of the lower eight ribs. The fibers pass inferiorly and anteriorly. Then the muscle fibers give way to dense fibrous tissue that forms an aponeurosis. The inferior border of the muscle is attached to the iliac crest, to the anterior superior iliac spine, and to the pubic tubercle. Between the spine and the tubercle the lower border has no bony attachment but forms a dense, strong band called the inguinal (Poupart's) ligament. Above the pubis the fibers of the aponeurosis of the external oblique of each side meet in the midline to form the linea alba. This is a white band of interlacing fibers extending from the pubis upward to the xiphoid process, thus helping to form a dense sheath covering the rectus abdominis muscle.

The umbilicus, or navel, is a scar in the midline, halfway between the xiphoid and symphysis pubis. At this point the umbilical cord of

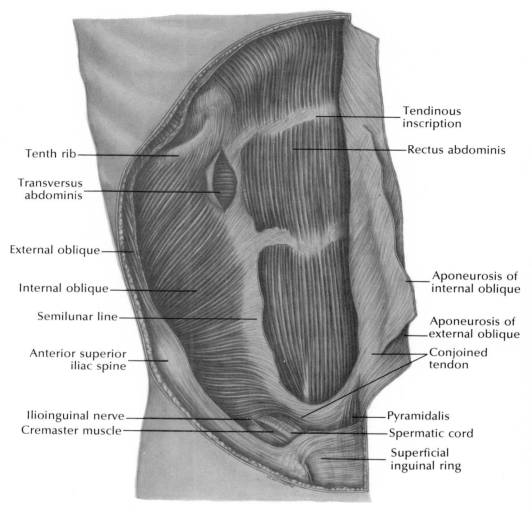

Tendinous inscription

Rectus abdominis

Tenth rib

Transversus abdominis

External oblique

Internal oblique

Semilunar line

Anterior superior iliac spine

Ilioinguinal nerve
Cremaster muscle

Aponeurosis of internal oblique

Aponeurosis of external oblique

Conjoined tendon

Pyramidalis
Spermatic cord
Superficial inguinal ring

Fig. 5-44. Muscles of abdominal wall. (Male, 57 years of age.)

the fetus was attached. The fibers of the linea alba strengthen this area.

The internal oblique muscle arises from the hinder part of the iliac crest and the deep fascia of the back and from the lateral half of the inguinal ligament. Its fibers pass superiorly at right angles to the direction of the fibers of the external oblique. It has a fanlike, tendinous insertion into the pubic bone, the linea alba, and the lower ribs and becomes a part of the sheath for the rectus abdominis muscle. A few fibers from the inferior border of the internal oblique form loops extending over the spermatic cord to become the cremaster muscle. 163

The transversus abdominis, or transverse abdominal muscle, lies deeper than the internal oblique and arises from the iliac crest, the inguinal ligament, the deep fascia of the back, and the lower ribs. Its fibers pass directly around the abdominal wall. Inferiorly, it is inserted into the pubis together with the internal oblique. This combined insertion may be either muscular or fibrous. If muscular, it is called the combined muscle; if fibrous, it is called the conjoined tendon or falx inguinalis. The transverse abdominal also has an insertion into the linea alba.

The pyramidalis muscle is inconstant and unimportant.

It is obvious that the oblique and transverse abdominal muscles form a triple muscular wall for the abdomen, and since the fibers run in three different directions, the wall is greatly strengthened. In an appendectomy the surgeon is careful to split each muscle layer parallel to the direction of its fibers so that the strength of the wall may be maintained (McBurney's incision).

The rectus abdominis, or straight abdominal muscle, arises from the upper border of the pubis and passes superiorly as a strong, heavy column of muscle to be inserted into the xiphoid and fifth, sixth, and seventh costal cartilages. There are three or four transverse bands of fibrous tissue (intersectiones tendineae) interrupting the muscular

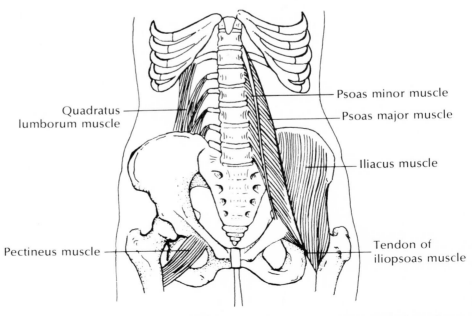

Fig. 5-45. Anterior view of iliopsoas, quadratus lumborum, and pectineus muscles.

bundles, which, therefore, do not extend the full length of the muscle itself.

The sheath of the rectus abdominis muscle requires some further description. The aponeurosis of the external oblique forms a complete anterior investment. When the aponeurosis of the internal oblique reaches the lateral border of the rectus, it splits; the anterior sheet blends with the aponeurosis of the external oblique, and the posterior sheet passes behind the rectus to form a posterior investment. The aponeurosis of the transverse abdominal helps to form the posterior portion of the sheath. However, the superior part of the rectus lies directly upon the anterior chest wall, and there are no aponeurotic investments posteriorly. In the lowest one fourth of the rectus the entire aponeurosis of the internal oblique and transverse passes in front of the rectus, and the only structure forming the posterior sheath is the anterior fascia outside the peritoneum (transversalis fascia).

The quadratus lumborum is a short, strong column of muscle arising from the hinder part of the iliac crest and transverse processes of the lower lumbar vertebrae and is inserted superiorly into the twelfth rib and transverse processes of the upper lumbar vertebrae.

The quadratus lumborum is innervated from branches of the upper three or four lumbar nerves; the anterior muscles of the abdominal wall are innervated from the lower six thoracic nerves.

It is evident from the description of the structure of the abdominal wall that the wall is a complex musculofibrous sheet. By altering the length of the muscle fibers, it is possible to adjust the wall to the varying size of the abdominal organs, and at the same time the tonus of the muscle fibers ensures that the general tension of the wall remains good. By voluntary contraction of the abdominal muscles it is possible to increase intra-abdominal pressure at will. If the abdominal wall were a rigid structure, it would be impossible to change the size of abdominal organs or to alter the pressure.

Inguinal canal. The inguinal canal is an oblique channel through the inferior part of the anterior abdominal wall just superior to the inguinal ligament. In a male the spermatic cord passes through the canal, and in a female the round ligament of the uterus lies in this channel. An inguinal hernia is an outpouching of the parietal peritoneum into this canal. The pouch is gradually lengthened and finally descends into the scrotum (or labium majus). Some portion of the abdominal organs, usually the omentum or a loop of the intestine, may also be pushed downward in this peritoneal tube. In an operation for repair of inguinal hernia the surgeon replaces these structures into the abdomen and attempts to obliterate the peritoneal pouch and

165

strengthen the abdominal wall by overlapping the ligaments, fascia, and muscles that form the canal.

As the spermatic cord passes from the anterior abdominal wall into the scrotum, it receives three investments: (1) the external spermatic fascia, derived from the aponeurosis of the external oblique

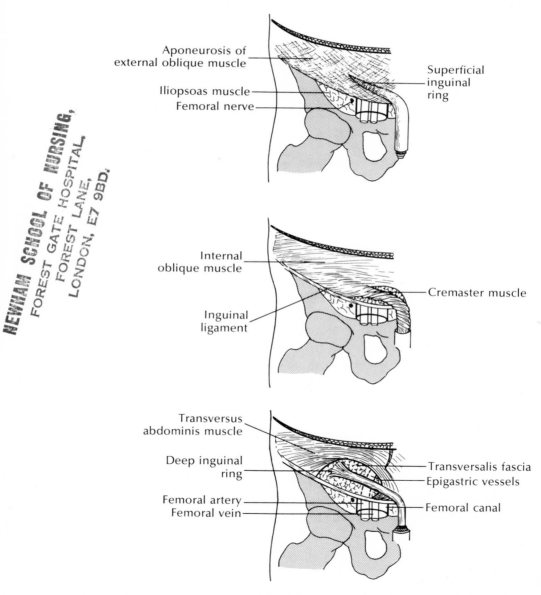

Aponeurosis of
external oblique muscle

Superficial
inguinal
ring

Iliopsoas muscle
Femoral nerve

Internal
oblique muscle

Cremaster muscle

Inguinal
ligament

Transversus
abdominis muscle

Deep inguinal
ring

Transversalis fascia
Epigastric vessels

Femoral artery
Femoral vein

Femoral canal

Fig. 5-46. Inguinal and femoral regions plus coverings of spermatic cord.

muscle, (2) the cremasteric fascia and cremaster muscle, derived from the internal oblique muscle, and (3) the internal spermatic fascia, which is continuous with the transversalis fascia, or connective tissue layer, lying external to the parietal peritoneum and beneath the transverse abdominal muscle (Fig. 5-46).

The opening in the transversalis fascia through which the spermatic cord leaves the abdominal cavity is the deep or abdominal inguinal ring, and the opening in the aponeurosis of the external oblique is the superficial or subcutaneous inguinal ring. In a healthy man the superficial ring is barely large enough to admit the tip of the little finger.

The inguinal canal is the site where there is most frequently weakening of the abdominal wall; hence, inguinal hernias are relatively common. However, areas of weakness are occasionally found about the umbilicus, in the linea alba above the umbilicus, in the femoral canal medial to the femoral vein, and in the lumbar region in the triangle between the iliac crest, latissimus dorsi, and external oblique, in the substance of the diaphragm, and beside the obturator artery as it leaves the pelvic cavity.

A hernia, which is a protrusion of a portion of the abdominal viscera through the body wall, may occur at any of the above sites. Inguinal hernias may be indirect, also called congenital, or direct, considered to be acquired. The difference in type assumes significance when surgery is needed to reduce the herniation. The indirect hernial sac enters the inguinal canal through the deep inguinal ring lateral to the inferior epigastric artery and veins (Fig. 5-46). If the sac extends the full length of the canal, it can pass through the superficial ring and into the scrotum or labium majus.

In a direct inguinal hernia the sac pushes into the posterior wall of the inguinal canal medial to the inferior epigastric vessels and inferior to the conjoined tendon. At that point the posterior wall of the canal is composed only of the transversalis fascia. However, because of the rather strong conjoined tendon, a direct hernia generally only causes a localized bulging of the wall of the inguinal canal. In extreme cases the sac may extend to and even through the superficial inguinal ring.

An inguinal hernia may be distinguished from a femoral hernia by the following criteria: an inguinal hernia is found superior to the inguinal ligament and medial to the pubic tubercle, whereas a femoral hernia is found inferior to the ligament and lateral to the tubercle. Inguinal hernias are more common in men than in women due, in part, to the weakness in the abdominal wall caused by the descending testis.

One malady, affecting both men and women and predisposing to hernias, is a sagging of the rectus abdominis because of a lack of tone in these muscles. Contrary to popular practice a straight-leg sit-up is not an effective means of strengthening these muscles, since in such an exercise the major movement occurs at the hip joint. As explained in Chapter 4, to cause movement at a joint, it is necessary to pass a muscle over the axis of rotation around which the movement occurs. The rectus abdominis does not pass over the transverse axis of the hip joint, but rather the iliopsoas does. Exercises that will effectively strengthen the rectus abdominis muscles are (1) straight-leg raises or (2) bent-knee curl-ups. Upon reflection, one may conclude that in a straight-leg raise primary movement still occurs at the hip and is accomplished by the iliopsoas (Fig. 5-45). This is correct; however, during a straight-leg raise the weight of the lower limbs and the action of the iliopsoas tend to tilt the pelvis forward, whereupon the rectus contracts to stabilize the pelvis. In a bent-knee curl the iliopsoas is shortened, and as one curls the chest towards the pubis, the major motive force is gained from contraction of the rectus abdominis muscles.

DEEP MUSCLES OF BACK

The deep muscles of the back are very numerous and variable. They consist of overlapping series of muscular columns arising from the sacrum and lower vertebrae and inserting into higher vertebrae. Some have long fibers and extend for long distances superiorly; others are short and connect adjacent bones. Some fibers go up and lateral, some up and medial, and some directly upward. The muscles of the back are usually divided into four groups or layers. All are innervated by the posterior rami of the spinal nerves. They extend the spinal column and produce various twisting and lateral movements of the trunk.

The first group consists of the serratus posterior superior, the serratus posterior inferior, and the splenius. The superior serratus arises from the spines of the last cervical and upper thoracic vertebrae, and the fibers pass inferiorly and laterally to be inserted into the third, fourth, and fifth ribs. The inferior serratus arises from the spinous processes of the last two thoracic and first two lumbar vertebrae, and the fibers pass laterally to be inserted into the last four ribs. These two muscles are usually very poorly developed. The splenius is a broad, flat muscle arising from the ligamentum nuchae and from the spines of the upper thoracic vertebrae. The fibers radiate superiorly and laterally to be inserted into the superior nuchal line of the occipital bone and into the transverse processes of the upper cervical vertebrae.

The second layer consists of the erector spinae (sacrospinalis), which is subdivided into the iliocostalis, the longissimus, and the spinalis. The various fibers of these muscles originate near the midline, are directed superiorly and laterally to be inserted into some portion of the axial skeleton above, and usually extend over several intervening bones.

The third group consists of the semispinalis and the multifidus. The fibers of these muscles are shorter than those of the second group and are directed superiorly and medially from origin to insertion.

The fourth and deepest group consists of the obliquus capitis superior and inferior, the rectus capitis posterior major and minor, the rotators, the interspinales, and the intertransversarii. These muscles have short fibers that originate from one member of the axial skeleton and usually pass directly upward to be inserted into the next bone above.

Certain muscles of the deep muscles of the neck and upper part of the back are inserted into the occipital bone behind the foramen magnum. The more important of these are the semispinalis, rectus capitis posterior major, rectus capitis posterior minor, and obliquus capitis superior muscles. These muscles produce extension of the head on the atlas, lateral movements of the head, and rotation of the atlas on the second cervical vertebra and, therefore, rotation of the head from side to side.

MUSCLES THAT MOVE THE HEAD

If one studies an articulated skeleton, one will see that the sacrum and the two hip bones form a heavy ring of bone that has a large central opening. In life the outlet of the pelvis is spanned by two fibromuscular sheets; the upper one is the pelvic diaphragm, which is attached to the medial aspect of the bones forming the pelvic girdle, and the lower one is the urogenital diaphragm, which is attached on either side to the conjoined ramus of pubis and ischium.

MUSCLES OF THE PELVIS AND PERINEUM

The pelvic diaphragm consists of two paired levator ani and coccygeus muscles. The levator ani muscle has two main portions; the pubococcygeal part arises from the medial surface of the pubis and passes posteriorly to be inserted into the coccyx, and the iliococcygeal part arises from the fascia covering the medial aspect of the obturator internus muscle and the inner surface of the ischium and is inserted into the coccyx. The coccygeus is a fan-shaped muscle that arises from the medial surface of the ischial spine and is inserted into the side of the sacrum and coccyx.

The connective tissue above these muscles and outside the peritoneum is quite dense and contains some smooth muscle fibers. In the space between the two pubococcygeus muscles the diaphragm is pierced by the urethra and the anal canal, and in women there is a

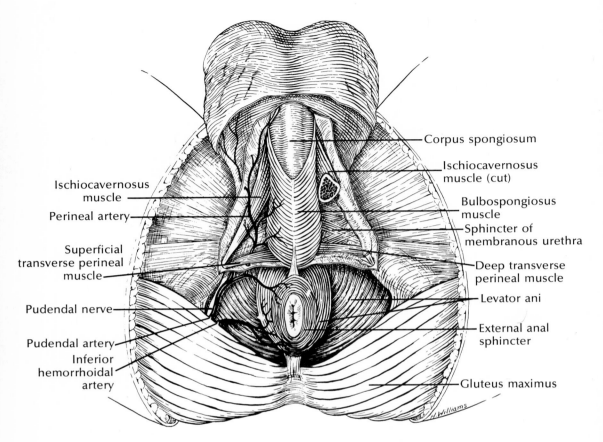

Corpus spongiosum

Ischiocavernosus
muscle (cut)

Bulbospongiosus
muscle

Sphincter of
membranous urethra

Deep transverse
perineal muscle

Levator ani

External anal
sphincter

Gluteus maximus

Ischiocavernosus
muscle

Perineal artery

Superficial
transverse perineal
muscle

Pudendal nerve

Pudendal artery

Inferior
hemorrhoidal
artery

Fig. 5-47. The male perineum. On the right the posterior portion of the right
crus of the penis and the perineal membrane (inferior fascia of the urogenital diaphragm) have been removed to show the muscles of the urogenital
diaphragm within the deep pouch. (Dissection by Dr. Frank Vecchio.)

third opening, the vagina. As these structures pass through the diaphragm, each tube receives attachments from the muscles and dense
fascia. These attachments are a major support of the pelvic viscera;
in addition, the muscles have a sphincteric action on the anal canal
and vagina.

An understanding of the perineum is necessary to visualize the
urogenital diaphragm. The perineum, the lowest portion of the trunk,
is a diamond-shaped area bounded on either side by the medial aspect
of the thigh and extending from the symphysis of the pubis anteriorly
to the coccyx posteriorly. It is subdivided into a posterior anal triangle
and an anterior urogenital triangle. The anus is located in the central
portion of the anal triangle, and on either side is a pyramidal-shaped

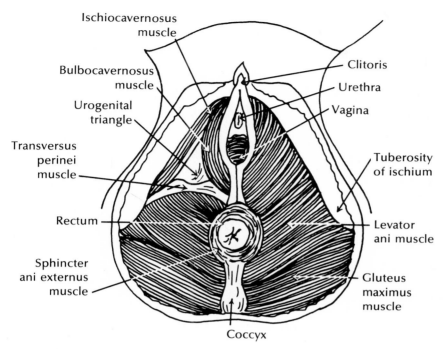

Ischiocavernosus muscle

Bulbocavernosus muscle

Urogenital triangle

Transversus perinei muscle

Rectum

Sphincter ani externus muscle

Clitoris

Urethra

Vagina

Tuberosity of ischium

Levator ani muscle

Gluteus maximus muscle

Coccyx

Fig. 5-48. The female perineum. The superficial structures have been omitted on the right side of the diagram (From Willson, J. R., Beecham, C. T., and Carrington, E. R.: Obstetrics and gynecology, ed. 4, St. Louis, 1971, The C. V. Mosby Co.)

space, called the ischiorectal fossa. The lateral wall of the fossa is the fascia covering the inner surface of the obturator internus muscle; the medial wall is the fascia covering the outer or lateral surface of the levator ani muscle; the posterior wall is the fascia covering the gluteus maximus muscle. In life the fossa is filled with fat and contains the pudendal vessels and nerves. The sphincter ani externus is the voluntary anal sphincter surrounding the inferior portion of the anal canal and anus. Some of its fibers blend with those of the levator ani, some pass into the central portion of the perineum, and other are attached to the tip of the coccyx (Figs. 5-47 and 5-48).

The urogenital triangle contains the external genitalia and the urogenital diaphragm and is subdivided into two spaces by layers of fascia. The superior fascia of the diaphragm is just below the levator ani muscle. The inferior fascia of the diaphragm (perineal membrane) is attached on either side to the conjoined ramus. The potential space thus formed is the deep perineal pouch and contains the deep group

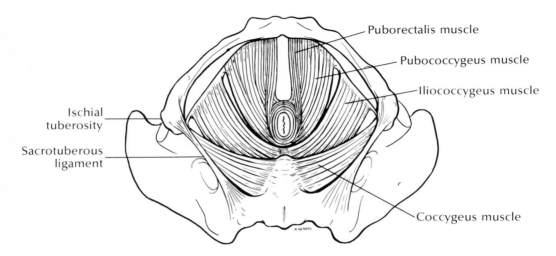

Puborectalis muscle

Pubococcygeus muscle

Iliococcygeus muscle

Ischial
tuberosity

Sacrotuberous
ligament

Coccygeus muscle

Fig. 5-49. Deep musculature of the pelvis, inferior view.

of perineal muscles. This group of muscles, together with the layer of fascia above and below, forms the urogenital diaphragm.

The deeper layer of fascia of the anterior abdominal wall is continued downward beneath the skin of the urogenital triangle as a thin fibrous sheet known as the superficial perineal (Colles') fascia. This sheet has firm attachments to the bone on either side and into the posterior edge of the urogenital diaphragm; it invests the scrotum and penis. The potential space between the inferior fascia of the urogenital diaphragm superiorly and the superficial perineal fascia inferiorly is the superficial perineal pouch. This space contains the proximal portions of the penis or clitoris and associated structures.

The muscles of the urogenital diaphragm (in the deep pouch) are the sphincter urethrae membranaceae and transversus perinei profundus. The muscles in the superficial pouch are the transversus perinei superficialis, the bulbospongiosus, and the ischiocavernosus.

The sphincter of the urethra arises from the inferior ramus of the pubis. Its fibers are directed medially and surround the urethra, forming a voluntary sphincter. The deep transverse perineal muscle arises from the ramus of the ischium and is inserted into the central portion of the perineum. These two muscles are not well separated from each other.

The superficial transverse perineal muscle is a small bundle that arises from the medial aspect of the ischial tuberosity and is inserted into the central point of the perineum. In a female it is usually very poorly developed. The bulbospongiosus arises from the central portion of the perineum and in men sweeps laterally surrounding the bulb of

172

Table 9. Important muscles

Name	Origin	Insertion	Nerve supply	Function
Sternocleidomastoid	Clavicle and sternum	Occiput	Spinal accessory	Extends head and flexes neck
Pectoralis major	Clavicle and sternum	Humerus	Lateral and medial pectoral	Flexes and adducts arm
Serratus anterior	Chest wall	Scapula	Long thoracic	Draws scapula forward
Trapezius	Upper vertebrae	Scapula and clavicle	Spinal accessory	Braces shoulder and elevates lateral angle of scapula
Latissimus dorsi	Lower vertebrae and ilium	Humerus	Thoracodorsal	Extends and adducts arm
Deltoid	Clavicle and scapula	Humerus	Axillary	Abducts arm
Triceps brachii	Humerus and scapula	Ulna	Radial	Extends arm and forearm
Biceps brachii	Scapula	Radius	Musculocutaneous	Flexes arm and forearm and supinates forearm
Flexors of forearm	Medial epicondyle of humerus, radius, and ulna	Wrist and fingers	Median (and ulnar)	Flex wrist and fingers
Extensors of forearm	Lateral epicondyle of humerus, radius, and ulna	Wrist and fingers	Radial	Extend wrist and fingers
Quadriceps femoris	Ilium and femur	Tibia	Femoral	Extends leg
Iliopsoas	Ilium and lumbar vertebrae	Femur	Lumbar nerves	Flexes thigh
Adductors of thigh	Ilium and pubis	Femur and tibia	Obturator	Adduct thigh
Gluteus maximus	Sacrum and ilium	Femur	Inferior gluteal	Extends thigh
Tensor fasciae latae	Ilium	Tibia	Superior gluteal	Abducts thigh
Hamstring group	Ischial tuberosity	Tibia and fibula	Sciatic	Flexes leg
Peroneus longus and brevis	Tibia and fibula	Foot	Peroneal	Plantar flex foot
Anterior tibial group	Tibia and fibula	Foot	Peroneal	Dorsiflexes or extends foot

Continued.

173

Table 9. Important muscles—cont'd

Name	Origin	Insertion	Nerve supply	Function
Posterior tibial group	Tibia and fibula	Foot	Tibial	Plantar flexes foot
Rectus abdominis	Pubis	Sternum and costal cartilages	Lower thoracic spinal nerves	Flexes trunk
Erector spinae	Vertebrae	Vertebrae and ribs	Spinal nerves	Extends trunk

the urethra and the corpus spongiosum to be inserted into the base of the penis. By its contraction, it aids in emptying the urethra. In women it is separated into two halves by the vagina, covers the bulb of the vestibule on either side, and acts as a sphincter of the vaginal opening. The ischiocavernosus arises from the tuberosity of the ischium, passes anteriorly over the crus of the penis, and is inserted into the pubis and corpus cavernosum penis. In women this muscle has similar relations but is smaller.

The muscles of the pelvis and perineum are innervated by branches from the pudendal nerve, which arise from the second through fourth sacral spinal cord segments.

OTHER GROUPS OF MUSCLES

The muscles of the eyeball are discussed in Chapter 7. The muscles of breathing and those associated with the larynx are discussed in Chapter 11; the muscles of chewing and swallowing, in Chapter 12.

Table 9 contains a summary of the more important muscles. If the function of each is opposed so that it contracts against resistance, the entire muscle will become firm and may be palpated beneath the skin from origin to insertion. Nearly all the muscles in the table may be identified in this manner, and the student should study their action in his own body.

REVIEW QUESTIONS

1. Name four large superficial muscles of the chest wall and shoulder; give one important function of each.
2. What are the bony attachments of the biceps brachii muscle? What functions does this muscle perform?
3. What is the main action of the triceps brachii muscle? What is its innervation?
4. Name four muscles on the volar aspect of the forearm. What does each do? What is the innervation of each?
5. Name four muscles on the dorsal aspect of the forearm. What does each do? What is the nerve supply?
6. What muscles abduct the fingers? What muscles adduct the fingers?
7. Describe the palmar aponeurosis.
8. What is the action of the iliopsoas muscle?
9. Describe briefly the quadriceps femoris muscle. What is its most important action?

10. Name the muscles that are located on the inner aspect of the thigh. What is their nerve supply?
11. Describe briefly the gluteus maximus muscle. What is its most important action?
12. What muscles are found in the hamstring group?
13. What are the three important muscles of the front of the leg? What is their nerve supply? Give one action that is common to all three.
14. Describe briefly the gastrocnemius muscle. Why is it so large in man?
15. Name the muscles that form the abdominal wall.
16. What is the inguinal canal? What passes through it in men? What passes through it in women?
17. What forms the pelvic diaphragm?
18. What is the musculotendinous cuff of the shoulder joint?
19. Name the muscles associated with the thumb.
20. What muscles join to form the calcaneal tendon?
21. Discuss direct versus indirect inguinal hernias.

CHAPTER 6

THE NERVOUS SYSTEM

The nervous system consists of the brain, the spinal cord, and the peripheral nerves. There are 31 pairs of spinal nerves and 12 pairs of cranial nerves. These connect all areas of the body with the central nervous system. Certain branches of these 43 nerves, connected with the viscera through outlying collections of nerve cells, or ganglia, form the autonomic nervous system.

CENTRAL NERVOUS SYSTEM

The brain and the spinal cord, parts of a continuous organ, are best discussed separately. Although developmental anatomy is beyond the scope of this book, Figs. 6-1 and 6-2 illustrate progressive stages in the early development of the caudal or spinal portion of the central nervous system. Shortly after formation of the germ layers, cells in the midline of the surface ectoderm thicken and form the neural plate, which invaginates to form the neural groove. As development proceeds, the neural groove deepens, forming the neural folds, which then pinch off to form the neural tube, the cells of which are called neuroepithelial cells. In the adult the cavity within the neural tube remains as the central canal of the spinal cord and as the ventricles of the brain. Cells adjacent to the neural groove form the neural crest, which gives rise to ganglia (dorsal root and autonomic), to some neuroglia, melanin-containing cells, as well as to the adrenal medulla.

The neural plate contains the precursors of four cell columns. Near the midline in an area named the basal plate, somatic and visceral motor neurons are found. Laterally, in the alar plate, visceral and somatic sensory neurons are located. The topographical relationship

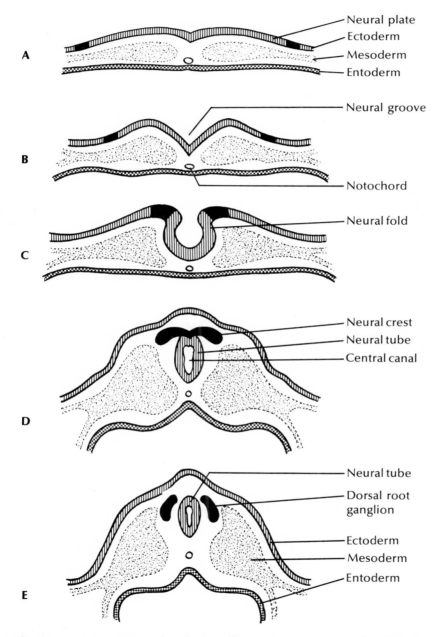

Fig. 6-1. Cross sections of embryos, illustrating progressive development of the caudal portion of the neural tube. **A,** Neural plate stage. **B,** Early neural groove stage. **C,** Advanced neural groove stage. **D,** Early neural tube stage. **E,** Advanced neural tube stage. (From DiDio, L. J. A.: Synopsis of anatomy, St. Louis, 1970, The C. V. Mosby Co.)

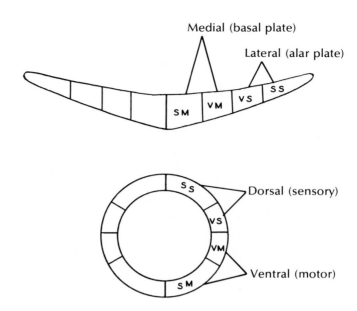

SM. Somatic motor cells

VM. Visceral motor cells

VS. Visceral sensory cells

SS. Somatic sensory cells

Fig. 6-2. The four columns of cells in the neural plate and in the neural tube. (From DiDio, L. J. A.: Synopsis of anatomy, St. Louis, 1970, The C. V. Mosby Co.)

of these cells to one another remains the same from the neural plate stage to the adult spinal cord (Fig. 6-2).

Shortly after formation of the three germ layers, the middle layer (mesoderm) assumes two different forms. In the head region it forms a loose mesh work, called the mesenchyme, which fills the spaces between the epithelial layers. In the body region the mesoderm condenses near the midline into segmental blocks, called somites, and a plate of mesoderm lateral to the somites. With further development the lateral plate splits into two laminae (Fig. 6-1). The dorsal layer comprises the somatic mesoderm, and the ventral layer forms the splanchnic mesoderm. The somatic mesoderm and ectoderm are closely associated and together form the somatopleure, which comprises the body wall. The splanchnic mesoderm and endoderm, jointly termed the splanchnopleure, are concerned mainly with development of the gut and its derivatives. Structures that arise from the somites or somatopleure (with the exception of hair follicles and sweat glands) are innervated by nerves classified as somatic. Structures that are derived from the splanchnopleure are innervated by nerve fibers classified as visceral.

The adult spinal cord is a column of nerve tissue extending from the foramen magnum to the level of the second lumbar vertebra. In the initial stages of intrauterine development the spinal cord and vertebral column are approximately the same length. After the third month of gestation the vertebral column grows relatively faster than the spinal cord. Thus, the nerves course more obliquely as their intervertebral foramina, through which they exit, are displaced caudally. This phenomenon, although present to a degree in all spinal nerves, is most marked in the lumbar and sacral nerves, which pass well below the conus medullaris, the caudalmost part of the spinal cord. Because of their nearly parallel course from the lower spinal cord segments and because of a fanciful resemblance to a "horse's tail," the nerve fibers in the lumbar cistern collectively are called the "cauda equina" (Figs. 6-3 and 6-4).

Spinal cord

The spinal cord is surrounded by several protective coverings, collectively called the meninges. The innermost covering is the thin, delicate, highly vascular pia mater, which is closely attached to the surface of the cord. Outside of this is the arachnoid, which is a delicate meshwork of fibrous tissue. The subarachnoid space between the pia mater and arachnoid is bridged by fine strands of connective tissue, the arachnoid trabeculae, and in life is filled with cerebrospinal fluid. The subdural space separates the arachnoid from a thick, relatively avascular outer connective tissue sheet, the dura mater. The spinal dura mater does not duplicate the intracranial arrangement, since the outer or periosteal layer of cranial dura becomes the independent periosteum for the vertebral bodies, while the inner layer of spinal dura is widely separated from the vertebral body by the fat and venous filled epidural space. The vertebral plexus of veins found in the epidural space is continuous superiorly with the dural venous sinuses (see Fig. 6-14).

The spinal cord has two indistinct spindle-shaped swellings: a cervical enlargement, extending from the level of the third cervical to that of the second thoracic vertebra, and a lumbar enlargement, extending from the level of the ninth thoracic to that of the first lumbar vertebra. The nerves to the extremities come from these two enlargements. Below the lumbar enlargement the cord quickly decreases in

179

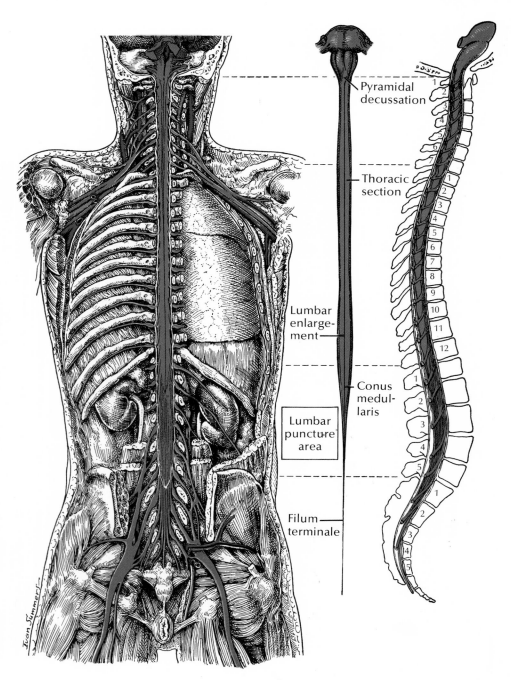

Fig. 6-3. Relation of the spinal cord, part of the brain, and some of the spinal nerves to surrounding structures. (From Mettler, F. A.: Neuroanatomy, ed. 2, St. Louis, 1948, The C. V. Mosby Co.)

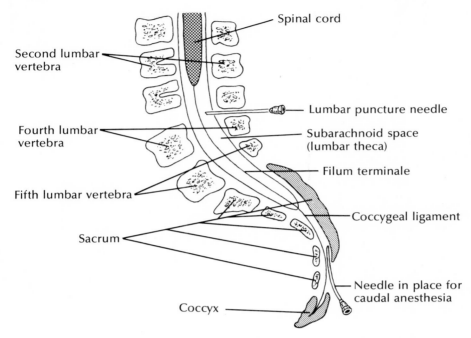

Fig. 6-4. Lumbar puncture, showing the needle inserted through the third lumbar intervertebral space, caudal to the termination of the spinal cord. (From DiDio, L. J. A.: Synopsis of anatomy, St. Louis, 1970, The C. V. Mosby Co.)

size to a cone-shaped termination (conus medullaris), from which is prolonged a slender thread of nonnervous tissue, the filum terminale, attached below to the coccyx (Fig. 6-3).

There are eight grooves extending along the cord. The median anterior fissure is deep and distinct for the entire length of the cord. The median posterior sulcus is quite shallow. The posterior lateral sulcus is an indistinct furrow along the line of attachment of posterior roots of the spinal nerves. The anterior lateral sulcus, marking the line of attachment of the anterior roots, is quite indistinct. In the upper segments of the cord there is another line, called the intermediate posterior sulcus, lying between the posterior median sulcus and the posterior lateral sulcus.

If a cross section of the cord is studied immediately after death, one will observe that it is composed of two kinds of tissue, one white and the other grayish pink. The white substance is composed largely of myelinated nerve fibers, whereas the gray substance is composed of nerve cells, neuroglia, blood vessels, and unmyelinated nerve fibers.

181

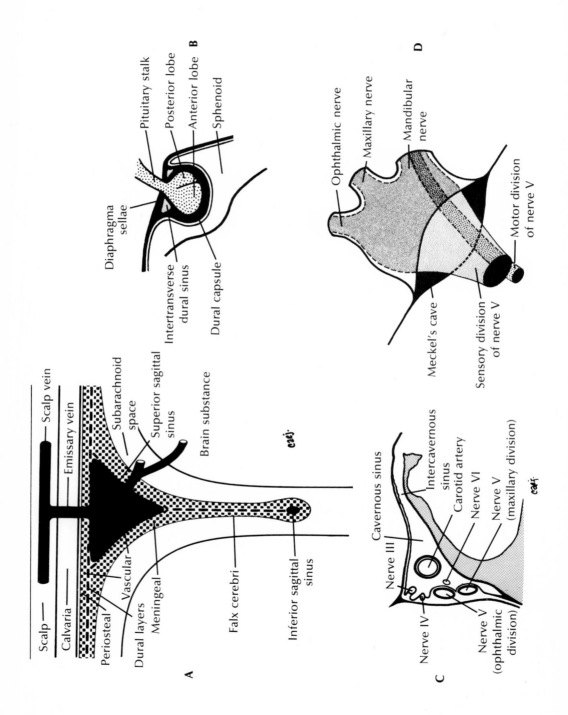

A

Scalp

Calvaria

Periosteal
Vascular
Dural layers
Meningeal

Falx cerebri

Inferior sagittal
sinus

Scalp vein

Emissary vein

Subarachnoid
space

Superior sagittal
sinus

Brain substance

B

Diaphragma
sellae

Intertransverse
dural sinus

Dural capsule

Pituitary stalk

Posterior lobe

Anterior lobe

Sphenoid

C

Nerve III

Nerve IV

Nerve V
(ophthalmic
division)

Cavernous sinus

Intercavernous
sinus

Carotid artery

Nerve VI

Nerve V
(maxillary division)

D

Ophthalmic nerve

Maxillary nerve

Mandibular
nerve

Motor division
of nerve V

Sensory division
of nerve V

Meckel's cave

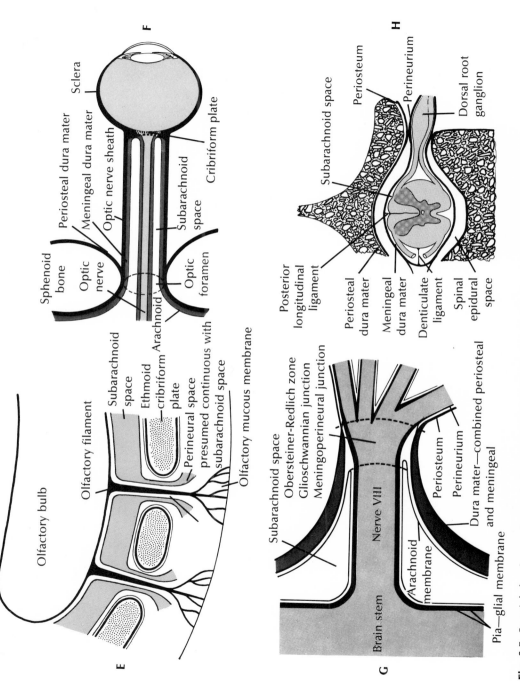

Fig. 6-5. Special dural complexes. **A,** Sagittal sinuses and falx. **B,** Diaphragma sellae. **C,** Cavernous sinus. **D,** Meckel's cave. **E,** Olfactory nerves. **F,** Optic nerve. **G,** Auditory nerve. **H,** Spinal root. (From Minckler, J.: Introduction to neuroscience, St. Louis, 1972, The C. V. Mosby Co.)

The gray substance in the cord is centrally located and, in cross section, somewhat resembles the letter H. In each half of the cord the gray substance is a comma-shaped mass united to the mass of the other side by a bar. The larger end of the comma, derived from the basal plate, forms the anterior horn and the tail of the comma, derived from the alar plate, the posterior horn. At the level of spinal cord segments first thoracic through second lumbar and second sacral through fourth sacral, a lateral or intermediate horn is interposed between the anterior and posterior horns. In a longitudinal section the masses are called the anterior and posterior columns, respectively. The neuroglial cells of various types form the supporting tissue of the cord.

The central canal of the cord lies within the central bar of gray matter, extends the entire length of the cord, and is continuous above with the fourth ventricle of the medulla. In an adult the caliber of the canal is extremely small, and it is usually blocked by the remnants of cells that originally lined the canal.

The nerve cells in the anterior horn are somatic motor in function, whereas those in the lateral horn are visceral motor in function (Fig. 6-2). Their processes form the anterior roots of the spinal nerves. The cells in the posterior horn receive sensory impulses that come in over the posterior roots and relay these impulses to the other parts of the central nervous system by means of synaptic transmission. A synapse is an area of functional contact between two neurons.

The white substance of the cord surrounds the gray and is composed of parallel longitudinal bundles of myelinated fibers. These columns in each half of the cord are grouped into three strands or funiculi. The posterior funiculus lies between the posterior median sulcus and the posterior lateral sulcus; the lateral funiculus lies between the posterior lateral sulcus and the anterior lateral sulcus; the anterior funiculus lies between the anterior lateral sulcus and the median anterior fissure. The funiculi are also called columns.

Within the white substance of the cord the fibers are arranged in definite groups or tracts. Fibers having a common origin or destination or both are found in close topographical relationships.

The general tracts of the spinal cord are the propriospinal, the long ascending, and the long descending tracts. Propriospinal tracts interconnect different levels of the spinal cord. The long ascending tracts contain sensory fibers and connect the spinal cord with the brain, whereas the long descending tracts contain motor fibers and connect the brain with the spinal cord. The location of the cells of origin and the distribution of the long tracts is often indicated by the names given the tracts. For example, fibers originating from cells in the spinal cord

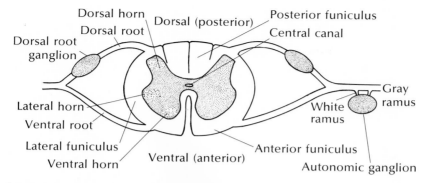

Fig. 6-6. Schematic cross section of spinal cord.

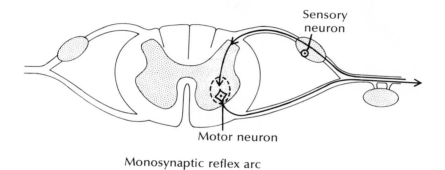

Monosynaptic reflex arc

Fig. 6-7. Two-neuron reflex arc. This type of arc found in knee-jerk reflex.

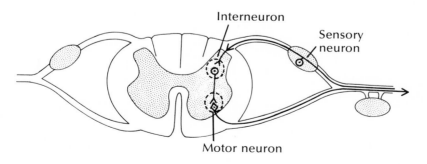

Polysynaptic reflex arc

Fig. 6-8. Three-neuron reflex arc. This type of arc produces many spinal reflexes.

and terminating in the thalamus are known as spinothalamic tracts.

Usually a fiber whose cell of origin is in a dorsal root ganglion does not go all the way to the brain. In the course of such a sensory fiber there is usually interposed at least one neuron whose cell of origin is in the gray matter of the cord. This intermediate or intercalated neuron also makes connections within the cord itself, thus making many spinal reflexes possible (Figs. 6-6 to 6-8).

The fibers in the posterior funiculus arise from cells in the dorsal ganglion of each spinal nerve. In cross sections of the cord the posterior funiculus increases in size from caudal to rostral. This is reasonable, since all the pathways connecting spinal cord and brain must be present at the highest cervical level and since only those required for a given level and below are present at successively lower segments. Sensory impulses of limb and body position, vibratory sensibility, and discrimination in light touch pass to the brain in the posterior or dorsal column on the same side of the body. Other fibers that carry sensory impulses for pain, temperature, and crude touch enter the cord via dorsal roots and terminate or synapse with other nerve cells in the spinal cord gray matter. Axons of the cells of the spinal cord gray matter cross over to the other side of the cord and pass to the brain in the anterior portion of the lateral funiculus.

The lateral funiculus contains a fiber tract called the lateral corticospinal tract. This bundle of nerve fibers conducts impulses from the cerebral cortex to the motor cells in the anterior horn of the spinal gray matter. Through this pathway we have conscious voluntary control over the movements of the skeletal muscles of the body. This pathway is also called the crossed pyramidal tract because the fibers arise

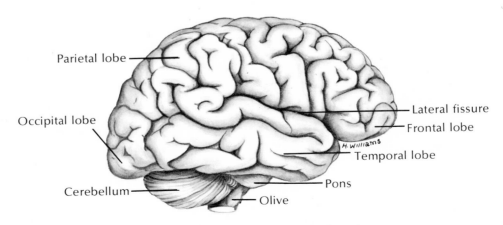

Fig. 6-9. Brain, lateral view. (Male, 45 years of age.)

mainly from pyramid-shaped cells of the cerebral cortex on one side of the brain, pass through the medullary pyramids, and as they pass downward, decussate or cross over to control movements of the opposite side of the body.

There are other bundles of fibers in the lateral and anterior funiculi that carry impulses to and from the brain for involuntary and reflex movements.

Brain

The brain is composed of three main parts: the brain stem, the cerebellum, and the cerebrum.

The brain stem begins at the foramen magnum as the upward continuation of the cervical spinal cord and is a mass of interlacing bundles of nerve fibers and nests of cells, called nuclei. It lies in the midline on the floor of the cranial cavity and extends forward to the level of the sella turcica of the sphenoid bone. The brain stem has the following main parts: medulla oblongata, pons, mesencephalon, and diencephalon.

The cerebellum consists of two lateral lobes and a central mass that is indistinctly separated from the lobes. It is placed in the posterior cranial fossa above the medulla and pons and is separated from the

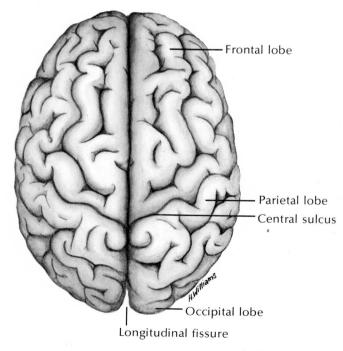

Fig. 6-10. Brain, superior view. (Male, 45 years of age.)

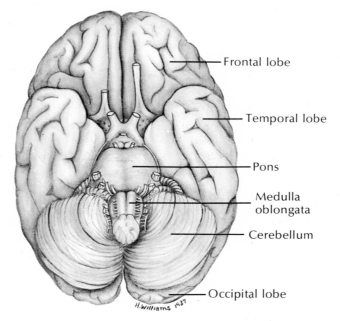

Frontal lobe

Temporal lobe

Pons

Medulla
oblongata

Cerebellum

Occipital lobe

H.Williams 1937

Fig. 6-11. Brain, inferior view. (Male, 45 years of age.)

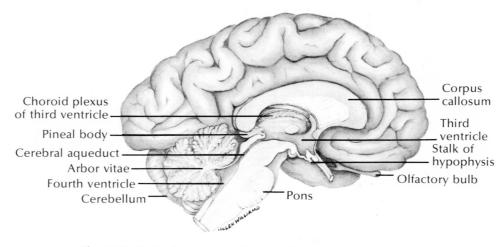

Choroid plexus
of third ventricle

Pineal body

Cerebral aqueduct

Arbor vitae

Fourth ventricle

Cerebellum

Pons

Corpus
callosum

Third
ventricle

Stalk of
hypophysis

Olfactory bulb

HELEN WILLIAMS

Fig. 6-12. Sagittal section of brain, showing medial aspect of left half of
brain.

188

posterior portion of the cerebrum above by a fold of dura mater, called the tentorium (see Fig. 6-36).

The cerebrum consists of two large hemispheres and a connecting bridge, the corpus callosum. In man the cerebral hemispheres are so large that they cover the other parts of the brain. When the brain is viewed from above, the cerebrum alone can be seen.

Medulla oblongata. The medulla oblongata is the portion of the brain stem that extends from the upper end of the spinal cord, just above the origin of the first cervical nerve, to the distinctly defined lower border of the pons. There is no such clear distinction from the spinal cord. The structures present in the cervical cord extend up into the medulla, gradually undergoing rearrangement in their course. The central gray matter is broken up into more or less distinct nests of cells or nuclear masses, with columns of white matter interwoven among the nuclei.

Important nuclei of the medulla are connected with the last four cranial nerves, that is, the ninth to the twelfth, inclusive. The taste fibers of the seventh and ninth make important connections in the medulla. On the posterior surface of the lower part of the medulla there are two nuclei on each side, the nucleus gracilis and the nucleus cuneatus. These receive the sensory impulses coming up in the posterior columns of the cord and relay them to the other side of the medulla, whence they pass upward to higher sensory nuclei and to the cerebral cortex. Nearly all sensory impulses received on one side of the body are registered finally on the opposite side of the brain. We have already pointed out that fibers carrying sensory impulses of pain and temperature cross in the cord. In the medulla there are also a number of centers for the regulation of essential activities of the body such as the respiratory center, cardiac center, vasomotor center, and centers for deglutition, vomiting, gastric secretion, and sweating.

On the side of the medulla there is a swelling formed by a nucleus, called, because of its shape, the olive. From the olive a large bundle of fibers arises that passes across the midline through the substance of the medulla and thence to the cerebellum. This bundle, together with fibers from the spinal cord, forms the bulk of the inferior cerebellar peduncle, or restiform body.

The dorsal surface of the medulla is at first an upward continuation of the cord, but it soon flattens out. The central canal becomes a widely dilated space, called the fourth ventricle, having the main substance of the medulla and pons in front and below and a thin roof behind and above.

The undersurface of the medulla is similar to that of the cord, but the midportion of the median anterior fissure is obliterated by an interlacing mass of crossing fibers known as the decussation of the pyramids. This marks the crossing of the corticospinal tract, which arises in the pyramidal cells of the cerebral cortex and ends in the anterior horn cells of the gray matter of the cord.

Pons. This portion of the brain stem lies ventral to the cerebellum, rostral to the medulla. It contains a large bundle of transverse fibers connecting with each half of the cerebellum and is the main mass of the middle cerebellar peduncle. These transverse fibers arise from cells embedded within the substance of the pons and relay impulses from the cerebral cortex to the cerebellum.

Deep in this transverse band and beneath the fourth ventricle there are longitudinal fiber bundles that carry impulses up and down the brain stem. The nuclei of the fifth, sixth, seventh, and eighth cranial nerves are located within the upper part of the pons. Sensory impulses received from the fifth and eighth nerves are relayed through these nuclei in their upward course to higher centers. Part of those for hearing and touch eventually reach the cerebral cortex, and others make reflex connections within the brain stem.

Mesencephalon. The mesencephalon is about 18 mm in length. In its center is the cerebral aqueduct (the aqueduct of Sylvius), a narrow canal connecting the fourth ventricle with the third ventricle.

The longitudinal bundles of the pons are continued upward into the mesencephalon. At its anterior end they form two prominent bands on the undersurface of the brain stem, the crura cerebri or cerebral peduncles, which are connected with the cerebral hemispheres. It is within these columns that most of the motor fibers pass down from the cerebrum to the lower parts of the nervous system. Large bundles of sensory fibers passing upward to the thalamus lie ventral to the cerebral peduncles.

The nuclei of the third and fourth cranial nerves are located in the ventral part of the mesencephalon. The anterior portion of the nucleus of the fifth nerve is also located there.

The red nucleus is an important mass in the mesencephalon. It is connected with the cerebellum by means of a band of fibers, called the brachium conjunctivum cerebelli or superior cerebellar peduncle. Fibers that pass downward into the cord from the red nucleus are important in certain reflex patterns.

On the upper surface of the mesencephalon are two pairs of small round swellings, called the colliculi. The inferior colliculi are relay stations for reflexes concerned with hearing, and the superior colliculi for reflexes concerned with sight.

Diencephalon. The diencephalon is that portion of the brain stem that surrounds the third ventricle. In the intact brain the upper surface is completely hidden by the overlying cerebral hemispheres. The pineal body is a small cone-shaped mass attached by a slender stalk to the upper surface of the diencephalon (see Chapter 8).

The undersurface of the diencephalon may be seen in the narrow space bounded behind by the cerebral peduncles and in front by the optic chiasm. The hypophysis is a small rounded body lying in the sella turcica and attached by a slender stalk to the diencephalon. The mammillary bodies, two small rounded masses seen just behind the stalk of the hypophysis, are a part of the hypothalamus.

The fibers carrying visual impulses leave the optic chiasm and sweep laterally under the cerebral peduncles; some pass to the superior colliculi for reflexes involving vision and others turn into the lateral part of the thalamus, where they are relayed up and back through the substance of each cerebral hemisphere to the back of the occipital lobe where visual impulses are registered on the cortex for conscious vision.

A very important group of nuclei lying within the substance of the diencephalon is the thalamus, which eventually receives nearly all the sensory impulses flowing into the central nervous system and relays them on to the cerebral cortex. That portion of the diencephalon lying ventral to and on either side of the third ventricle is called the hypothalamus and has extremely important and diverse reflex functions. Experimental evidence indicates that there are centers here that have to do with the regulation of many essential functions such as temperature control, water and fat metabolism, sleep, sexual activity, and emotional control.

Cerebellum. The cerebellum is a solid mass of tissue consisting of a core of white matter and a rather thin continuous layer of gray matter on the surface. The gray matter is of uniform thickness and is thrown into a series of more or less parallel folds. In a sagittal section it can be seen as primary, secondary, and tertiary folds, with branches of white matter projecting into the folds, forming a treelike pattern, thus suggesting the term arbor vitae. These folds are also known as laminae.

Buried within the white matter of each cerebellar hemisphere is the dentate nucleus, the most important nuclear mass of the cerebellum.

The cerebellum is connected with the rest of the brain by three pairs of nerve bundles, or peduncles, already mentioned. The inferior cerebellar peduncle, or restiform body, brings nerve fibers from the nuclei of the medulla and some from the spinal cord. The middle cerebellar peduncle, or brachium pontis, brings nerve fibers from the nuclei of the pons. The superior cerebellar peduncle, or brachium conjunctivum cerebelli, carries impulses from the dentate nucleus of the

191

cerebellum to the red nucleus of the mesencephalon and thalamus. The cerebellum is a coordination center for muscular activity, particularly for the muscles used in walking.

Cerebrum. The cerebrum has an outer layer of gray matter, and each hemisphere has a large central cavity called a lateral ventricle (Fig. 6-16). The surface has many complex folds called gyri, separated from each other by depressions called fissures or sulci. The pattern of these folds is fairly stable, but the detail differs greatly from brain to brain and indeed on the two sides of the same brain. There are certain well-marked fissures that may be distinguished in every brain.

The longitudinal fissure separates the two hemispheres. Passing almost at right angles to this fissure outward and downward over the side of each hemisphere is the central sulcus. On the lateral side of the hemisphere, below the end of the central sulcus, is the lateral fissure, or sulcus, which begins on the undersurface of the brain and passes out and back along the side of the brain.

On the undersurface of the front of the cerebrum there is the olfactory sulcus, in which lies the olfactory tract, and on each side are two long prominent grooves, the collateral and inferior temporal sulci.

On the medial surface of each hemisphere there are two important grooves, the sulcus cinguli, curving around the corpus callosum, and posterior to this, the calcarine sulcus.

Each hemisphere is arbitrarily divided into several lobes. The frontal lobe lies above the lateral fissure and in front of the central sulcus. Behind the central sulcus lies the parietal lobe, and below the lateral fissure lies the temporal lobe. The posterior pole of the cerebrum, called the occipital lobe, extends from the parietooccipital fissure inferiorly to the preoccipital notch. The calcarine sulcus lies on the medial surface of the occipital lobe.

The interior of the cerebrum contains large bundles of fibers that connect various portions of the same hemisphere, various parts of the two hemispheres with each other by way of the corpus callosum, and the cortex of each hemisphere with sensory and motor nuclei in lower parts of the nervous system. Within the substance of the cerebrum and in close contact with these interlacing bands of fibers are the basal ganglia, or corpus striatum, a group of nuclei that serves as a coordinating center for sensory and motor impulses.

Cerebral localization. Certain areas of the cerebral cortex are specialized for definite functions. The precentral gyrus of the frontal lobe anterior to the central sulcus is specialized for voluntary motor movements. Each part of the body is represented by groups of pyramidal cells, the order being that illustrated in Fig. 6-13. The area for the foot is nearest the longitudinal fissure, often actually on the medial surface of the hemisphere. The rest of the body is represented in order, the face being the last—just above the lateral fissure. The left cerebral hemisphere governs movements of the right side of the body; the right hemisphere governs those of the left side of the body.

The motor area governing speech is in the left frontal lobe of right-handed persons in the angle between the central sulcus and lateral fissure. In left-handed persons it is the right frontal lobe, which governs speech. This is a condition known as cerebral dominance.

That area of the parietal lobe just behind the central sulcus is set aside for conscious perception of such sensations as touch, heat, vibration, limb position, and cold. Areas are assigned to the specific parts of the body for sensations just as for movements, and corresponding areas are placed side by side.

The occipital cortex on both sides of the calcarine sulcus receives impulses of vision.

Auditory impulses are received in the temporal lobe just inferior to the middle of the lateral fissure (Fig. 6-13).

In man the portion of the cortex that receives sensations of smell appears small. It is on the undersurface of the temporal lobe in a rolled-in convolution of the brain called the hippocampus. This is lateral to the mammillary bodies of the diencephalon.

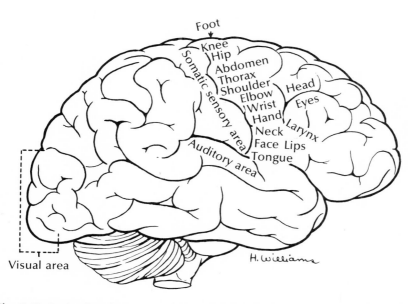

Fig. 6-13. Brain showing areas of cerebral localization. Same brain as shown in Fig. 6-9. Somatic sensory area is the portion of cortex receiving impulses from all parts of the skin.

These areas just mentioned, devoted to motor outflow and to sensory reception, occupy only a small portion of the entire cerebral cortex. The rest, the so-called association areas, are devoted to such functions as motor patterns, memory, and attention and to building composite concepts from various sensory impulses. It is probable that the portion of the frontal lobe anterior to the primary motor area is devoted to the motor patterns involved in such activities as walking, writing, and playing musical instruments. Concepts of word-hearing are in the temporal lobe, and those of word-seeing are in the occipital lobe.

Coverings of the brain (meninges). Like the cord, the brain has three coverings, the pia mater, arachnoid, and the dura mater. The

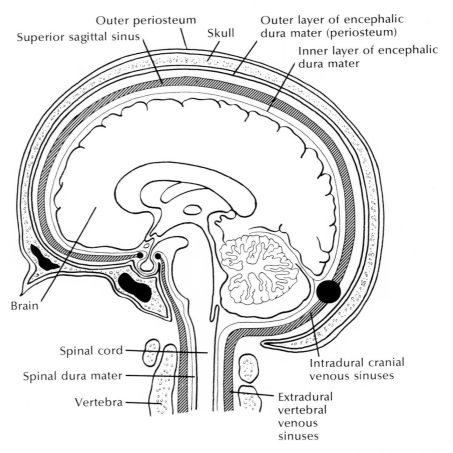

Fig. 6-14. The two layers of the cranial dura mater. Note that only its inner layer is continuous with the spinal dura mater. (From DiDio, L. J. A.: Synopsis of anatomy, St. Louis, 1970, The C. V. Mosby Co.)

thin and delicate pia is closely applied to the surface of the brain, passing into the depth of the various sulci, or fissures, and protruding into
the ventricles. The arachnoid, a thin meshwork between dura and pia,
bridges over the sulci but does not enter them. The meshes in the pia-
arachnoid complex contain cerebrospinal fluid and networks of blood
vessels. The dura is a tough fibrous sheet, which within the cranium
is divided into two layers. The outer layer, or periosteal dura, is closely
adherent to the inner surface of the brain case. The inner layer, or
meningeal dura, which corresponds to dura mater of the cord, forms
the outermost covering of the brain. It also forms various septa, or
partitions: (1) the falx cerebri, which extends into the longitudinal
fissure between the cerebral hemispheres (see Fig. 6-5, A), (2) the
tentorium cerebelli between the cerebellum and the occipital lobes
(see Fig. 6-36), (3) falx cerebelli between the cerebellar hemispheres,
and (4) the diaphragma sellae, which bridges over the depression in
the sphenoid bone, the sella turcica (see Fig. 6-5, B).

Between the two layers of dura there is a system of venous sinuses
that receives blood from the brain and empties it into the internal
jugular veins in the neck (Figs. 9-29 and 9-30). The cranial dura
mater receives most of its blood supply from the middle meningeal
artery, which enters the skull through the foramen spinosum in the
sphenoid bone. The artery then runs upward grooving the inner surface of the temporal and parietal bones. Fractures of these bones tend
to tear the vessel, and the bleeding that occurs leads to the formation

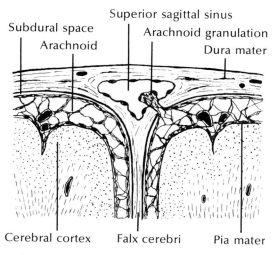

Superior sagittal sinus

Subdural space   Arachnoid granulation

Arachnoid   Dura mater

Cerebral cortex   Falx cerebri   Pia mater

Fig. 6-15. Coronal section of skull showing coverings of brain and superior
sagittal sinus. (After Weed.)

of a rather localized extra or epidural hemorrhage or hematoma. A subdural hematoma, usually caused by a venous tear, tends to spread over the surface of the brain deep to the dura mater.

Ventricles of the brain. The central canal of the cord extends upward into the brain where it undergoes certain changes and enlargements. In each cerebral hemisphere is a large lateral ventricle consisting of a central part with three outpouchings, or horns. The anterior horn extends into the frontal lobe; the posterior horn, into the occipital lobe; and the inferior horn, into the temporal lobe. The central part of each lateral ventricle communicates with the third ventricle by a small opening, the interventricular foramen, or foramen of Monro (Fig. 6-18).

The third ventricle is a small cleftlike cavity in the center of the diencephalon. It is continuous behind with the cerebral aqueduct, which leads into the fourth ventricle.

The fourth ventricle lies beneath the cerebellum on the upper surface of the pons and anterior half of the medulla. The fourth ventricle communicates with the spaces of the arachnoid by means of three small openings, or foramina. There is one opening in the midline of the posterior part of the roof of the ventricle and one lateral opening from each lateral recess of the ventricle (Figs. 6-16 and 6-17). There are folds of pia mater, each with a plexus of blood vessels pushing into the ventricles. These folds are called choroid plexuses.

Cerebrospinal fluid. The ventricles of the brain, the central canal of the spinal cord, and the subarachnoid space (between the dura-arachnoid complex and the pia mater) are all filled with a clear colorless fluid qualitatively similar to blood plasma. This fluid is formed for

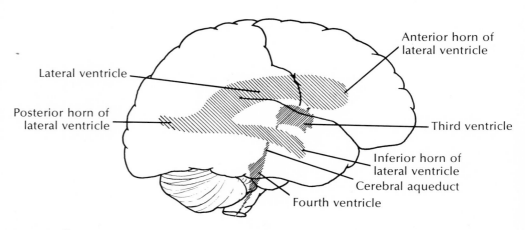

Anterior horn of lateral ventricle

Lateral ventricle

Posterior horn of lateral ventricle

Third ventricle

Inferior horn of lateral ventricle

Cerebral aqueduct

Fourth ventricle

Fig. 6-16. Ventricles of brain.

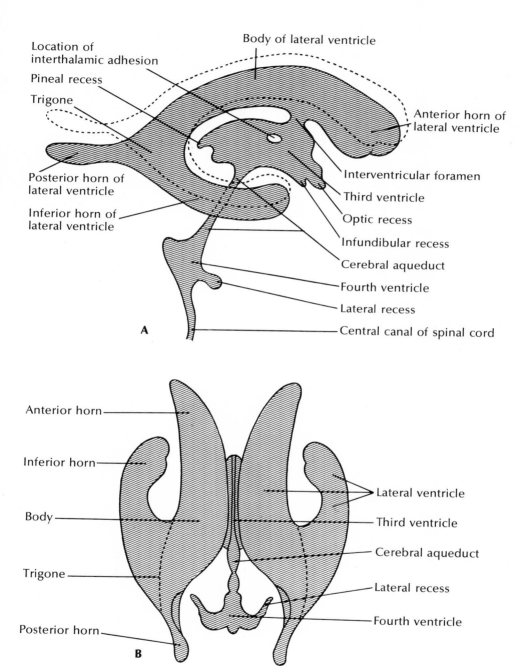

Fig. 6-17. The ventricular system. **A,** Viewed from the right side. **B,** Viewed from above. (From DiDio, L. J. A.: Synopsis of anatomy, St. Louis, 1970, The C. V. Mosby Co.)

197

the most part by the choroid plexuses in the ventricles of the brain and
to a lesser extent by the cells that line the ventricles and central canal
of the spinal cord. It passes out into the subarachnoid space through
three openings in the roof of the fourth ventricle. In a normal adult,
approximately 150 ml of cerebrospinal fluid is present at any one time,
whereas on an average, 450 ml of fluid is formed per day. The obvious
need for replacement requires a slow circulation and resorption (Fig.
6-18). The fluid in the subarachnoid space passes up over the cerebral
hemispheres and is resorbed via fingerlike projections of the arachnoid

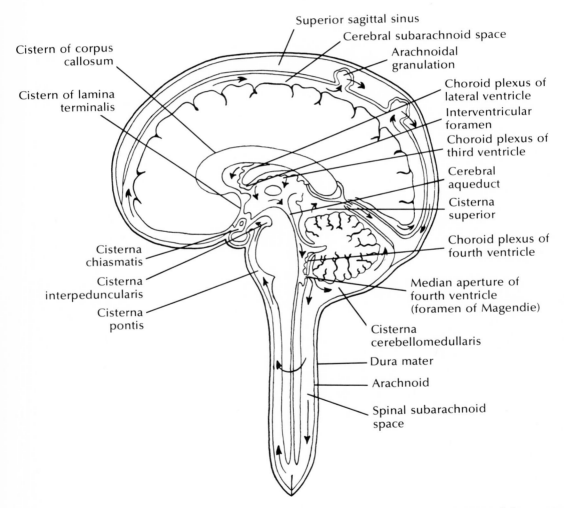

Fig. 6-18. Main sites of formation, circulation, and absorption of the cerebrospinal fluid. (From DiDio, L. J. A.: Synopsis of anatomy, St. Louis, 1970,
The C. V. Mosby Co.)

(arachnoid villi or arachnoid granulations) into the dural venous sinuses (especially the superior sagittal sinus). The functions of the cerebrospinal fluid are as follows: (1) mechanical support, since the fluid buoys up the brain and acts as a water cushion around the brain and spinal cord, (2) protection of the brain from sudden physical shocks that might crush the brain against the cranium, and (3) maintenance of the ionic environment around the nerve cells.

Hydrocephalus. Mechanical obstruction of cerebrospinal fluid circulation, either within the ventricular system or in the subarachnoid space, leads to raised cerebrospinal fluid pressure and to progressive dilation of the ventricular system. Such dilation causes pressure upon the surrounding brain tissue, which becomes compressed. In infancy, because the brain case still retains sutures of fibrous tissue, increased pressure will cause enlargement and thinning of the brain case.

Lumbar puncture. Lumbar puncture is the introduction of a needle through the midline ligaments between the third through fifth lumbar vertebrae into the lumbar cistern (see Fig. 6-4). This procedure can be used to (1) remove cerebrospinal fluid for examination or (2) introduce selected drugs or anesthetics. Nerve fibers in the dural sac, which form the cauda equina, are floating in the cerebrospinal fluid and, therefore, normally are pushed aside by the tip of the needle.

Growth of the brain. The brain grows very rapidly during the first few years of life. Although a small percentage of nerve cells, specifically microneurons, form after birth, the growth is due mainly to an increase in size of cells already present, to proliferation and growth of nonnervous cells (glia), to development of synaptic contacts and dendritic branching, and to myelination of the various fiber tracts. The cortex, particularly that of the parietal and frontal lobes, grows more rapidly in the first two years, with the pattern becoming increasingly complex up to about 6 years of age.

The various fiber tracts of the central nervous system do not develop myelin sheaths at the same time. The afferent and efferent fibers of the spinal nerves show myelin after the fifth fetal month, but

Table 10. Volume of the brain at different ages

Age	Approximate volume
Birth	350 cc
1 year	750 cc
2 years	900 cc
4 years	1,000 cc
20 years	1,200 cc

the corticospinal tracts do not become fully myelinated until the second year of life. This in part explains the fact that babies have a definite pattern of developmental activity, and we cannot expect them to be able to walk, for example, until the nervous system is mature enough to enable the child to perform that function.

**PERIPHERAL
NERVOUS SYSTEM**

The peripheral nervous system is composed of fibers that conduct efferent (motor) or afferent (sensory) impulses between the central nervous system and nonnervous tissue. Peripheral nerves, for descriptive purposes, are said to belong to two groups, spinal and cranial nerves.

Spinal nerves

A nerve leaving the spinal cord through a corresponding intervertebral foramen is generally named for the vertebral body below which it exits. In the cervical region, however, the first cervical nerve passes between the occiput and the first cervical vertebra; hence, there are eight pairs of cervical nerves. There are 12 thoracic, five lumbar, five sacral, and one coccygeal for a total of 31 spinal nerves. That portion of the cord that corresponds and gives rise to a pair of nerves is known as a segment. Therefore, there are 31 segments in all (see Fig. 6-3).

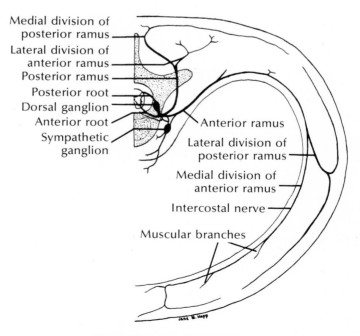

Medial division of posterior ramus
Lateral division of anterior ramus
Posterior ramus
Posterior root
Dorsal ganglion
Anterior root
Sympathetic ganglion
Anterior ramus
Lateral division of posterior ramus
Medial division of anterior ramus
Intercostal nerve
Muscular branches

Fig. 6-19. A typical spinal nerve.

A typical spinal nerve. All 31 pairs of spinal nerves with the exception of the first and last (first cervical and coccygeal) are constructed upon a common plan: two roots on each side, an anterior and posterior, attach the nerve to the spinal cord (Figs. 6-6 and 6-19). The posterior or dorsal root possesses a small swelling, or ganglion, containing cell bodies of sensory nerve cells. The posterior root is often missing in the first cervical and coccygeal; hence, sensory fibers are absent in these nerves. The anterior or ventral root has no ganglion.

The anterior root of every spinal nerve is composed of motor nerve fibers coming from nerve cells that lie within the gray matter of the spinal cord. Such a cell body with its processes is an efferent neuron. Neurons in the ventral horn are classified as somatic motor, whereas those in the lateral horn subserve visceral functions. These fibers carry motor impulses to the structures (muscles and glands) innervated by that nerve. The posterior root contains sensory nerve fibers that pass from the nerve cells in the dorsal root ganglion; these are afferent pathways. These fibers carry impulses from the peripheral distribution of the nerve, whether it be from skin or from underlying tissue (somatic or visceral structures). A typical spinal nerve therefore contains four functional components: somatic motor, somatic sensory, visceral motor, and visceral sensory. Sensory receptors for temperature, touch, and pain are located in the skin. Sensory receptors in the deeper structures such as muscles, tendons, and joint capsules are for vibration, pain, position, and tension. The sensations that arise from stimuli within the body are just as important as those arising from external stimuli, although we are not usually as conscious of them. All sensory impulses enter the cord through the dorsal root and ganglion. The two roots unite in the intervertebral foramen to form a common trunk. Just outside the foramen the trunk divides into a posterior or dorsal ramus and an anterior or ventral ramus. The anterior ramus is usually much the larger. The posterior ramus divides into medial and lateral divisions or branches. The anterior ramus also divides into lateral and medial divisions or branches.

A nerve trunk contains both sensory and motor fibers. The cutaneous branches are typically sensory; the muscular branches must carry motor fibers but, in addition, include many sensory fibers conveying sense of position and muscle tension.

The spinal nerves, from the second thoracic to the twelfth thoracic, inclusive, follow the pattern of a typical nerve. They lie in the substance of the body wall between the ribs and send motor branches to intercostal muscles and sensory branches to the skin.

The remaining spinal nerves require further description. The anterior rami of the upper four cervical nerves (cervical plexus) innervate the anterior region of the neck; the anterior rami of the lower four cervical and first thoracic nerves (brachial plexus) are reserved for the innervation of the upper extremity; the anterior rami of the lumbar and upper four sacral nerves (lumbosacral plexus) are used for the innervation of the lower extremity; the anterior rami of the fifth sacral and coccygeal nerves (coccygeal plexus) innervate the perineal region.

Cervical plexus. The anterior rami of the first four cervical nerves form the cervical plexus from which the following three groups of nerves arise:

1. Three ascending sensory branches: the lesser or smaller occipital, the great auricular, and the transverse cutaneous nerve of the neck

2. Three descending sensory branches: the medial (anterior), in-

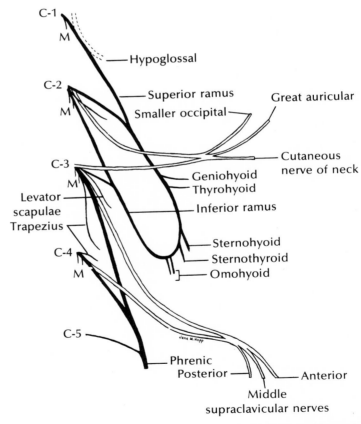

Fig. 6-20. Left cervical plexus. The cutaneous branches are drawn in black outline and the muscular branches in solid black. Fibers, *M*, go to deep muscles of neck.

termediate (middle), and lateral (posterior) supraclavicular nerves

3. Branches to numerous neck muscles and communicating branches to phrenic, vagus, accessory, and hypoglossal nerves

Fig. 6-20 is a simple diagram of the cervical plexus. The first cervical nerve usually has no sensory fibers and therefore no dorsal ganglion. The second and third cervical nerves carry sensory fibers from the back of the scalp, from the region posterior and inferior to the ear, and from the front of the neck inferior to the mandible. The fourth cervical nerve has sensory fibers from the lower portions of the neck down to the level of the collar bone and from the skin of the upper portion of the shoulder. Fibers arise from the anterior rami and go directly to the deep muscles lying in front of the cervical vertebrae. Some fibers also go to the sternocleidomastoid and trapezius muscles, but the chief nerve supply for these two muscles is from the accessory nerve. From a loop between the first and second cervical nerves, motor fibers go to the rectus capitis lateralis and rectus capitis anterior. Other fibers from this loop are, for a time, incorporated within the sheath of the hypoglossal nerve and were formerly called the descendens hypoglossi but are now called the superior ramus of the ansa cervicalis. From a loop between the second and third cervical nerves comes the inferior ramus (descendens cervicalis), which unites with the superior ramus to form the ansa cervicalis, from which are innervated the sternohyoid, sternothyroid, and omohyoid muscles. The superior ramus also sends motor fibers to the geniohyoid and thyrohyoid muscles. Some nerve fibers from the upper cervical segments of the cord pass upward through the foramen magnum into the skull and back out through the jugular foramen as the spinal portion of the eleventh cranial nerve.

The phrenic nerve supplies the diaphragm, which in early embryonic life lies in the cervical region. This nerve arises from the third, fourth, and fifth cervical nerves but derives most of its fibers from the fourth. In the neck it lies upon the anterior scalene muscle and is accessible to the surgeon in this position, where he may cut or remove the nerve to paralyze the diaphragm in treatment of certain diseases of the chest.

The posterior rami of the upper four cervical nerves supply the deep muscles of the back of the neck. The second, third, and fourth have sensory fibers from the back of the neck and head in the greater and third occipital nerves.

Brachial plexus. The four lower cervical nerves and the first thoracic nerve supply the upper limb. After their emergence from the intervertebral foramina, anterior rami of these five nerves undergo an interweaving, known as the brachial plexus, from which originate the various nerves supplying the shoulder, arm, forearm, and hand. Fig. 6-21 shows a diagram of this plexus. There are three cords, named from their relation to the brachial artery: one lateral, one medial, and one posterior.

The nerves arising from the brachial plexus are the following:

1. The suprascapular and dorsal scapular nerves course over the scapula to supply muscles attached to the superficial aspect of that bone. The suprascapular nerve supplies the supraspinatus and infraspinatus muscles; the dorsal scapular nerve supplies the rhomboideus major and rhomboideus minor muscles and some fibers to the levator scapulae muscle.

2. The medial and lateral anterior thoracic nerves, penetrating

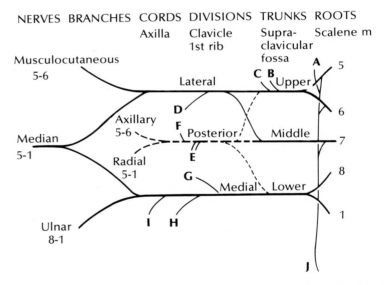

Fig. 6-21. Brachial plexus and nerves arising directly from its roots, trunks, and cords. Anterior divisions, solid lines; posterior divisions, broken lines. The three posterior divisions join to form the posterior cord (broken line). Upper plexus: *A*, dorsal scapular n (levator scapulae, rhomboid m); *B*, subclavian n (subclavius m); *C*, suprascapular n (supraspinatus and infraspinatus m); *D*, lateral anterior thoracic n (pectoral m). Middle plexus: *E*, subscapular n (subscapular and teres major m); *F*, thoracodorsal n (latissimus dorsi m). Upper and middle plexus: *J*, long thoracic n (serratus anterior m). Lower plexus: *G*, medial anterior thoracic n (pectoral m); *H*, medial cutaneous n of arm; *I*, medial cutaneous n of forearm. (From Willis, W., and Grossman, R.: Medical neurobiology, St. Louis, 1973, The C. V. Mosby Co.)

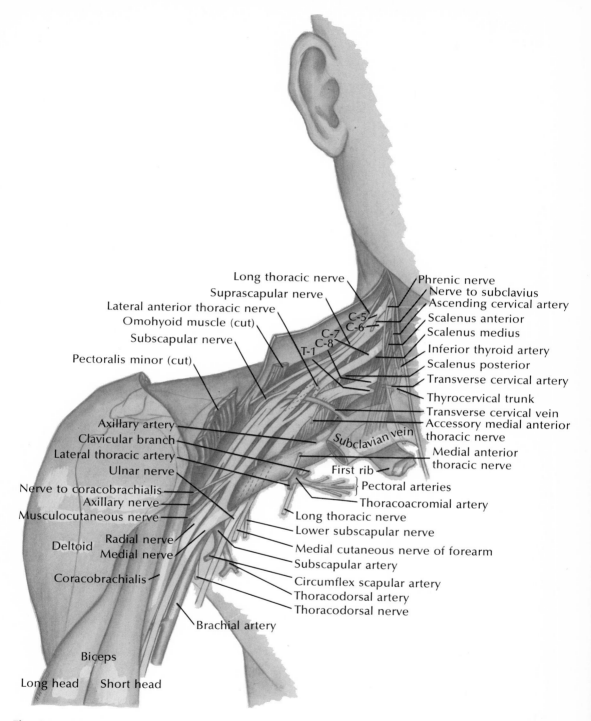

Fig. 6-22. Right brachial plexus. In this specimen there were two medial anterior thoracic nerves; no medial cutaneous nerve of the arm could be found. Minor variations from the typical pattern are very common. (Male, 87 years of age.)

the costocoracoid membrane or the pectoralis minor, supply that muscle and the pectoralis major.

3. The long thoracic nerve runs down the lateral chest wall to the serratus anterior muscle.

4. The thoracodorsal nerve and two subscapular nerves pass inferiorly and posteriorly through the armpit (axilla). The thoracodorsal nerve supplies the latissimus dorsi muscle and the two subscapular nerves supply the subscapularis and the teres major muscles.

5. The axillary (circumflex) nerve supplies the deltoid and teres minor muscles and is also distributed to the skin over the deltoid muscle. After the axillary nerve arises from the posterior cord of the brachial plexus it passes posteriorly around the shaft of the humerus just below the tubercles, enters the deltoid on the deep surface of the muscle, and is accompanied by the posterior humeral circumflex artery.

6. The musculocutaneous nerve supplies the muscles on the anterior aspect of the upper arm, the biceps brachii, coracobrachialis, and brachialis. It is the sensory supply for the skin on the lateral side of the forearm.

7. The ulnar nerve supplies the flexor carpi ulnaris and ulnar part of the flexor digitorum profundus in the forearm. It supplies the muscles of the hand except the lumbricals of the second and third digits and the opponens, short flexor, and short abductor of the thumb. It is sensory to the medial side of the hand, the little finger, and the medial (ulnar) half of the ring finger. The ulnar nerve is rather superficial where it passes behind the medial epicondyle of the humerus, and when it is hit in this position, it gives rise to a sensation of pin and needle pricks in the area of its sensory distribution.

8. The median nerve supplies the remaining muscles of the anterior aspect of the forearm and hand. Its cutaneous fibers are distributed to the volar surface of the thumb, index, and long fingers.

9. The radial nerve winds posteriorly around the humerus, supplying the triceps in its course. It also supplies all the muscles on the posterior aspect of the forearm and sends sensory branches to the skin on the posterior aspect of the forearm and hand. As the radial nerve passes around the humerus, it is accompanied by the profunda artery of the arm. The radial nerve lies very close to the humerus and may be seriously injured in fracture of the midshaft of the bone.

10. The medial cutaneous nerve of the upper arm and the medial

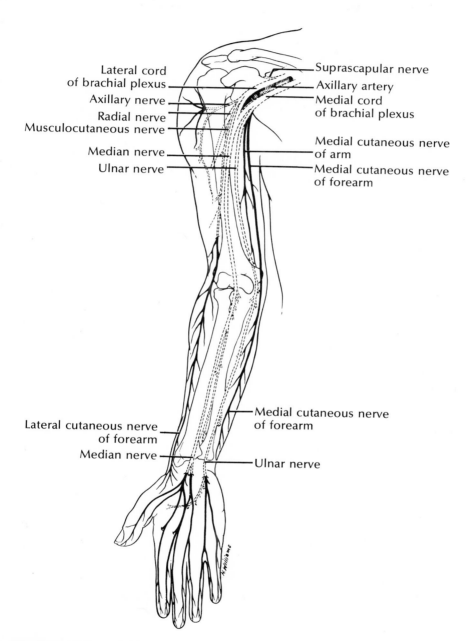

Lateral cord
of brachial plexus

Axillary nerve

Radial nerve

Musculocutaneous nerve

Median nerve

Ulnar nerve

Suprascapular nerve

Axillary artery

Medial cord
of brachial plexus

Medial cutaneous nerve
of arm

Medial cutaneous nerve
of forearm

Medial cutaneous nerve
of forearm

Lateral cutaneous nerve
of forearm

Median nerve

Ulnar nerve

Fig. 6-23. Nerves of the right arm. Cutaneous branches are shown in solid black; deeper branches are shown in dotted outline.

cutaneous nerve of the forearm have sensory fibers for the medial side of the upper arm and forearm, respectively.

Fig. 6-23 shows the distribution of these nerves in an outline drawing of the upper extremity. The sensory branches transmit impulses giving rise to sensations of pain, touch, temperature, pressure, position, vibration, and muscle tension inward to the cord; the muscular branches carry nerve impulses outward from the cord to the muscles.

The posterior rami of the lower four cervical nerves and the first thoracic nerve are smaller than the anterior rami and send branches to the deep muscles of the upper part of the back and to the skin over them.

CLINICAL CONSIDERATIONS. To locate a lesion of the brachial plexus or one of its branches, it is necessary to check each muscle and to analyze the nerve supply of affected muscles. Injury to the entire brachial plexus is uncommon; however, injuries to radial, musculocutaneous, ulnar, or median nerves are clinically important. The radial nerve supplies all the muscles of the posterior or extensor compartment of the arm, forearm, and hand. A significant clinical finding of radial nerve damage is wrist drop. The musculocutaneous nerve is the major but not sole supply to muscles on the anterior aspect of the arm that are the flexors of the elbow. If the nerve is damaged, flexion of the elbow can be obtained but against only light resistance. If the median nerve is damaged, wrist flexion is weak, ulnar deviation occurs, and the thumb cannot be opposed. With damage to the ulnar nerve the hand assumes a characteristic clawed appearance. The fourth and fifth fingers are hyperextended at the metacarpophalangeal joints and flexed at the interphalangeal joints (see Figs. 5-24 and 5-25).

Lumbosacral plexus. The anterior rami of the five lumbar and upper four sacral nerves form a plexus that gives rise to nerves supplying the lower limb and perineum (Fig. 6-26).

The following are the nerves originating in the lumbosacral plexus:

1. The iliohypogastric nerve is sensory to the anterior abdominal wall and sends motor fibers to muscles of the same area.
2. The ilioinguinal nerve is sensory to the anterior abdominal wall and external genitalia and has motor fibers for muscles of the abdominal wall. The iliohypogastric and ilioinguinal nerves may be fused.
3. The genitofemoral nerve is sensory to the skin of the inguinal area and the external genitalia and motor to the cremaster muscle.

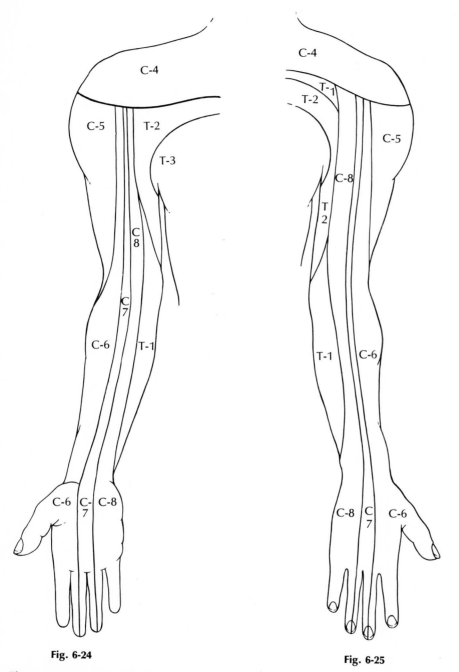

Fig. 6-24

Fig. 6-25

Fig. 6-24. Segmental sensory distribution of arm, anterior view. *C,* Cervical
segments; *T,* thoracic segments. (After Collier and Purves-Stewart.)
Fig. 6-25. Segmental sensory distribution of arm, posterior view. *C,* Cervical
segments; *T,* thoracic segments. (After Collier and Purves-Stewart.)

209

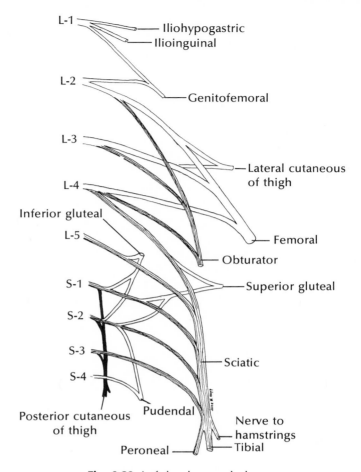

Fig. 6-26. Left lumbosacral plexus.

4. The lateral cutaneous nerve of the thigh is sensory to the lateral side of the thigh.

5. The femoral nerve is motor to the quadriceps, sartorius, pectineus, and iliacus muscles and sensory both to the anterior aspect of the thigh and to the medial side of the leg below the knee (saphenous nerve).

6. The obturator nerve is motor to the adductor muscles of the inner or medial portion of the thigh and has some sensory fibers from the same area.

7. The tibial nerve (medial popliteal) is motor to the muscles and sensory to the skin of the calf of the leg and to the sole of the foot.

8. The peroneal nerve (lateral popliteal) is motor to the muscles

210

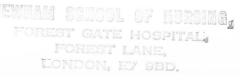

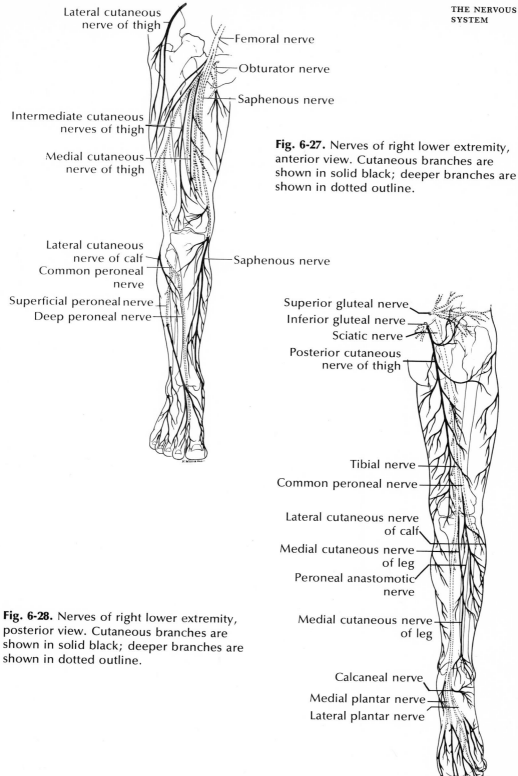

Lateral cutaneous
nerve of thigh

Femoral nerve

Obturator nerve

Saphenous nerve

Intermediate cutaneous
nerves of thigh

Medial cutaneous
nerve of thigh

Fig. 6-27. Nerves of right lower extremity,
anterior view. Cutaneous branches are
shown in solid black; deeper branches are
shown in dotted outline.

Lateral cutaneous
nerve of calf
Common peroneal
nerve
Superficial peroneal nerve
Deep peroneal nerve

Saphenous nerve

Superior gluteal nerve
Inferior gluteal nerve
Sciatic nerve
Posterior cutaneous
nerve of thigh

Tibial nerve
Common peroneal nerve

Lateral cutaneous nerve
of calf

Medial cutaneous nerve
of leg
Peroneal anastomotic
nerve

Medial cutaneous nerve
of leg

Fig. 6-28. Nerves of right lower extremity,
posterior view. Cutaneous branches are
shown in solid black; deeper branches are
shown in dotted outline.

Calcaneal nerve
Medial plantar nerve
Lateral plantar nerve

that evert and dorsiflex the foot and sensory to the lateral side of the leg and dorsal surface of the foot. The peroneal nerve is quite near the surface as it passes lateral to the neck of the fibula; it is frequently injured when a person falls sideways and may be severely damaged in this location by pressure from a plaster cast that is too tight.

The sural or medial cutaneous nerve of the leg is formed from sensory branches of the tibial and peroneal nerves and is sensory to the calf of the leg and lateral side of the foot.

9. The nerve to the hamstring muscles is motor to the muscles of the posterior aspect of the thigh.

The three nerves just named, tibial, peroneal, and nerve to the hamstrings, are usually enclosed in a common sheath in the upper thigh. Thus is constituted the sciatic nerve, which emerges through the greater sciatic foramen and passes inferiorly on the posterior aspect of the thigh for a short distance before splitting into its component parts. The sciatic is the largest nerve of the body.

10. The superior gluteal nerve supplies the gluteus medius, gluteus minimus, and tensor fasciae latae muscles; the inferior gluteal nerve supplies the gluteus maximus muscle.

11. The posterior cutaneous nerve of the thigh is sensory to the skin of the buttock, and the posterior aspect of thigh and leg.

12. The pudendal nerve is motor to the muscles and sensory to the skin of the perineum.

Figs. 6-27 and 6-28 are outlines of the lower limb showing the cutaneous distribution of the nerves.

Frequently for purposes of description the lumbosacral plexus is divided into three parts: the lumbar, sacral, and pudendal. The lumbar plexus includes the anterior rami of the upper three lumbar nerves and that part of the anterior ramus of the fourth lumbar nerve that goes to the femoral and obturator nerves. The sacral plexus is formed from the rest of the anterior ramus of the fourth lumbar nerve, the anterior rami of the fifth lumbar and first sacral nerves, and part of the anterior rami of the second and third sacral nerves. The remaining parts of the anterior rami of the second and third sacral nerves and part of the anterior ramus of the fourth sacral nerve form the pudendal plexus.

Coccygeal plexus. The coccygeal plexus is formed from the anterior rami of the fifth sacral and the coccygeal nerves and a part of the anterior ramus of the fourth sacral nerve. It sends fibers to the coccygeus and levator ani muscles and receives fibers from the skin over the coccyx.

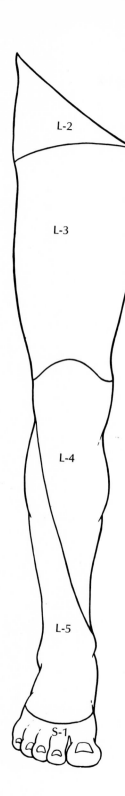

Fig. 6-29. Segmental sensory distribution to anterior aspect of lower extremity. *L,* Lumbar segments; *S,* sacral segments. (After Collier and Purves-Stewart.)

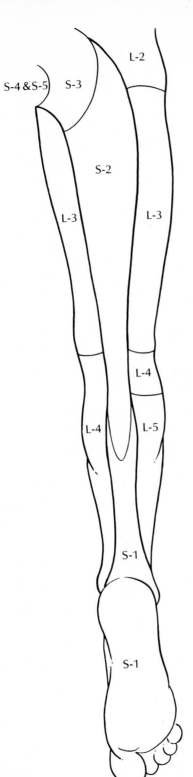

Fig. 6-30. Segmental sensory distribution to posterior aspect of lower extremity. *L,* Lumbar segments; *S,* sacral segments. (After Collier and Purves-Stewart.)

The posterior rami of the lumbar, sacral, and coccygeal nerves supply the deep muscles of the lower part of the back, the skin of the small of the back, and the medial portion of the buttocks.

Segmental sensory distribution. All of the sensory nerves from a given skin area ultimately come into a specific segment of the spinal cord, although they may pass inward from the surface along more than one nerve. This fact is of great importance when a physician is attempting to determine the exact site of an injury to or a disease of the spinal cord. The segmental distribution of the various segments of the spinal cord is shown in Figs. 6-24, 6-25, and 6-29 to 6-32.

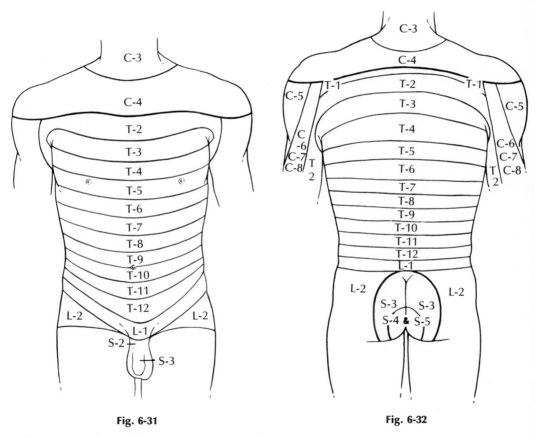

Fig. 6-31   **Fig. 6-32**

Fig. 6-31. Sensory distribution to anterior aspect of torso. *C*, Cervical segments; *T*, thoracic segments; *L*, Lumbar segments; *S*, sacral segments. (After Collier and Purves-Stewart.)

Fig. 6-32. Sensory distribution of nerves to posterior aspect of torso. *C*, Cervical segments; *T*, thoracic segments; *L*, lumbar segments; *S*, sacral segments. (After Collier and Purves-Stewart.)

215

Table 11. Cranial nerves

Nerve number and name	Site of exit from skull	Functional components	Structures innervated
I. Olfactory	Cribriform plate of ethmoid bone	Special sensory (smell)	Nasal mucosa
II. Optic	Optic canal	Special sensory (sight)	Retina
III. Oculomotor	Superior orbital fissure	Somatic motor	Extraocular muscles
		Visceral motor (parasympathetic)	Iris and ciliary body
IV. Trochlear	Superior orbital fissure	Somatic motor	Superior oblique muscle
V. Trigeminal			
1. Ophthalmic	Superior orbital fissure	Sensory	Orbit plus skin of face
2. Maxillary	Foramen rotundum	Sensory	Nasal cavity plus skin of face
3. Mandibular	Foramen ovale	Sensory	Oral cavity plus skin of face
		Somatic motor	Muscles of mastication plus accessory muscles
VI. Abducent	Superior orbital fissure	Somatic motor	Lateral rectus muscle
VII. Facial	Stylomastoid foramen	Somatic motor	Muscles of facial expression
		Visceral motor (parasympathetic)	Lacrimal and salivary glands
		Special sensory (taste)	Anterior two thirds of tongue
		Sensory	External ear
VIII. Vestibulocochlear	Remains within cranium	Special sensory (balance and hearing)	Semicircular canals; cochlea
IX. Glossopharyngeal	Jugular foramen	Somatic motor	Stylopharyngeal muscle
		Visceral motor (parasympathetic)	Parotid gland
		Special sensory (taste)	Posterior third of tongue
		Sensory	Walls of pharynx
X. Vagus	Jugular foramen	Somatic motor	Muscles of larynx
		Visceral motor (parasympathetic)	Smooth muscle of gut
		Special sensory (taste)	Root of tongue
		Sensory	Larynx and gut
XI. Accessory	Jugular foramen	Somatic motor	Sternocleidomastoid and trapezius muscles
XII. Hypoglossal	Hypoglossal canal	Somatic motor	Muscles of tongue

There are 12 pairs of nerves attached to the brain stem. They **Cranial nerves** emerge through special openings in the skull (Table 11). These nerves are named in order beginning with the most anterior.

Note that several nerves, specifically the fourth, sixth, eleventh, and twelfth, although supplying striated muscles, do not contain any demonstrable sensory fibers. It is generally accepted that sensory fibers from these muscles are conveyed to the central nervous system by branches of the fifth, or trigeminal, nerve. Because of its widespread sensory distribution, both superficial and deep, the trigeminal is often called "the great sensory nerve of the head."

Olfactory nerve. The nerve of smell arises by a number of fine bundles from the olfactory area situated in the nasal cavity, partly on the upper portion of the septum and partly on the superior concha or turbinate. In each nostril there are about 20 nerve bundles that pass through the cribriform plate of the ethmoid bone into the olfactory bulb (see Fig. 6-5, *E*). Relays of fibers carry sensory impulses back along the olfactory tract to the substance of the cerebrum.

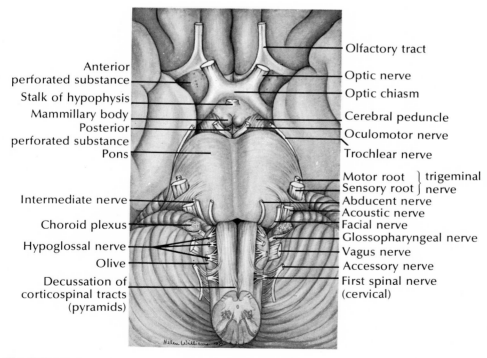

Fig. 6-33. Brain stem, inferior view, to show attachment of cranial nerves. (Male, 45 years of age.)

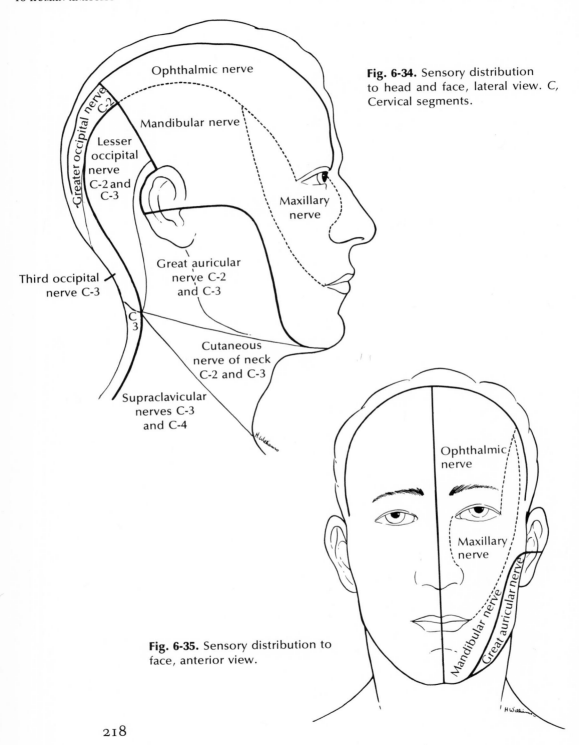

Ophthalmic nerve

Greater occipital nerve
C-2

Mandibular nerve

Lesser
occipital
nerve
C-2 and
C-3

Maxillary
nerve

Third occipital
nerve C-3

Great auricular
nerve C-2
and C-3

C
3

Cutaneous
nerve of neck
C-2 and C-3

Supraclavicular
nerves C-3
and C-4

Fig. 6-34. Sensory distribution
to head and face, lateral view. C,
Cervical segments.

Ophthalmic
nerve

Maxillary
nerve

Mandibular nerve

Great auricular nerve

Fig. 6-35. Sensory distribution to
face, anterior view.

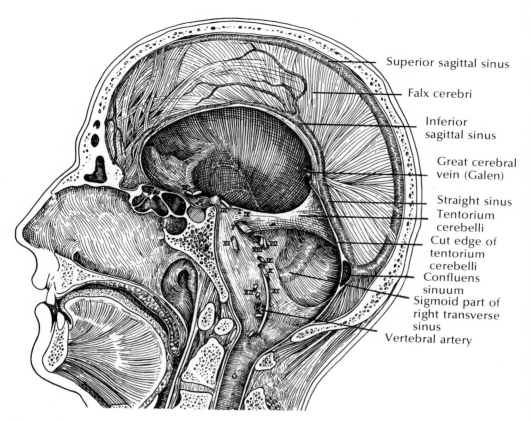

Superior sagittal sinus

Falx cerebri

Inferior
sagittal sinus

Great cerebral
vein (Galen)

Straight sinus
Tentorium
cerebelli
Cut edge of
tentorium
cerebelli
Confluens
sinuum
Sigmoid part of
right transverse
sinus
Vertebral artery

Fig. 6-36. Sagittal section of head showing medial aspect of right half of skull. The brain and spinal cord have been removed, but the dura mater has been left intact. The second to seventh cranial nerves are shown at their point of exit from the cranial cavity.

Optic nerve. The nerve of sight arises from cells in the retina of the eye. The nerve emerges from the back of the eyeball and passes into the skull through the optic canal, after which it joins the nerve from the other eye at the optic chiasm. Here the fibers from the nasal half of each retina cross over to the other side. The fibers from the temporal half of each retina do not cross but continue in the optic tract of the same side (see Fig. 7-10). From the chiasm the optic tracts carry the sensory impulses of vision to the brain stem, and eventually the fibers reach the visual cortex at the back of the occipital lobe. In reality the retina is an outgrowth of a portion of the brain wall, and the optic nerve is the distal part of a brain tract whose cells of origin lie in the retina and whose fibers end in the brain stem. The optic nerve is covered by three sheaths derived from the three coverings of the brain.

219

The outer sheath, which is a prolongation of the dura mater, is quite dense and fibrous and blends with the sclera of the eyeball (see Fig. 6-5, *F*).

Oculomotor nerve. The oculomotor nerve arises from the under-surface of the brain stem in front of the pons, passes forward into the orbit through the superior orbital fissure, and supplies the levator palpebrae superioris, superior rectus, medial rectus, inferior rectus, and inferior oblique muscles of the eyeball. If this nerve is damaged, the upper lid droops, and the eyeball has a downward and outward cast; inward, upward, and directly downward movements of the eyeball are impossible. The oculomotor nerve also supplies the smooth muscles of the iris and ciliary body (cranial autonomic outflow). If these fibers are destroyed, the pupil remains dilated and there is difficulty in accommodation for near and far vision.

Trochlear nerve. The trochlear nerve arises from the dorsal surface of the midbrain and passes around the side of the brain stem and then forward into the orbit through the superior orbital fissure to supply the superior oblique muscle of the eye. If this muscle is paralyzed, the eyeball has an upward and outward cast.

Trigeminal nerve. The trigeminal nerve has two roots, a sensory and a motor, attached close together to the side of the pons. On the sensory root as it passes laterally into the middle fossa of the skull there is a large ganglion called the trigeminal (gasserian) ganglion. There are three large sensory branches bringing fibers into this ganglion: (1) the ophthalmic, bringing sensory impressions from the orbit, upper eyelid, bridge of the nose, and scalp as far as the crown of the head, (2) the maxillary, bringing sensory impressions from the lower eyelid, the lower portions of the nose, the upper cheek, upper lip, jaw, and palate, and (3) the mandibular, bringing sensory impressions from the lower lip and jaw, tongue, lower part of the face and cheek, and front of the ear. The ophthalmic nerve passes through the superior orbital fissure; the maxillary, through the foramen rotundum; and the mandibular, through the foramen ovale.

The motor root of the trigeminal lies beneath the trigeminal ganglion and is continued into the mandibular nerve as it emerges through the foramen ovale. The motor fibers go to the muscles of mastication, namely, the medial and lateral pterygoid muscles, the masseter muscle, and the temporal muscle. For this reason the motor part of the trigeminal is frequently called the masticator nerve. The motor root also supplies two muscles in the neck, the anterior belly of the digastric and the mylohyoid, and the tensor veli palatini and tensor tympani muscles. The tensor veli palatini and tensor tympani muscles are supplied by fibers from the branch going to the medial pterygoid muscle.

The fifth nerve carries sensory fibers for heat, cold, pain, and touch, but not for taste.

Abducent nerve. The abducent nerve arises from the undersurface of the brain stem just behind the pons and passes forward through the superior orbital fissure to supply the lateral rectus muscle of the eyeball. If this nerve is damaged, there is an internal squint (toward the nose).

Facial nerve. The facial nerve arises from the side of the brain stem just behind the pons very close to the origin of the eighth nerve. Together with the eighth nerve, the seventh nerve enters the internal acoustic meatus. It then continues through the facial canal, passes over the inner ear, changes its direction to course downward in the

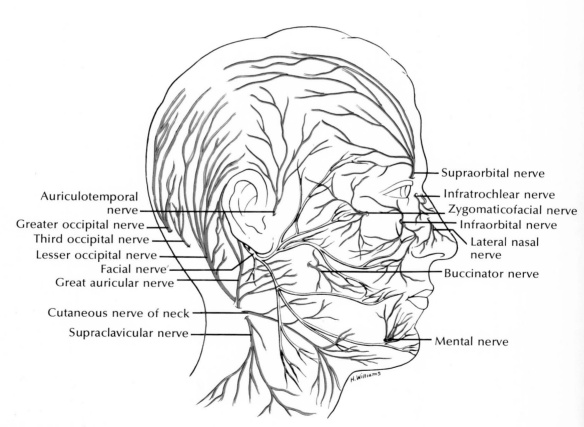

Fig. 6-37. Nerves of the face and head. Sensory nerves in red; facial nerve in black outline.

221

mastoid process, and emerges through the stylomastoid foramen. Its fibers are then distributed to the muscles of facial expression. If the facial nerve is damaged, paralysis of muscles on that side of the face results in a masklike expression. The eyelid on the affected side cannot be closed voluntarily, and the corner of the mouth droops. The facial nerve is also motor to the posterior belly of the digastric muscle, the stylohyoid muscle, and the stapedius muscle.

Within its sheath the facial nerve, essentially motor, also carries sensory fibers from the taste buds of the anterior two thirds of the tongue. These sensory fibers have their nuclei in the geniculate ganglion, which is a small oval swelling present on the facial nerve in the facial canal. The sensory fibers reach the nerve in the facial canal by a branch called the chorda tympani, which crosses the middle ear cavity in its course from the mandibular nerve to the facial. The facial nerve also carries sensory fibers from the muscles of facial expression. The facial nerve, in addition, contains secretory fibers (cranial autonomic outflow) to the submandibular and sublingual salivary glands, and there are other secretory fibers that reach the lacrimal gland by a complicated pathway. As the taste and secretory fibers are traced toward the brain from the geniculate ganglion, they form a separate bundle between the main part of the seventh nerve and the eighth nerve, and this bundle is called the intermediate nerve (pars intermedia). The intermediate nerve and the chorda tympani nerve are successive parts of a single visceral nerve conveying secretory fibers to the submandibular and sublingual salivary glands in addition to sensory fibers from the taste buds of the anterior two thirds of the tongue.

Vestibulocochlear nerve. The eighth cranial nerve was formerly called the acoustic nerve, but since it has two distinct sensory parts, vestibular and auditory, it has now been given a name that emphasizes this fact. Vestibular fibers arise in cells located within the semicircular canals, which are organs of balance intimately associated with the inner ear and located within the petrous part of the temporal bone. The auditory fibers arise from the hair cells of the organ of Corti, the essential receptive organ of hearing located within the cochlea of the inner ear. These two parts, enclosed in a single sheath, form the eighth nerve, which emerges from the petrous portion of the temporal bone and reaches the brain stem behind the pons.

Glossopharyngeal nerve. The glossopharyngeal nerve joins the side of the medulla just behind the eighth nerve and in front of the tenth nerve. It passes out of the skull through the jugular foramen into the neck. The trunk has two swellings, the superior (jugular) and inferior (petrous) ganglia, which are analogous to the dorsal root ganglia of spinal nerves. It carries motor fibers to the stylopharyngeus muscle. Fibers from the ninth, tenth, and eleventh cranial nerves and from the superior cervical ganglion of the sympathetic send branches to the side wall of the pharynx where the pharyngeal plexus is formed. All the muscles of the pharynx and soft palate (except stylopharyngeus, tensor tympani, and tensor veli palatini) are innervated from this plexus. It also carries sensory fibers from the mucosa of the pharynx and back of the tongue. There is a component conveying sensory fibers from the taste buds of the back of the tongue and secretory fibers to the parotid gland (cranial autonomic outflow). This nerve receives important sensory fibers by way of the carotid ramus, from the carotid sinus and carotid body; these fibers are very important in reflexes controlling blood pressure.

Vagus nerve. The vagus nerve arises from the side of the medulla just behind the ninth nerve and leaves the skull through the jugular foramen. There are two ganglia, the superior (jugular) and inferior (nodose), which are analogous to the dorsal root ganglia of spinal nerves. Immediately after it enters the neck it is joined by a large branch from the eleventh cranial nerve carrying motor fibers that are distributed to muscles of the larynx and pharynx (pharyngeal plexus). The vagus has sensory fibers from the mucosa of the larynx and also a few from the external ear. The visceral fibers of the vagus are distributed to the heart, lungs, bronchi, esophagus, stomach, and intestine.

Accessory nerve. The accessory nerve has two portions, the cranial, arising from the medulla behind the vagus, and the spinal, arising from the upper five or six cervical segments in the cord. The nerve passes through the jugular foramen where its cranial portion joins the vagus and is distributed to the muscles of the larynx and pharynx (pharyngeal plexus).

The spinal portion forms a nerve trunk that passes through the foramen magnum to enter a common sheath with the part arising from the medulla. On emerging through the jugular foramen, the spinal fibers are distributed to the sternocleidomastoid and trapezius muscles.

Hypoglossal nerve. The hypoglossal nerve arises from the medulla posterior to the eleventh nerve, leaves the skull through the hypoglossal canal, and supplies the muscles of the tongue.

The autonomic nervous system regulates visceral function. Viscera, plural of the latin word *viscus,* meaning internal organ, in a broad sense encompasses the following systems and their associated tissues (cardiac muscle, smooth muscle, and glands):

**AUTONOMIC
NERVOUS SYSTEM**

1. Digestive
2. Respiratory
3. Urinary

4. Genital
5. Endocrine
6. Vascular

With the exception of the sweat glands and the smooth muscle of the hair follicles found in the skin, all of the tissues that are included under the term visceral are found in conjunction with the six visceral systems. Motor nerve fibers, which innervate tissue of these six systems, are classified as visceral to delimit them from somatic fibers, which innervate skeletal (striated) muscle.

Although the autonomic nervous system classically is described as a motor system, afferent or sensory fibers from the viscera take part in reflex arcs in the nerves of the autonomic nervous system. These afferent fibers are called visceral afferents to distinguish them from somatic afferents. The somatic afferents convey sensory modalities from skeletal muscle, tendons, bones, joints, skin, and subcutaneous tissue.

The following are special features of the autonomic nervous system:

1. Two motor neurons interposed between the central nervous system and peripheral effector organs
2. Ganglia (site of synapses between preganglionic and postganglionic neurons) that must be clearly differentiated from dorsal root ganglia that are sensory
3. Nerve trunks and plexuses so formed

The autonomic nervous system may be considered a system of twos. It can be divided into the peripheral autonomic nervous system and the central control centers. The peripheral system may be further subdivided on the basis of structure and function into the thoracolumbar (sympathetic) and craniosacral (parasympathetic) divisions.

There are several general functions that can be ascribed to the two divisions of the autonomic nervous system as follows:

1. Sympathetic:
   a. Vasomotor: constriction of blood vessels in skin and gut
   b. Sudomotor: secretion of sweat glands
   c. Pilomotor: erection of hair follicles by arrector pili muscles

The sympathetic portion of the autonomic nervous system has been called the "fight or flight" system. This simply means that the body is mobilized to defend itself. Such mobilization necessitates increased blood flow to the heart, lungs, as well as to skeletal muscles, which move the body. Blood vessels in the above areas are dilated rather than constricted by the sympathetic nerve fibers, whereas vessels in the skin and gut are constricted.

2. Parasympathetic: peristalsis of the gastrointestinal tract from the mouth to anal canal plus secretion of glands that empty into and thereby augment peristalsis. Such innervation includes glands from the lacrimal (in the orbit) to mucous glands in the wall of the anal canal.

Thoracolumbar outflow. On each side of the vertebral column there lies a chain of ganglia connected with each other by short nerve trunks. The chain begins below the base of the skull, with the large, superior cervical ganglion, and extends inferiorly through the neck, thoracic cavity, and abdominal cavity into the pelvic cavity where each chain ends by joining its fellow in a very small ganglion, the ganglion impar, lying on the anterior surface of the coccyx. There are usually three cervical ganglia on each side, but in the thoracic, lumbar, and

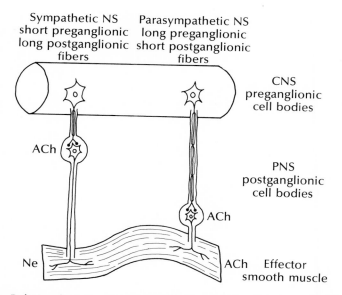

Fig. 6-38. Relative lengths of preganglionic and postganglionic fibers of sympathetic and parasympathetic nervous system and neural transmitters. The preganglionic neurons of the sympathetic nervous system have axons of relatively short length, whereas the postganglionic axons are relatively long. The situation is reversed in the parasympathetic nervous system, where the preganglionic axons are long and the postganglionic axons short. The synaptic transmitter used by both systems at the junction between preganglionic and postganglionic neurons is acetylcholine. The postganglionic neuron of the sympathetic nervous system uses norepinephrine as its transmitter (usually), whereas the parasympathetic postganglionic neuron uses acetylcholine. (From Willis, W., and Grossman, R.: Medical neurobiology, St. Louis, 1973, The C. V. Mosby Co.)

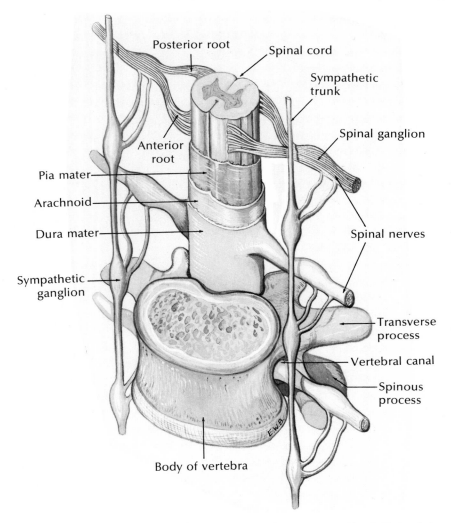

Fig. 6-39. Diagram of the spinal cord showing meninges, formation of the spinal nerves, and relations to a vertebra and to the sympathetic trunk and ganglia. (From Anthony, C. P., and Kolthoff, N. J.: Textbook of anatomy and physiology, ed. 8, St. Louis, 1971, The C. V. Mosby Co.)

sacral regions there is typically a ganglion associated with each spinal nerve (Fig. 6-39). However, in the lumbar and sacral regions the number of ganglia is quite variable. The entire chain is frequently called the paravertebral ganglionated trunk.

A typical thoracic nerve is connected with its autonomic ganglion by means of white and gray rami. In the white ramus are myelinated nerve fibers that come from cells located within the spinal cord and

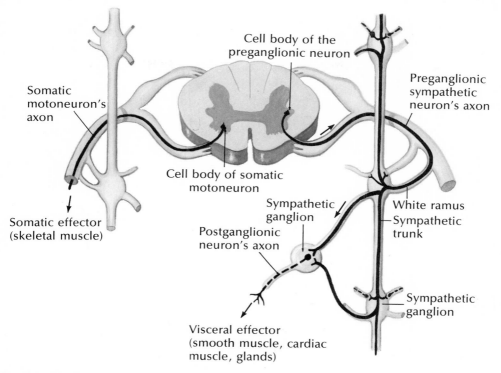

Cell body of the
preganglionic neuron

Somatic
motoneuron's
axon

Preganglionic
sympathetic
neuron's axon

Cell body of somatic
motoneuron

Somatic effector
(skeletal muscle)

Sympathetic
ganglion

Postganglionic
neuron's axon

White ramus

Sympathetic
trunk

Sympathetic
ganglion

Visceral effector
(smooth muscle, cardiac
muscle, glands)

Fig. 6-40. Diagram showing difference between the neural pathways from
the central nervous system to visceral effectors and to somatic effectors.
A relay of two autonomic neurons—preganglionic and postganglionic—
conduct from cord (or brain stem) to visceral effectors. Note that, in contrast, only one somatic motoneuron (anterior horn neuron) conducts from
cord to somatic effectors with no intervening synapses. Note the location
of the preganglionic neuron's cell in lateral or intermediate body and
axon. Where are the postganglionic neuron's cell body and axon located?
(From Anthony, C. P., and Kolthoff, N. J.: Textbook of anatomy and physiology, ed. 8, St. Louis, 1971, The C. V. Mosby Co.)

are known as preganglionic fibers. The preganglionic fibers synapse
with the processes of nerve cells located in the autonomic (sympathetic) ganglion. The gray ramus contains fibers having little or no
myelin that come from the ganglion cells and are known as postganglionic fibers. The thoracic spinal nerves and the upper two lumbar
spinal nerves have white rami, and since the white rami come only
from these segments of the spinal cord, this part of the autonomic
nervous system is called the thoracolumbar outflow. The white and
gray rami are also called rami communicantes or communicating
rami.

227

However, not all the fibers in the white rami associated with a given spinal nerve end in the autonomic ganglion attached to that nerve. In the upper thoracic region many fibers turn upward in the ganglion-ated chain to synapse in the cervical ganglia. In the middle and lower thoracic regions many preganglionic fibers pass out along certain nerve trunks, the splanchnic nerves, to ganglia located in plexuses near the origin of the great arteries, which supply the abdominal viscera. These are the celiac ganglion, the superior mesenteric ganglion, and the inferior mesenteric ganglion, or collectively, the collateral ganglia. From the lower thoracic and lumbar regions, certain other fibers turn inferiorly in the ganglionated chain to synapse in the lower lumbar and sacral ganglia (Fig. 6-40).

All the ganglia give rise to many gray rami. The gray rami from a single paravertebral ganglion may go to several peripheral nerves, either spinal or cranial. Also fibers in gray rami frequently travel along the course of blood vessels; this is particularly true of the superior cervical ganglion, which sends fibers along the branches of the carotid artery. From the collateral ganglia postganglionic fibers travel along the visceral arteries within the abdomen.

A single white ramus bringing efferent impulses from a cell in a given spinal segment of the spinal cord synapses with a number of ganglion cells located in one or more autonomic (sympathetic) ganglia, and in turn the gray rami from these cells have a widespread distribution. For example, impulses originating in the first thoracic segment of the spinal cord go to sweat glands, pilomotor muscles, and the smooth muscle of blood vessels of the head, as well as to certain specific smooth muscles within the eyeball, and to the heart.

The distribution of the thoracolumbar outflow is shown by red lines in Fig. 6-41.

From the cervical ganglia many nerve fibers pass to the blood vessels associated with the head, thus forming numerous small plexuses. Other postganglionic fibers from the cervical ganglia go to the cervical nerves and on to the smooth muscle of blood vessels, sweat glands, and pilomotor muscles of the upper extremity. From the thoracic ganglia, fibers are given off that form esophageal, pulmonary, and cardiac plexuses. Many fibers from the vagus nerves are intermingled in the thoracic plexuses.

The superficial cardiac plexus is small and is located below the arch of the aorta. The deep cardiac plexus is larger and has two halves, one lying on either side of the aorta and trachea. The pulmonary and coronary plexuses are a continuation of the deep cardiac plexus. Below the deep cardiac plexus the two vagus nerves leave the plexus and pass inferiorly on either side of the esophagus but soon subdivide to

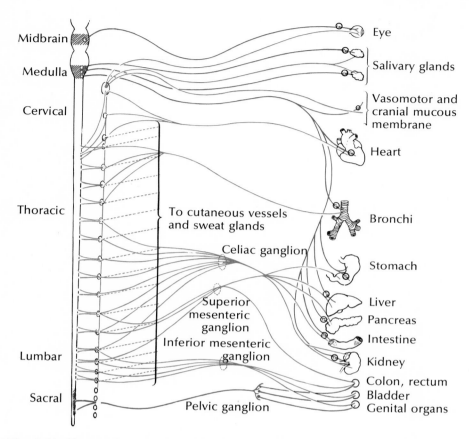

Fig. 6-41. The autonomic nervous system. Craniosacral outflow in blue lines. Thoracolumbar outflow to cutaneous vessels and sweat glands in dotted red lines and to other structures in solid red lines. (After Meyer and Gottlieb.)

form the esophageal plexus. At the esophageal opening of the diaphragm two nerve bundles are formed, the anterior and posterior vagal trunks.

There are large networks of nerve fibers lying about the collateral ganglia, forming the celiac, superior mesenteric, and inferior mesenteric plexuses. The gastric, hepatic, splenic, phrenic, adrenal, and renal plexuses are derived from the celiac plexus. The vagus nerves also send fibers to the celiac and mesenteric plexuses. The intermesenteric nerves are inferior continuations of the celiac plexus to the mesenteric plexuses. The downward continuation below the inferior mesenteric plexus is called the superior hypogastric plexus. Since it lies anterior to the sacrum, it is sometimes known as the pre-

229

sacral nerve. As the superior hypogastric plexus passes into the pelvis, it divides into right and left hypogastric nerves, which in turn enter the pelvic nerve plexuses (inferior hypogastric plexuses). The sacral nerves also send fibers to the pelvic plexuses. Therefore, each pelvic plexus consists of postganglionic thoracolumbar outflow fibers, preganglionic sacral parasympathetic fibers, and visceral sensory fibers. Each pelvic organ has a small nerve plexus derived from the pelvic plexuses.

The greater splanchnic nerve receives fibers from the fifth to the ninth or tenth sympathetic ganglia, and its fibers pass to the celiac ganglion. The lesser splanchnic nerve arises from the ninth to the eleventh ganglia, and its fibers pass to the aorticorenal ganglion. The lowest splanchnic nerve arises from the last thoracic ganglion, and its fibers pass to the renal plexus. The splanchnic nerves contain involun-

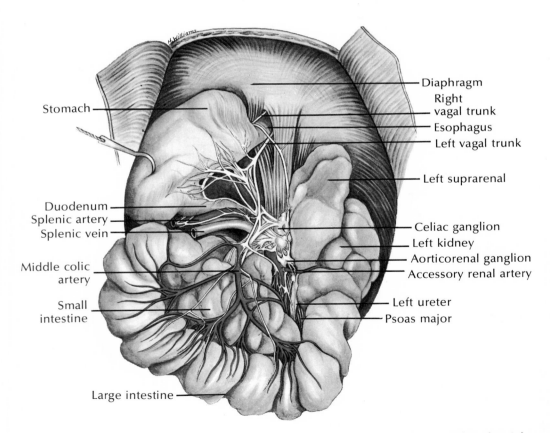

Fig. 6-42. Celiac plexus. The stomach has been turned up and to the right, and the transverse colon has been pulled inferiorly. (Dissection by Dr. R. W. Machamer.) (Term fetus.)

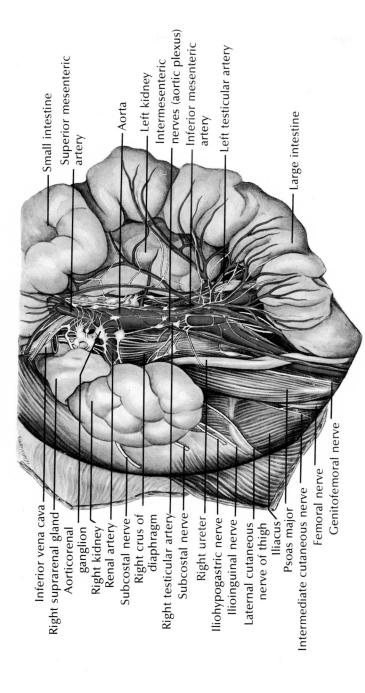

Small intestine
Superior mesenteric artery
Aorta
Left kidney
Intermesenteric nerves (aortic plexus)
Inferior mesenteric artery
Left testicular artery
Large intestine

Inferior vena cava
Right suprarenal gland
Aorticorenal ganglion
Right kidney
Renal artery
Subcostal nerve
Right crus of diaphragm
Right testicular artery
Subcostal nerve
Right ureter
Iliohypogastric nerve
Ilioinguinal nerve
Lateral cutaneous nerve of thigh
Iliacus
Psoas major
Intermediate cutaneous nerve
Femoral nerve
Genitofemoral nerve

Fig. 6-43. Inferior and superior mesenteric plexuses. The posterior parietal peritoneum and inferior vena cava have been removed. (Dissection by Dr. R. W. Machamer.) (Term fetus.)

231

tary motor fibers passing from the thoracic cord to the viscera and also many afferent fibers carrying sensory impulses to the spinal cord. The afferent fibers make their way into the cord by way of the dorsal roots.

The thoracolumbar outflow is characterized by (1) being the involuntary outflow from the thoracic and lumbar regions of the central nervous system, (2) having ganglia relatively near the central nervous system, and (3) having short preganglionic fibers (white) and long postganglionic fibers (gray) (Fig. 6-38).

Craniosacral outflow. The craniosacral outflow is the involuntary outflow coming from the two ends of the central nervous system. From the brain are fibers passing out with the third, seventh, ninth, and tenth cranial nerves; from the second, third, and fourth sacral nerves is an outflow to the pelvic region. In Fig. 6-41 the craniosacral division is indicated in blue lines.

The ganglia of the craniosacral outflow are always located in or very close to the organ innervated. The preganglionic fibers come from cells located within the central nervous system, and the postganglionic fibers arising in the ganglia go to the particular structure innervated. With the cranial nerves are the following four autonomic ganglia located in the head:

1. The ciliary ganglion of the third nerve, which sends visceral motor fibers to the ciliary muscle and the sphincter muscle of the iris
2. The pterygopalatine (sphenopalatine) ganglion of the seventh nerve, which sends visceral motor fibers to the lacrimal gland and to glands located in the nasal and pharyngeal mucosa
3. The otic ganglion of the ninth nerve, which sends visceral motor fibers to the parotid gland
4. The submandibular (submaxillary) ganglion of the seventh nerve, which sends visceral motor fibers to the submandibular and sublingual salivary glands

Sensory fibers of the trigeminal nerve pass through these ganglia; therefore, they are frequently described with the fifth nerve, although functionally they are not part of it. Sensory fibers pass through the ciliary ganglion to join the ophthalmic branch. Sensory fibers from the submandibular and sublingual salivary glands pass through the submandibular ganglion to the lingual branch of the mandibular division. Sensory fibers from the nasal mucosa pass through the pterygopalatine ganglion to the maxillary division. Sensory fibers from the parotid gland pass through the otic ganglion to the auriculotemporal branch of the mandibular division. Gray fibers from the superior cervical ganglion also pass through these ganglia. Only the fibers of the parasympathetic system synapse in the ganglia.

232

The autonomic fibers of the vagus have a very widespread distribution. In the thorax they go to the heart and smooth muscle of the esophagus and respiratory tract. In the abdominal cavity the fibers are intermingled with the plexuses of the thoracolumbar outflow and go mainly to the glands and smooth muscle of the digestive tube down to about the middle of the transverse colon.

The sacral autonomic outflow comes from sacral nerves two, three, and four, and the fibers are intermingled with the thoracolumbar fibers of the pelvic plexuses. The fibers go to the distal colon, rectum, and pelvic viscera (Fig. 6-44).

The craniosacral outflow is characterized by (1) being the involuntary outflow from the two ends of the central nervous system, (2) hav-

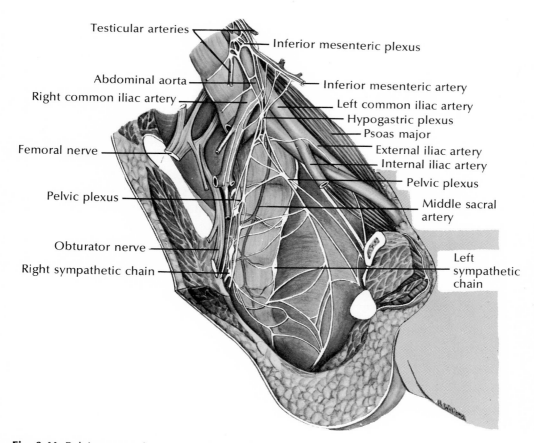

Fig. 6-44. Pelvic nerve plexuses. The parietal peritoneum has been stripped away and the right hip bone has been removed by an oblique cut. (Dissection by Dr. R. W. Machamer.) (Term fetus.)

233

ing ganglia close to the organ supplied, and (3) having long preganglionic fibers and short postganglionic fibers.

There are other distinctions between the two divisions of the autonomic nervous system. Many structures receive postganglionic fibers from both divisions, which functionally have opposite actions.

Some of the more important functional distinctions are presented in Table 12.

Sweat glands, arrector pili (pilomotor) muscles, and peripheral blood vessels are innervated by the thoracolumbar outflow and not by the craniosacral outflow.

In the nerves supplying viscera, glands, and blood vessels are fibers that carry sensory impulses from these structures to the central nervous system. Many of these fibers pass through the various plexuses and ganglia of the autonomic system. They leave the ganglia by passing in the white rami to the dorsal root ganglia and then by way of the posterior roots into the spinal cord. Although these sensory fibers pass through the autonomic nervous system, they do not synapse with any of the cells within that system. Sensory nerve fibers synapse only within the central nervous system. Most of these sensory impulses never reach conscious levels, and those that do are poorly localized and rather indefinite, producing sensations of general discomfort or comfort. Even sensations of pain, which at times may be extremely severe, are not sharply localized. Nevertheless, the sensory impulses arising in the viscera play essential parts in reflexes that control such functions as digestion, circulation, and reproduction.

Clinical considerations. An example of autonomic dysfunction is seen when damage occurs to the carotid plexus, the collection of post-

Table 12. Contrasted functions of craniosacral and thoracolumbar outflows

	Craniosacral	*Thoracolumbar*
Pupil of eye	Constricts	Dilates
Heart rate	Slows	Increases
Bronchi	Constricts	Dilates
Salivary glands	Causes increased flow of thin, watery saliva	Causes thick, viscid saliva
Peristalsis of intestine	Augments	Lessens
Sphincters of intestine	Relaxes	Contracts
Urinary bladder	Promotes emptying	Inhibits emptying
Genitalia	Promotes erection	Promotes ejaculation
Sweat glands	Absent	Promotes secretion
Peripheral blood vessels	Absent	Constricts
Adrenal medulla	Absent	Promotes secretion

ganglionic sympathetic fibers passing to the head region with branches of the carotid artery. Firstly, the three general functions of the sympathetic system, vasomotor, sudomotor, and pilomotor, are disturbed. The face on the affected side will be flushed, but the skin will be dry. Sympathetic fibers also pass to the smooth muscles in the upper eyelid and the iris. The eyelid will droop, and the pupil will be constricted by the parasympathetically controlled sphincter of the pupil. This combination of disturbances collectively is called Horner's syndrome.

REVIEW QUESTIONS

1. Discuss early development of the caudal portion of the spinal cord.
2. Discuss somatic versus visceral neurons and the structures they innervate.
3. In an adult the spinal cord extends between what two vertebral levels?
4. What structures are found in the white matter of the cord?
5. What comprises the gray matter of the cord? Where is the gray matter located?
6. Describe the meningeal coverings of the cord.
7. What is the cauda equina?
8. Discuss reflex arcs, monosynaptic and polysynaptic.
9. Name the subdivisions of the brain.
10. Name the four lobes of the cerebrum.
11. Where is the motor area of the cerebral cortex?
12. Where is the area of cerebral cortex that governs speech?
13. Where are the areas of conscious perception for the following sensations: touch, vision, hearing, and smell?
14. What are association areas? Give two examples.
15. What is meant by cerebral dominance?
16. What is one important function of the cerebellum?
17. What are the main subdivisions of the brain stem?
18. Describe the coverings of the brain.
19. Where is cerebrospinal fluid formed? Where is it resorbed?
20. Discuss hydrocephalus.
21. Discuss lumbar puncture.
22. What is the approximate volume of the brain at birth and at 20 years of age?
23. How many pairs of spinal nerves are there? How may they be grouped? How many are there in each group?
24. Describe briefly a typical nerve and its functional components.
25. Describe the phrenic nerve.
26. What forms the brachial plexus? List and give functions for the nerves that arise from the plexus.
27. Describe the ulnar nerve.
28. List the nerves arising from the lumbosacral plexus.
29. Describe the sciatic nerve.
30. List the cranial nerves.
31. Name four sensory ganglia associated with the cranial nerves.
32. List the cranial nerves that are purely sensory.
33. List the cranial nerves that are purely motor.
34. Describe the trigeminal nerve.
35. Describe the vagus nerve.
36. What are the two main subdivisions of the autonomic nervous system?
37. What are the anatomical characteristics of the thoracolumbar outflow?
38. What are the anatomical characteristics of the craniosacral outflow?
39. List the general functions of both the thoracolumbar and craniosacral outflows.

235

CHAPTER 7

THE SPECIAL SENSE ORGANS

T he special sense organs include the olfactory mucosa of the nose, the taste buds of the mouth, the eye, the ear, and the receptors in skin, muscle, and tendon.

OLFACTORY CELLS   The olfactory epithelium of the nose is limited to a small irregular area on the medial surface of the superior turbinate and the adjacent surface of the nasal septum. In living persons this area is more yellow in color than the surrounding pink respiratory mucosa.

In the olfactory mucosa there are two types of cells, the olfactory cells and the supporting cells. The supporting cells are columnar in shape and contain a yellow pigment that gives the yellowish tinge to the olfactory region. The olfactory cells are bipolar nerve cells whose axons pass through the cribriform plate of the ethmoid as the fibers of the olfactory, or first cranial, nerve (see Fig. 6-5, *E*). The dendrites reach the surface of the mucosa by passing between the supporting cells, and each divides into many fine, hairlike processes. These processes receive the olfactory stimuli directly without any intervening sense organ. The cell bodies are analogous to the cells of the dorsal root ganglia of the spinal nerves, but there is no true ganglion associated with the first cranial nerve.

TASTE BUDS   Each taste bud is a small onion-shaped nest of cells in the mucosa of the mouth; the free end of each bud opens on the surface as a gustatory pore. The supporting cells are spindle-shaped and are arranged

236

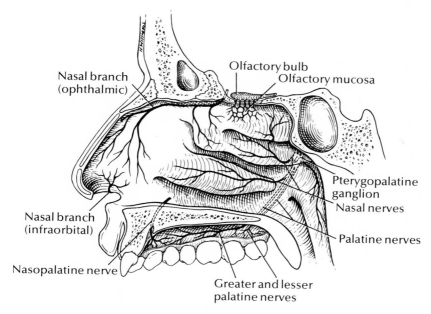

Fig. 7-1. Lateral wall of the right nostril. The pterygopalatine ganglion is drawn in dotted lines to show its position.

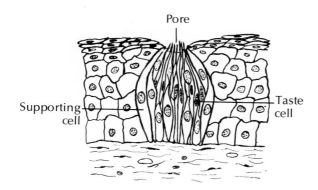

Fig. 7-2. A taste bud.

about the outside, forming the sheath of the bud; a few are within the bud. The taste cells, modified supporting cells, are long and slender, and each ends as a fine hair at the surface level of the pore.

The hair (taste) cells have no axons and are considered to be epithelial cells. The first nerve cell bodies subserving taste are found in the dorsal root ganglia of the seventh, ninth, and tenth cranial nerves. These cells send long dendrites to the taste buds, where they end as fine branches about the bases of the hair cells. The hairs of the taste

237

cells are stimulated by the presence of various chemicals. This stimulation is transmitted to the nerve cell dendrites, which transform the stimuli into nerve impulses and conduct them to the nerve cell bodies located in the ganglia. The axons of the ganglion cells then transmit the impulse to the nuclear center of taste in the medulla. The sense of taste from the anterior two thirds of the tongue is mediated by way of the facial nerve and from the posterior third by the glossopharyngeal. Taste from the root of the tongue and epiglottis is mediated by the vagus.

THE EYE

The eyeball is almost spherical. It lies in the orbital cavity and is protected anteriorly by the eyelids. With it must be considered the lacrimal glands and the nasolacrimal duct.

The eyeball is considerably smaller than the bony orbit, and the space between is filled with connective tissue and fat. In this tissue are lodged the extrinsic ocular muscles, the blood vessels, and the various nerves associated with the eye.

The two layers of cranial dura are prolonged through the optic canal into the orbit (see Fig. 6-5, *F*). The meningeal, or inner layer, envelops the optic nerve and is fused anteriorly with the sclera at the point of entry of the optic nerve fibers. The periorbital, or outer layer of dura, forms the outer lining, or periosteum, of the orbital bone and is also reflected onto the six extraocular muscles as muscle sheaths. At the anterior end of the muscles, the sheath thickens and spreads laterally forming a continuous layer (the orbital fascia or capsule of Tenon). Posteriorly the capsule is attached to the sclera at the entrance of the optic nerve and anteriorly is attached at the sclerocorneal junction. Between these two sites of attachment the capsule is connected to the sclera only by fine but numerous bands of connective tissue.

When an eyeball is removed, the capsule formed by the reflection of the muscle sheaths can serve as a socket for a prosthetic device. An additional advantage is that the capsule, since it is continuous with the sheath of the extraocular muscles, moves with their contractions, thereby moving the prosthetic device. The sheaths for the medial and lateral rectus muscles are strong and form the medial and lateral check ligaments; they are thought to prevent overfunction of these muscles. Below the eyeball the fascia spreads out like a hammock to form the suspensory ligament of the eyeball (Figs. 7-3 and 7-4).

Extrinsic muscles of the eye. The four rectus muscles and the levator palpebrae superioris muscle arise from a common circular tendon of fibrous tissue surrounding the optic nerve at its emergence from the optic canal. The four rectus muscles, called superior, inferior,

238

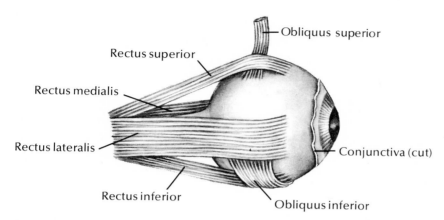

Rectus superior

Obliquus superior

Rectus medialis

Rectus lateralis

Conjunctiva (cut)

Rectus inferior

Obliquus inferior

Fig. 7-3. Extrinsic muscles of right eye, lateral view. The muscle belly of the superior oblique muscle has been removed, leaving only the distal portion of the tendon and its insertion into the eyeball.

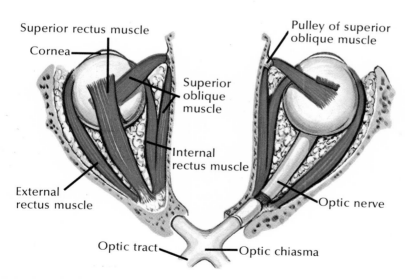

Superior rectus muscle

Cornea

Pulley of superior oblique muscle

Superior oblique muscle

Internal rectus muscle

External rectus muscle

Optic nerve

Optic tract

Optic chiasma

Fig. 7-4. Illustration of relationship of four extrinsic eye muscles of left and right eyeballs. Inferior rectus and inferior oblique muscles of each eye are situated below eyeball and are not visible. (From Schottelius, B. A., and Schottelius, D. D.: Textbook of physiology, ed. 17, St. Louis, 1973, The C. V. Mosby Co.)

239

lateral or external, and medial or internal because of their relation to the eyeball, pass anteriorly to their insertions into the eyeball, a short distance behind the margin of the cornea (Fig. 7-7).

The superior oblique muscle arises from the bone, just above the common circular tendon. It passes anteriorly on the nasal side of the medial rectus over the eyeball to the margin of the orbit, where it becomes tendinous and passes through a fibrous pulley. The tendon then turns laterally and posteriorly to an insertion into the eyeball behind its equator and between the levels of insertion of the superior and lateral rectus muscles. Contraction of the superior oblique muscle rotates the eyeball downward and outward.

The inferior oblique muscle arises from the floor of the orbit on the medial side. The muscle passes laterally beneath the eyeball to an insertion behind the equator and between the levels of insertion of the inferior and lateral rectus muscles. This muscle rotates the eye upward and outward. The need for the oblique muscles, which direct the eyeball outward, is clear when one remembers that, from their origin in the common circular tendon, the superior and inferior recti course forward and outward. Unopposed by the oblique muscles, the superior rectus, on contraction, would direct the eyeball inward as well as upward, and the inferior rectus would turn the eyeball inward and downward. The inferior oblique and the superior rectus acting together rotate the eyeball directly upward; the superior oblique and inferior rectus turn it directly downward. The lateral rectus turns the eyeball directly outward (laterally), and the medial rectus turns the eyeball inward (medially).

The orbital muscle is a small mass of smooth muscle fibers found in the back of the orbit. It bridges across the inferior orbital fissure, the cleft in the lower lateral part of the back of the orbit.

Eyelids. The eyelids are two fibromuscular curtains, one placed in front of each eye. In addition to having fibers of the orbicularis oculi muscle, which are the chief muscle bundles of the lids, the upper lid is provided with a special muscle, the levator palpebrae superioris, which arises from the common circular tendon surrounding the optic nerve and is innervated by the third cranial nerve. In each eyelid the levator splits into two laminae, the deeper or posterior lamina constitutes the layer of smooth muscle that inserts into the tarsal plate. Innervation of the smooth muscles is by sympathetic nerve fibers from the carotid plexus, damage to which causes drooping of the eyelid.

The connective tissue framework of the eyelid is called the orbital septum or palpebral fascia. This is a sheet of connective tissue attached all around to the bony margin of the orbital cavity. At the margin of each eyelid the septum is condensed into a fibrous plate, the

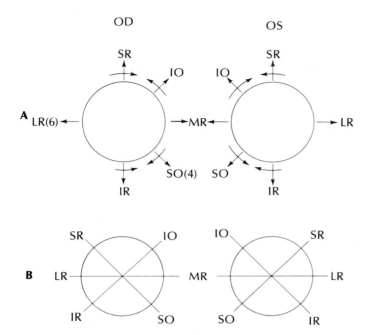

Fig. 7-5. Actions of the extraocular muscles. From the primary position, the *SO* and the *IO* each abduct the eye; however, their major functional use is as shown. **A,** Deviations *(centrifugal arrows)* and torsions *(circumferential arrows)* produced by individual muscles. **B,** Major muscles used for moving each eye in the six cardinal directions of gaze. Abbreviations: *SR,* superior rectus; *IR,* inferior rectus; *MR,* medial rectus; *IO,* inferior oblique; *SO,* superior oblique; *LR,* lateral rectus; *OD* right eye; *OS,* left eye. (From Willis, W., and Grossman, R.: Medical neurobiology, St. Louis, 1973, The C. V. Mosby Co.)

tarsus. The tarsus of the upper lid is shaped like a half oval; the tarsus of the lower lid is smaller and rod-shaped. The medial and lateral extremities of each tarsus are anchored to the margin of the orbit by the medial and lateral palpebral ligaments.

The eyelashes are short hairs projecting from the free margins of the eyelids; the upper ones curve upward, and the lower ones curve downward. In the lids there are numbers of small sebaceous and sweat glands that empty by minute openings along the free margin. Inflammation of one or more of the sebaceous glands results in a condition known as a sty (see Fig. 14-3).

Eyebrows. The eyebrows are a pair of arches of thickened skin, one placed above each orbit and closely studded with short, coarse hairs. Fibers of the muscles of expression, particularly fibers of the frontalis and orbicularis oculi, are interlaced beneath this thickened area of skin.

Conjunctiva. The conjunctiva is a layer of mucous membrane covering the inner surface of the eyelids (palpebral conjunctiva) and the surface of the sclera (bulbar conjunctiva). The epithelium is stratified columnar in type and changes to stratified squamous at the lid margins, where it is continuous with the skin of the lids. At the margin of the cornea the bulbar conjunctiva is continuous with the stratified squamous epithelium covering the cornea. Conjunctivitis, often called "pink eye," is an inflammation of the vessels supplying the conjunctiva.

Lacrimal apparatus. The lacrimal gland, a small organ the size and shape of an almond, lies in the upper, lateral portion of the orbit. Its function is to secrete tears, which are then emptied by several small ducts onto the conjunctiva behind the lateral half of the upper lid (Fig. 7-6).

The small openings, or puncta lacrimalia, of the lacrimal canaliculi are visible near the medial end of each eyelid. The lacrimal sac is formed by the union of the canaliculus of each eyelid; the sac drains by way of the nasolacrimal duct into the inferior meatus of the nose, beneath the inferior turbinate. The canaliculi are limited by their small caliber and can carry only a small amount of secretion; consequently, when the lacrimal gland is stimulated, via parasympathetic

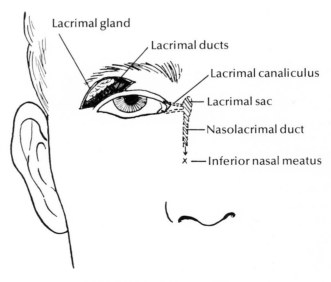

Fig. 7-6. Lacrimal apparatus.

fibers carried with the facial nerve, excess tears overflow onto the cheek.

Wall of the eyeball. The wall of the eyeball is composed of three coats. The outer is called the sclera; it is thick and strong and is opaque posteriorly, whereas anteriorly it is transparent and is called the cornea. The sclera is continued posteriorly and blends with the meningeal dura mater of the brain, which forms the outer sheath of the optic nerve. The visible portion of the sclera is the white part of the eyeball.

The middle coat is the choroid; it is heavily pigmented and vascular. Anteriorly the choroid is replaced by the iris, a colored disc behind the cornea. The amount of melanin and its location in the iris determine the color of the eye. If the melanin is present only in its posterior aspect, the iris appears blue; if pigment is scattered throughout the iris, the color of the iris appears brown. In the center of the iris there is an opening, called the pupil, through which light is admitted into the interior of the eye. The iris is contractile, and by varying the size of the pupil, the eye adjusts itself to varying intensities of light.

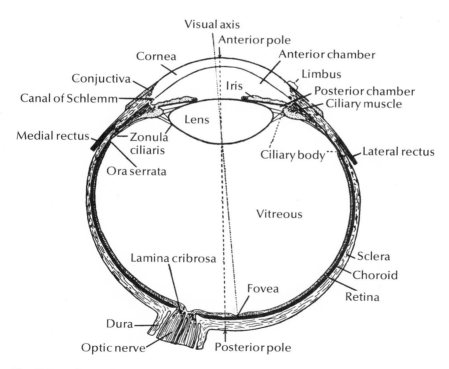

Fig. 7-7. Schematic horizontal meridional section of right eye. (Redrawn and modified from Salzmann; from Bevelander, G., and Ramaley, J.: Essentials of histology, St. Louis, 1974, The C. V. Mosby Co.)

The iris contains many smooth muscle fibers. Part of these are arranged in a circular fashion about the pupil and form the sphincter of the pupil, the function of which is to constrict the pupil. The rest of the smooth muscle cells are arranged in a radial fashion, and their contraction causes dilatation of the pupil. The sphincter fibers are innervated by parasympathetic fibers of the third cranial nerve, whereas the dilator fibers are innervated by sympathetic fibers from the superior cervical ganglion. Attaching the iris to the choroid is the ciliary body, which contains bundles of smooth muscle (ciliary muscles) arranged in a radial manner and innervated by parasympathetic fibers from the third cranial nerve. The crystalline lens, which focuses the entering light rays on the retina, is suspended behind the pupil by a suspensory ligament attached at its periphery to the ciliary body. The ciliary muscle controls the shape of the lens. As the ciliary muscle contracts, it relaxes the suspensory ligament allowing the elastic lens to enlarge, or become more convex, an accommodation necessary for near vision. It is to be noted then that muscular contraction is required for closeup viewing, one reason why reading "tires" the eyes more than viewing distant objects does.

The innermost layer of the eyeball is called the retina; it is a thin delicate membrane composed of ten layers named as follows:

1. Pigmented epithelium
2. Rods and cones
3. External limiting membrane
4. Outer nuclear (granular) layer
5. Outer plexiform (molecule) layer   (see Fig. 7-8)
6. Inner nuclear (granular) layer
7. Inner plexiform (molecule) layer
8. Ganglion cell layer
9. Nerve fiber layer
10. Internal limiting membrane

Within the retina there are ganglion cells that are analogous to the dorsal root ganglion cells of a spinal nerve.

Interior of eyeball. That portion of the interior of the eyeball between the cornea and iris is the anterior chamber, and the small portion between the iris and lens is the posterior chamber. A thin, transparent fluid, called the aqueous humor, fills both the anterior and posterior chambers. An over accumulation of aqueous humor creates an increase in intraocular pressure, a condition known as glaucoma. It may be acute or chronic or primary or secondary to some other condition such as tumor or inflammation. Pain and distortion of vision accompany this condition. The vitreous body is a transparent jellylike substance that fills the interior of the eyeball behind the lens.

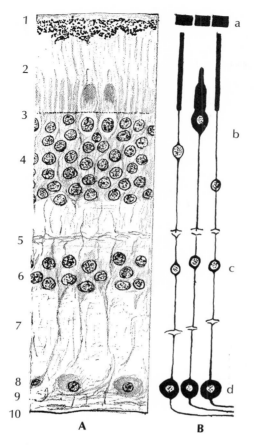

1
2
3
4
5
6
7
8
9
10

a
b
c
d

A   B

Fig. 7-8. Human retina. **A,** Section of retina. **B,** Isolated cells, diagrammatically presented. Numbers to left of illustration and letters to right correspond to numbers and letters in outline on opposite page. (From Bevelander, G., and Ramaley, J.: Essentials of histology, ed. 7, St. Louis, 1974, The C. V. Mosby Co.)

By use of an instrument called an ophthalmoscope, it is possible to look directly at the retina. This is an examination of the eyegrounds, or fundus, of the eye. The physician directs a light through the pupil, thus illuminating the interior of the eye. Fig. 7-9 is an illustration of what he sees. The retina is red because of the rich blood supply of the underlying choroid. Numerous small blood vessels are visible running over the inner surface of the retina. Toward the nasal side of the back of the eye there is a depressed white area, called the optic disc or papilla nervi optici. Here the filaments of the optic nerve receive a myelin sheath as they leave the eyeball, thus producing the white color seen here. The optic disc is also known as the blind spot because

245

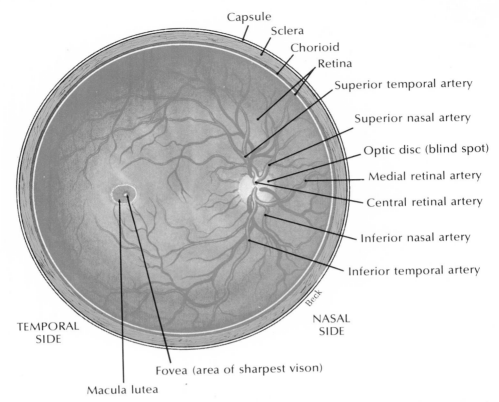

Capsule
Sclera
Chorioid
Retina
Superior temporal artery
Superior nasal artery
Optic disc (blind spot)
Medial retinal artery
Central retinal artery
Inferior nasal artery
Inferior temporal artery

TEMPORAL
SIDE

NASAL
SIDE

Fovea (area of sharpest vison)
Macula lutea

Fig. 7-9. The right eyeground (fundus) showing vessels, optic disc, macula lutea, and layers of the eyeball. (From Anthony, C. P., and Kolthoff, N. J.: Textbook of anatomy and physiology, ed. 8, St. Louis, 1971, The C. V. Mosby Co.)

light rays focused on the ensheathed nerve cannot be seen. The retinal artery enters the eyeball within the optic disc, and the retinal veins leave. A few millimeters lateral to the disc and directly behind the pupil is a small yellow area, called the macula lutea, containing a central depression, called the fovea centralis. The fovea is the area of most distinct vision.

The eye acts like a camera. Light rays pass through the transparent cornea at the front of the eyeball, through the pupil, and through the lens, which focuses light rays upon the nerve cells of the retina. The light rays pass entirely through the transparent retina to the deepest layer, the rod and cone cells. These receive the stimulus and generate nerve impulses that are transmitted through the retinal layers to a layer of large ganglion cells. The axons from the ganglion cells

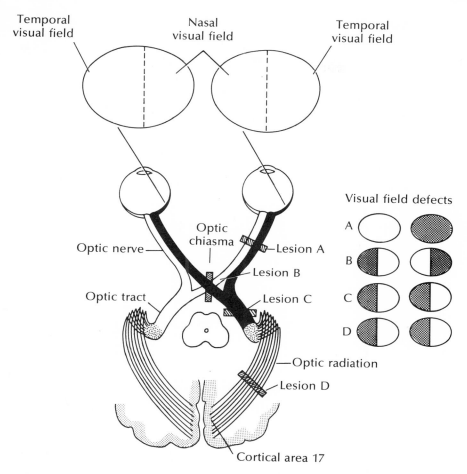

Temporal
visual field

Nasal
visual field

Temporal
visual field

Visual field defects

Optic
chiasma

Optic nerve

Lesion A

Lesion B

Optic tract

Lesion C

Optic radiation

Lesion D

Cortical area 17

A

B

C

D

Fig. 7-10. Visual pathway and visual field defects that result from lesions at different levels. Right optic nerve destruction causes complete blindness in the same eye. A lesion in the optic chiasm causes blindness in the temporal visual fields of both eyes. Right optic tract interruption causes blindness in the nasal visual field of the right eye and in the temporal visual field of the left eye, a condition that also occurs following complete destruction of the optic radiation on the right side.

pass out of the retina in the optic nerve and carry impulses to the visual centers of the brain.

Rods contain a substance, rhodopson, which is extremely light sensitive. The breakdown of rhodopsin produces a chemical change that initiates a nerve impulse. Cones also contain light sensitive material that, however, appears to be relatively less sensitive to light. Rods, therefore, are considered to facilitate vision in dim light as well as

247

adaptation to darkness. Rods are absent in the fovea centralis but increase in density towards the periphery. Cones, the sensory receptors for color vision as well as discriminative sight, occupy exclusively the fovea centralis but decrease in density towards the periphery. Since the fovea contains the greatest number of cones, clearest vision in good light is attained when the image is focused directly on the fovea. To see an object better in dim light, we look slightly to the side of the object, thereby focusing the image nearer the periphery of the retina, where the rods are concentrated.

The ophthalmic artery, a branch of the internal carotid, passes into the orbital cavity through the optic canal inferior to the optic nerve. The central artery of the retina, a branch of the ophthalmic, pierces the sheath of the optic nerve about 12 mm behind the eyeball and runs in the center of the optic nerve to supply the retina. Immediate and total blindness of the eye will occur if its retinal artery is obstructed. The veins of the orbit form two main trunks, the inferior and superior ophthalmic veins, which empty into the anterior end of the cavernous sinus. The inferior veins communicate with the venous plexuses, around the pterygoid muscles, whereas the superior veins communicate freely with the facial vein. Since neither the superior veins nor the facial vein contains valves, the superior ophthalmic may readily conduct infected clots (thrombi) from the superficial aspect of the face, resulting in cavernous sinus thrombosis, usually occlusive (see Fig. 9-30). Such occlusion, or blockage, may lead to marked congestion, stasis, edema, meningitis, and possibly even ischemic necrosis of surrounding tissues. The functional effects of venous occlusion on the brain are similar to those of arterial occlusion. Although different parts of the brain react at different rates to ischemia, cortical tissue will not generally recover normal function if subjected to more than five minutes of complete ischemia. The stasis produced by venous occlusion may lead to an abrupt rise in intracranial pressure and hemorrhage from the capillaries of the brain.

The central vein of the retina accompanies the central artery into the center of the optic nerve. Since the nerve is surrounded by the meninges, an increase in intracranial pressure can be transmitted to the subarachnoid space around the optic nerve, causing compression and engorgement of the venous and lymphatic channels, a condition known as papilledema. Papilledema produces an enlargement of the blind spot, caused by swelling of the optic nerve head, resulting in a decrease in visual acuity.

THE EAR   The organ of hearing has the following three subdivisions: (1) the external ear, (2) the middle ear, and (3) the inner ear.

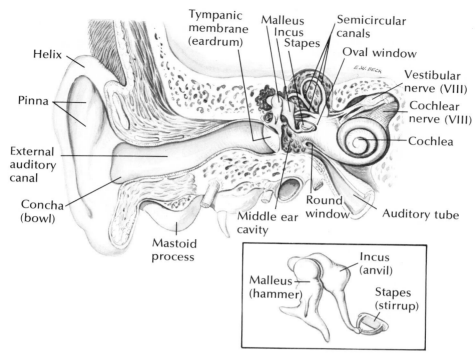

Fig. 7-11. Illustration showing anatomy of external, middle, and inner ear. Auditory ossicles are shown enlarged in box. (From Schottelius, B. A., and Schottelius, D. D.: Textbook of physiology, ed. 17, St. Louis, 1973, The C. V. Mosby Co.)

External ear. The external ear has two parts, the auricle, or pinna, and the external auditory meatus, or canal. The auricle is a shell-shaped organ attached to the side of the head. It is composed of an irregular plate of elastic cartilage covered with skin. It varies greatly in size and shape, and it is usually smaller in women than in men. The angle of its attachment to the head varies greatly. A number of vestigial muscles are associated with the auricle, but rarely is any functional muscle found.

The external auditory canal, a bent tube about 35 mm long and varying in diameter, is the connecting passageway between the auricle and the middle ear. The lateral third of its wall is cartilaginous, and the remainder is bony. The skin over the cartilaginous portion contains many fine hairs, sebaceous glands, and special glands for the secretion of ear wax. The external canal receives sensory nerve fibers from the mandibular division of the trigeminal, the vagus, and the great auricular nerve, a branch from the cervical plexus (see Fig. 249

6-20). The vagus is also sensory to the mucosa of the larynx, and for this reason, stimulation of the auricular branch frequently causes a tickling sensation in the throat and a desire to cough.

Middle ear. The middle ear, or the tympanic cavity, a small air chamber within the temporal bone, may be likened to a six-sided box. The lateral wall is the tympanic membrane, or eardrum, which separates the middle ear from the external ear. The eardrum is a thin, translucent disc of fibrous tissue placed at the medial end of the external canal, sealing it off from the cavity of the middle ear.

The posterior wall of the middle ear has a small opening communicating with the mastoid air cells. It is this opening that transmits the infections that travel from the middle ear to the air cells and produce mastoiditis.

The anterior wall of the middle ear has the opening of the auditory tube (eustachian tube), which connects the middle ear with the nasopharynx. By means of this tube the air pressure in the middle ear is equalized with atmospheric pressure. Infections may pass from the nasopharynx to the middle ear along this tube. The medial, or pharyngeal, end of the auditory tube is cartilaginous, and the lateral end is bony. The cartilaginous part is about 25 mm long, and the bony part about 10 mm long. The medial orifice of the auditory tube is located in the lateral wall of the nasopharynx about 10 mm directly behind the inferior turbinate. From the medial end the tube is directed laterally, superiorly, and posteriorly to the middle ear.

The floor of the middle ear is a thin sheet of bone that separates the ear cavity from the jugular fossa.

The roof of the middle ear, also a thin sheet of bone, separates the ear cavity from the middle cranial fossa.

The medial wall of the middle ear consists of dense bone in which there are two openings, a round and an oval window, communicating with the inner ear. The foot piece of the stapes fits into the oval window. Inferior to the oval window is the round window, which is closed over by a small fibrous disc, called the secondary drum membrane (Figs. 7-11 to 7-13).

Extending across the middle ear cavity is a chain of three ossicles, the malleus (hammer), incus (anvil), and stapes (stirrup). It is by means of these bones that sound waves are transmitted from the outer to the inner ear.

The chorda tympani nerve, a branch of the facial nerve, which transmits taste sensation from the anterior two thirds of the tongue and which carries secretomotor fibers to the salivary glands, crosses the cavity of the middle ear, passing between the malleus and the incus.

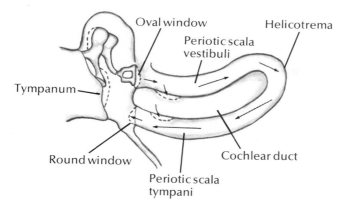

Fig. 7-12. Coronal diagram relating oval window to vestibule and vestibular periotic space, and round window to tympanic periotic space. Dotted lines show effects of movement of tympanum and ossicular chain on membranes of oval and round windows. Represented is effect of high frequency vibration on basal turn area. (From Minckler, J.: Introduction to neuroscience, St. Louis, 1972, The C. V. Mosby Co.)

The tensor tympani muscle lies in a bony canal superior to the auditory tube. Its tendon is inserted on the long process of the malleus, which in turn is firmly attached to the center of the medial surface of the tympanic membrane; thus, the muscle regulates tension in the membrane. It is innervated by the motor part of the trigeminal nerve. The stapedius muscle is inserted on the stapes. It is a tiny muscle arising within the temporal bone in the posterior wall of the middle ear and is innervated by the facial nerve. It assists in regulating pressure on the foot piece of the stapes in the oval window by dampening movement of the ossicles.

The middle ear cavity is lined with mucous membrane continuous with that of the auditory tube and nasopharynx and with that of the mastoid air cells. The ossicles and chorda tympani nerve are all covered with the same tissue. The mucous membrane of the middle ear receives its sensory innervation from the glossopharyngeal nerve.

Inner ear. The inner ear lies within the petrous portion of the temporal bone; it consists of complex bony passages, called the osseous labyrinth and the membranous labyrinth. The inner ear is also called the vestibulocochlear organ to emphasize its dual function of equilibrium and hearing (Figs. 7-13 and 7-14).

The osseous labyrinth consists of a central portion, called the vestibule, which communicates with the three semicircular canals and with the cochlea. Each semicircular canal forms two thirds of a circle. The three canals on each side are placed at right angles to each

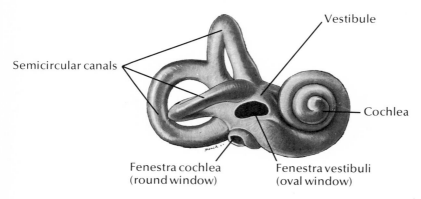

Semicircular canals

Vestibule

Cochlea

Fenestra cochlea
(round window)

Fenestra vestibuli
(oval window)

Fig. 7-13. External view of right bony labyrinth, diagrammatic.

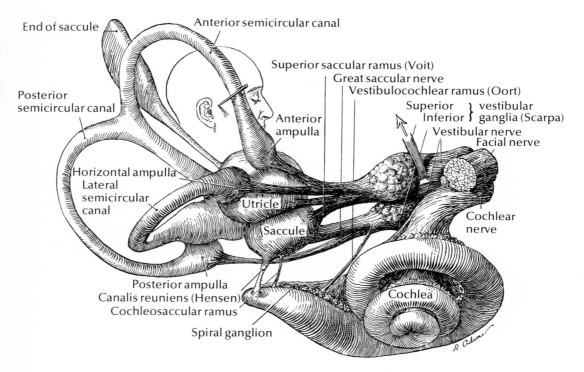

End of saccule

Anterior semicircular canal

Superior saccular ramus (Voit)
Great saccular nerve
Vestibulocochlear ramus (Oort)

Posterior
semicircular canal

Anterior
ampulla

Superior } vestibular
Inferior } ganglia (Scarpa)
Vestibular nerve
Facial nerve

Horizontal ampulla
Lateral
semicircular
canal

Utricle

Saccule

Cochlear
nerve

Posterior ampulla
Canalis reuniens (Hensen)
Cochleosaccular ramus

Cochlea

Spiral ganglion

Fig. 7-14. Diagram of the membranous labyrinth and the eighth cranial
nerve (from a dissection by Max Brödel). The cochlea has been turned
laterally and inferiorly and the superior branch of the vestibular nerve has
been elevated. (From Mettler, F. A.: Neuroanatomy, ed. 2, St. Louis, The
C. V. Mosby Co.)

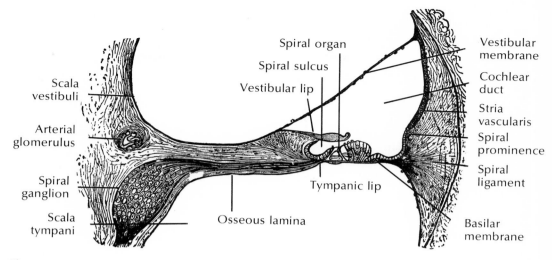

Scala vestibuli

Arterial glomerulus

Spiral ganglion

Scala tympani

Osseous lamina

Spiral organ

Spiral sulcus

Vestibular lip

Tympanic lip

Vestibular membrane

Cochlear duct

Stria vascularis

Spiral prominence

Spiral ligament

Basilar membrane

Fig. 7-15. Radial section through one of the coils of the cochlea. (×50.) (From Toldt, C.: Atlas of human anatomy, ed. 2, New York, The Macmillan Co.)

other. A canal of each ear is parallel to a canal in the ear of the opposite side. The cochlea is a coiled tube that makes two and one-half turns around a central pillar, called the modiolus. There is a thin shelf of bone winding around the modiolus that divides the tube of the cochlea into two portions, a scala tympani and scala vestibuli. These two portions communicate with each other through a small opening at the apex of the modiolus, known as the helicotrema (Fig. 7-12).

The membranous labyrinth is a closed sac within, but not nearly filling, the bony labyrinth; it contains a clear fluid, called endolymph, secreted by cells of the cochlea. The clear fluid outside the membrane wall but within the bony labyrinth is called perilymph. Perilymph is similar in composition to, communicates with, and is presumed to arise in conjunction with cerebrospinal fluid. The endolymph and perilymph do not mingle, each being in a closed compartment.

The utricle and saccule, two saclike portions of the membranous labyrinth, lie within the bony vestibule and communicate with each other. Three membranous semicircular ducts, one for each bony canal, are connected with the utricle; each duct has a dilatation, called an ampulla, near one end. The cochlear duct, or scala media, is connected with the saccule by means of a tiny duct, the canalis reuniens. The cochlear duct coils up within the cochlea between the scala tympani and scala vestibuli. The end of the saccule is drawn out into a   253 long diverticulum, the endolymphatic duct, which lies in a tiny canal, the aqueduct of the vestibule, extending from the vestibule through the temporal bone to the subarachnoid space in the posterior fossa of the skull.

The eighth cranial nerve enters the cranial cavity on its emergence from the internal acoustic meatus of the temporal bone. Within the canal the trunk is composed of two parts, a cochlear and a vestibular portion (Fig. 7-14).

The bipolar ganglion cells of the cochlear nerve are located in the spiral ganglion within the modiolus. The dendrites are distributed around the bases of the receptor cells, the hair cells of the organ of Corti, and the axons form the cochlear nerve. A discussion of the transmission of sound is beyond the scope of this book; however, it is clear that movements of the tympanic membrane (eardrum) are transmitted via the ossicles to the perilymph in the vestibule of the inner ear (Fig. 7-12). Movements of the perilymph in the scala vestibuli are transmitted through the vestibular membrane, the endolymph of the cochlear duct, and basilar membrane into the perilymph of the scala tympani. With displacement of the basilar membrane, the position of the hair cells in the organ of Corti in relation to the tectorial membrane is altered. The hairlike processes of the hair cells are bent or sheered creating an impulse that is passed on to the dendrites, or afferent endings, of the spinal ganglion cells. The impulse is

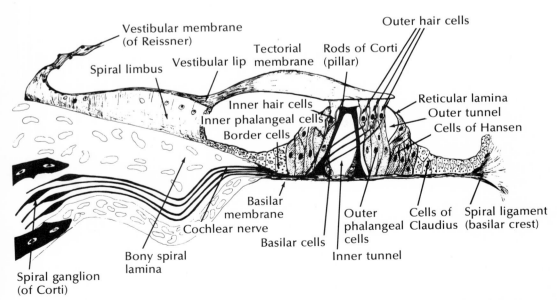

Fig. 7-16. Diagram of organ of Corti. (From Minckler, J.: Introduction to neuroscience, St. Louis, 1972, The C. V. Mosby Co.)

transmitted via the ganglion cell axons to the auditory center of the brain stem. From the auditory center the impulses are relayed to the auditory cortex.

Vestibular apparatus. The vestibular apparatus, composed of two groups of sensory receptors, the otolith organs and the semicircular canals, relays information to the central nervous system regarding head position as well as acceleration of the head.

There are two otolith organs, the utricle and saccule (Fig. 7-14). The sensory epithelium in both organs, called the macula, is composed of supporting and sensory hair cells. The sensory hair cells have cilia on their free surface that project into the otolithic membrane, a gelatinous membrane that contains imbedded crystals of calcium carbonate, called otoconia. The afferent fibers of the utricle or saccule are affected whenever the otolithic membrane is shifted with respect

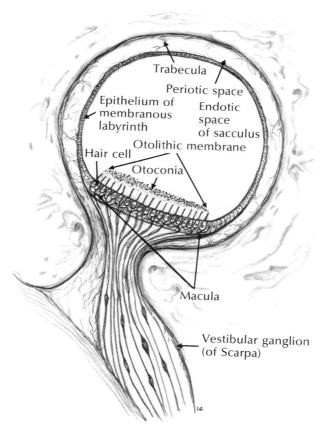

Fig. 7-17. Macula—diagram of histology. (From Minckler, J.: Introduction to neuroscience, St. Louis, 1972, The C. V. Mosby Co.)

255

to the sensory epithelium. Most of the afferents show a spontaneous discharge when the head is upright. With a change in head position the otolithic membrane changes position, thereby shifting the cilia of the hair cells. A given afferent fiber will discharge more frequently when the cilia on its hair cell are bent in one direction and less frequently when they are bent in the opposite direction. Thus any tilt of the head will result in a patterned response from each otolith organ, with some afferents increasing and others decreasing their discharges.

There are three semicircular ducts in each labyrinth, and the ducts on the two sides of the head form pairs oriented in the same plane. The sensory epithelium of the semicircular ducts is located within the ampulla, the dilated portion of the duct near its junction with the utricle (Fig. 7-14). The sensory epithelium of the semicircular ducts, called the crista, contains supporting cells and hair cells. The hair cells have cilia, which in each crista are polarized in the same direction. The cilia of the hair cells project into a gelatinous structure known as the cupula. The cupula and crista are oriented at right angles to the plane of the semicircular ducts. When the head rotates, the inertia of the endolymph within one or more pairs of the ducts causes a relative movement of the endolymph opposite to that of the head. The movement of the endolymph causes the cupula to bend in the direction of flow, thereby distorting the cilia on the hair cells,

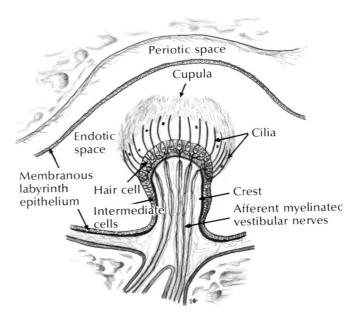

Fig. 7-18. Crest in ampulla of semicircular canal. (From Minckler, J.: Introduction to neuroscience, St. Louis, 1972, The C. V. Mosby Co.)

which either increases or decreases the rate of impulse discharge in the afferent fibers (Fig. 7-18).

The vestibular afferents have their cell bodies in the vestibular ganglion, which is located in the internal auditory meatus (Fig. 7-14). The central processes of these bipolar nerve cells travel in the eighth cranial nerve to terminate either in the vestibular nuclei of the brain stem or the cerebellum.

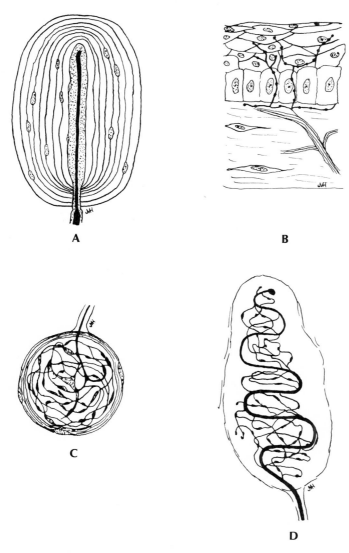

Fig. 7-19. Various types of sensory nerve endings. **A,** Pacinian corpuscle.
B, Free nerve endings. **C,** Corpuscle of Krause. **D,** Corpuscle of Meissner.   257

SENSORY NERVE ENDINGS IN SKIN, MUSCLE, AND TENDON

The cutaneous nerves end in a variety of ways among the cells of the layers of the skin. Some terminate as free nerve endings, part of which serve as receptors for the sense of pain. Other nerve fibers terminate in specialized end organs, which vary greatly in form. These are usually microscopic structures. Different nerve endings are specialized for the reception of special stimuli, such as heat, cold, pressure, vibration, and the size and shape of objects.

Fig. 7-19 illustrates various kinds of sensory nerve endings. A represents a pacinian corpuscle. This type has many consecutive layers of fibrous tissue for a capsule, and the entire structure is just visible to the unaided eye. Pacinian corpuscles are found in the deeper layers of the skin of the palms of the hands and the soles of the feet, in the areolar tissue of the posterior abdominal wall, and near joints. B illustrates free nerve endings in stratified squamous epithelium. Free nerve endings are abundant in skin and mucous membranes, and a few are found about the roots of hair and in serous membranes. C illustrates a corpuscle of Krause, which is found in the conjunctiva, in the mucosa of the lips and tongue, and in the synovial membranes. Large corpuscles of this variety are found in the glans of the penis and clitoris. D illustrates an oval corpuscle of Meissner. This type is found in the skin of the palms of the hands and the soles of the feet and in the tips of the fingers and toes.

There are spindle-shaped structures associated with voluntary muscles and tendons. These have a capsule of connective tissue and a core of fibers that is partly nervous and partly muscular.

The pacinian corpuscles are probably the sensory receptors for pressure. The end organs of Krause, in some areas at least, may be stimulated by temperature changes; Meissner's corpuscles are associated with touch. The neuromuscular spindle bundles, associated with muscles and tendons, are receptors for sense of position, balance, and muscle tension.

REVIEW QUESTIONS

1. Where are the end organs for sense of smell located?
2. Describe a taste bud.
3. What cranial nerves contain fibers carrying the sensation of taste?
4. List the extrinsic muscles of the eyeball and give the nerve supply of each.
5. What is the anterior chamber of the eye?
6. Describe the eyelids.
7. Describe the lacrimal apparatus.
8. Name the three coats of the eyeball.
9. What are the three subdivisions of the ear?
10. What is the sensory innervation of the external auditory meatus?
11. What is the sensory innervation of the mucosa of the middle ear?
12. What are the subdivisions of the osseous labyrinth?
13. Where is perilymph found? Where is endolymph found?
14. What two kinds of sensory fibers are found in the eighth cranial nerve?

15. Name three types of sensory end organs found in the skin.
16. What is the optic disc?
17. What is the function of the tensor tympani muscle?
18. What structures pass through the optic canal?
19. Discuss visual field defects following optic nerve, chiasm, and optic tract de-struction.
20. Discuss location and function of rods and cones.
21. Discuss importance of anastomosis between ophthalmic and facial veins.

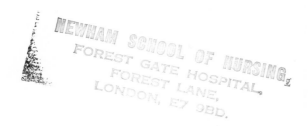

CHAPTER 8

THE ENDOCRINE SYSTEM

Glands that secrete a substance directly into the blood stream are known as endocrine glands, whereas glands that secrete a substance through a duct onto a surface are known as exocrine. Some glands have both endocrine and exocrine functions; this explains why certain glands, such as the pancreas, are included in the endocrine system. The secretions of the endocrine group are called hormones. Hormones control the orderly functioning of the body, not by initiating new reactions but rather by acting as catalysts, or accelerators, in a wide range of physiochemical reactions. Life usually will continue when a hormone is deficient, although its quality may be altered. Severe adrenal cortical deficiency, however, is incompatible with life, and it is obvious that normal gonadal function controls the continuation of life for succeeding generations. Each hormone is a complex chemical substance, the action of which will be described briefly under the appropriate gland.

Functionally each gland may be studied from (1) its dysfunction, hypoactivity or hyperactivity, (2) the consequences of its removal, (3) the results of the injection of extracts of the glands, and (4) the result of the administration of a purified or synthetic hormone.

HYPOPHYSIS *Anatomy.* The hypophysis, or pituitary body, is a small oval mass about the size of a pea lying in the sella turcica of the sphenoid bone and attaching by a slender stalk to the undersurface of the brain, just posterior to the optic chiasm (see Fig. 6-33). The sella is lined with dura mater. A sheet of the same tissue, stretched over the fossa, forms the diaphragm of the sella in which there is a small central hole

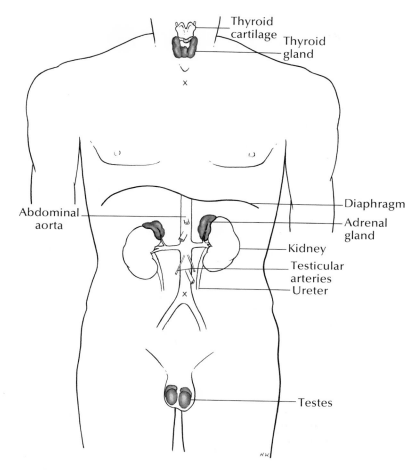

Fig. 8-1. Diagram showing general position of certain ductless glands in the male: the thyroids, suprarenals, and testes. The upper X marks the position in the infant of the thymus, and the lower X that of the aortic paraganglia.

through which the stalk passes (see Fig. 6-5). The pituitary gland also has coverings derived from the arachnoid and the pia mater. It is supplied by small vessels that arise from the internal carotid arteries and from the arterial circle of Willis at the base of the brain.

The pituitary is surrounded by a venous circle composed of the two cavernous sinuses laterally and the anterior and posterior inter-cavernous sinuses (Fig. 8-3). The veins from the gland drain into these sinuses. Since the third, fourth, sixth, and part of the fifth cranial nerves pass through the cavernous sinus, it is obvious that many very important structures are in close relation to the pituitary.

261

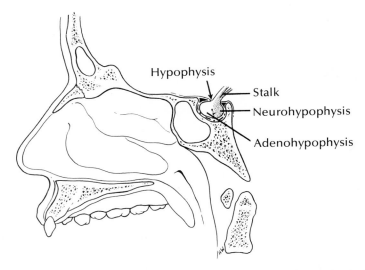

Hypophysis

Stalk

Neurohypophysis

Adenohypophysis

Fig. 8-2. Diagram of sagittal section of skull to show the hypophysis in the sella turcica.

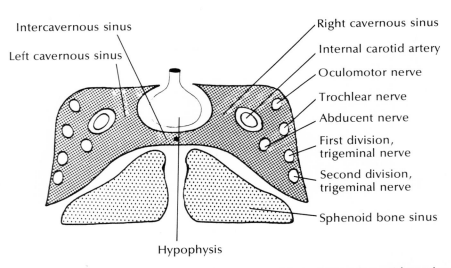

Intercavernous sinus

Left cavernous sinus

Right cavernous sinus

Internal carotid artery

Oculomotor nerve

Trochlear nerve

Abducent nerve

First division, trigeminal nerve

Second division, trigeminal nerve

Sphenoid bone sinus

Hypophysis

Fig. 8-3. Diagram of the cavernous sinuses, with the internal carotid arteries and the third, fourth, fifth, and sixth cranial nerves within. (From DiDio, L. J. A.: Synopsis of anatomy, St. Louis, 1970, The C. V. Mosby Co.)

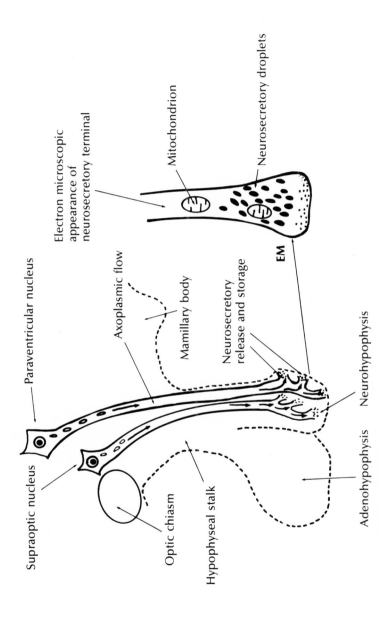

Fig. 8-4. Hypothalamus-neurohypophyseal tract. (From Minckler, J.: Introduction to neuroscience, St. Louis, 1972, The C. V. Mosby Co.)

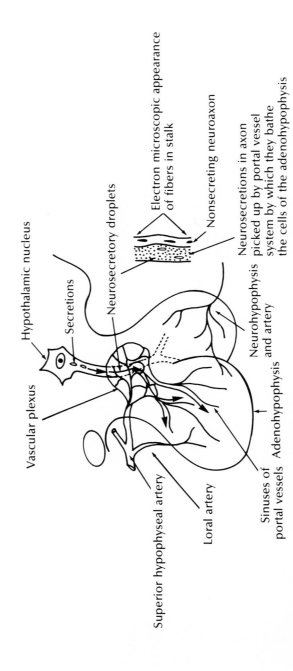

Fig. 8-5. Hypothalamoadenohypophyseal portal system. (From Minckler, J.: Introduction to neuroscience, St. Louis, 1972, The C. V. Mosby Co.)

264

In tumors of this gland there are usually visual distrubances due to pressure on the optic chiasm or the optic tract, but there may be disturbances of the other nerves or of circulation. An enlarged pituitary would initially impinge upon the medial aspect of the optic tract, or the posterior aspect of the optic chiasm. Crossover fibers from both nasal retinae run in these parts of the visual pathway. Since nasal retina receives impulses from the temporal or lateral visual field, interruption of normal conduction in the crossover fibers would cause an initial narrowing of the visual field, a condition known as tunnel vision.

The hypophysis is divided into a large anterior lobe and a smaller posterior lobe by a thin sheet of tissue, the intermediate part, lying between the two lobes. In man the intermediate part is very thin, and the two lobes are not sharply separated. From the anterior lobe there is a thin, upward extension along the stalk, called the tuberal part. Embryologically, the posterior lobe is a derivative of the brain, and the remainder of the gland comes from the epithelial lining of the oral cavity. The posterior lobe and the stalk are frequently referred to as the neurohypophysis, and the remainder of the gland is referred to as the adenohypophysis.

Many nerve fibers enter the pituitary from the plexus of sympathetic nerve fibers surrounding the internal carotid artery. The function of these fibers is to control the vascular supply to the gland. There are also bundles of nerve fibers connecting the neurohypophysis with nuclei in the diencephalon (Figs. 8-4 and 8-5).

The production of pituitary hormones is under the control of "releasing factors" produced by the hypothalamus. This production is controlled in various ways: (1) by the level of circulating pituitary hormones reaching the hypothalamus by way of the blood stream (short feedback), (2) by the level of target gland hormone reaching the hypothalamus (long feedback), and (3) by cells of the hypothalamus producing releasing factors in response to stimuli from other areas of the brain or peripheral receptors, for example, visual stimuli. Often the sight of a hungry infant is enough to start milk dripping from the mother's breasts. The visual stimuli travel via nerve impulses from the retina to the hypothalamus and then via hormone release from hypothalamus to pituitary (Fig. 8-6).

Functions. In man the intermediate part has no function. The adenohypophysis is known to secrete at least seven hormones as follows: (1) somatotropin, or growth hormone (GH), is essential for normal body growth. Underproduction of this substance during childhood results in a dwarf. Overproduction in childhood results in a giant, and overproduction in adult life produces acromegaly, a condition charac-

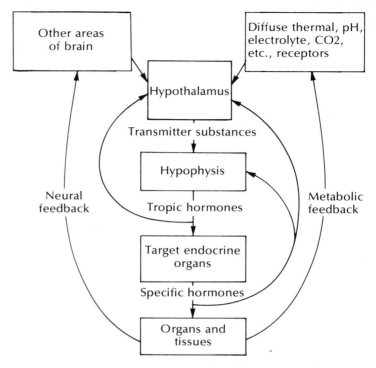

Fig. 8-6. Prototype of neuroendocrine function and feedback systems. (From Minckler, J.: Introduction to neuroscience, St. Louis, 1972, The C. V. Mosby Co.)

terized by enlargement of the extremities and coarsening of the facial features (Fig. 8-7), (2) thyrotropin, or thyroid stimulating hormone (TSH), increases the growth and activity of thyroid cells, (3) corticotropin, or adrenocorticotropic hormone (ACTH), regulates the growth and function of the adrenal cortex and is especially important in the production and release of glucocorticoid hormones such as cortisol, (4) melanocyte stimulating hormone (MSH) in humans increases skin pigmentation by dispersing melanin granules in the melanocytes, (5, 6, and 7) the three gonadotropins are follicle stimulating (FSH), luteinizing (LH), and prolactin (PR), or lactogenic hormones. In women, FSH enlarges the graafian follicle to the point of rupture, and LH in concert with FSH causes ovulation. In men, FSH in conjunction with LH stimulates spermatogenesis. Prolactin is one of the group of hormones necessary for breast development and milk secretion. If gonadotropin production fails before puberty, sexual maturity does not take place; if production fails after puberty, there is a regression of secondary sexual characteristics.

266

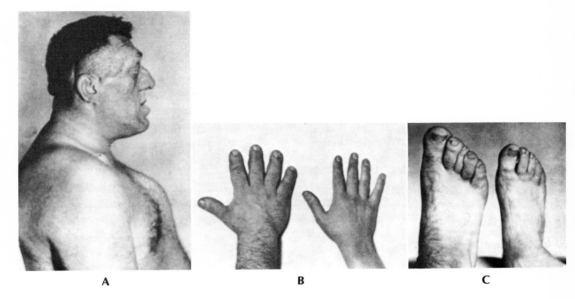

A   B   C

Fig. 8-7. A, Acromegalic patient showing protruding sternum, kyphosis, heavy coarse features, and prognathus. **B,** and **C,** Comparison of acromegalic hand and foot with those of a normal adult male (on the right of each figure). (From Lisser, H., and Escamilla, R. F.: Atlas of clinical endocrinology, ed. 2, St. Louis, 1962, The C. V. Mosby Co.)

The neurohypophysis contains a substance, vasopressin, called the antidiuretic hormone, which is needed for the kidneys to concentrate urine properly and thus to conserve water in the body. If this hormone is deficient, diabetes insipidus results. Another secretion associated with the neurohypophysis, oxytocin, stimulates the contraction of uterine musculature especially during childbirth and also is responsible for the ejection of milk from the breast. Both hormones, elaborated in the neurosecretory cells of the hypothalamus, pass via axons and are released into the circulation of the neurohypophysis (Fig. 8-4).

Because of the large number of hormones produced by the hypophysis, the gland is sometimes referred to as the "master" gland.

Anatomy. The thyroid gland, a horseshoe-shaped mass clasping the upper part of the trachea, lies in the lower part of the neck. It has a large lobe on each side and a median bar, the isthmus, which lies anterior to the upper rings of the trachea (usually the second, third, and fourth). The ultimo-branchial body, an integral part of the thyroid, in man is represented by the parafollicular or C cells.

THYROID GLAND

267

The superior thyroid artery, a branch of the external carotid, enters the gland at the superior end of each lobe, and the inferior thyroid artery, a branch of the thyrocervical trunk from the subclavian, enters the inferior end of each lobe. Sympathetic nerve fibers from the superior and middle cervical ganglia enter with and supply the blood vessels of the gland (Fig. 8-8).

The gland is enclosed within a fibrous capsule that fuses on each side with the fascia surrounding the carotid artery and is intimately united to that of the trachea. In front of the thyroid are the sternohyoid and sternothyroid muscles; these muscles must be pulled aside or cut in operations on the gland. Posterior and lateral to each lobe is the carotid sheath, which contains the jugular vein, the carotid artery, the vagus nerve, and the recurrent laryngeal branch of the vagus (the motor nerve to the vocal folds). Usually during surgery the sur-

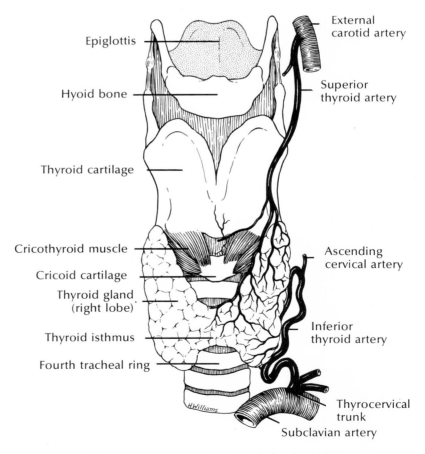

Fig. 8-8. Anterior view of thyroid gland and larynx.

geon does not disturb the posterior inferior portion of either lobe so that he may avoid these structures as well as the parathyroid glands (see Fig. 12-5).

Functions. The thyroid gland produces three hormones: thyroxine, triiodothyronine, and thyrocalcitonin. Thyrocalcitonin, produced by the parafollicular cells, reduces plasma calcium levels by a direct rapid and transient inhibition of bone resorption. The other thyroid hormones have a marked effect on cellular metabolism.

Hypothyroidism (underactivity) results in a decrease in the basal metabolic rate, and hyperthyroidism (overactivity) results in an increase. Iodine is essential for the formation of thyroid hormones.

Goiter, an enlargement of the gland, can be caused by a deficiency of iodine, which prevents the formation of adequate amounts of thyroid hormones. Feedback to the pituitary is reduced resulting in a further release of TSH, which causes hypertrophy of the thyroid cells and eventually of the entire gland. The size of the gland also increases in adolescence, menstruation, and pregnancy.

Hypothyroidism, if it occurs in infancy, leads to a condition known as cretinism. The child fails to grow and is imbecile and infantile. If treatment is not delayed too long, the administration of thyroid hormones will improve the condition. The disease may be the result of an inadequate iodine intake by the mother and occurs most commonly in districts in which the soil contains little iodine.

Hypothyroidism appearing in an adult produces myxedema. A person with this condition takes on a bloated appearance. The skin is sallow and dry, and the senses are dulled. The patient is lethargic and mentally slow. Again, thyroid hormones will alleviate the symptoms.

A person with hyperthyroidism is nervous, restless, and irritable; the heart rate is increased, and the blood pressure is elevated. Despite a very good appetite the patient loses weight. The eyes frequently become protuberant. Removal of part of the gland and administration of certain antithyroid drugs alleviates the disease.

Anatomy. On the back of the thyroid gland and usually embedded within its capsule are several small, round, granular bodies, called the parathyroid glands. There are usually two pairs, but there may be more or fewer. There is also a great variation in size, but commonly they resemble grains of wheat. Each gland is supplied by a single artery that may arise from any branch of the superior or inferior thyroid arteries (Fig. 8-9).

**PARATHYROID
GLANDS**

Functions. The parathyroids are concerned with the regulation of the calcium content of the blood. Calcium is important in the construction of bones and teeth, and the calcium level of the blood is im-

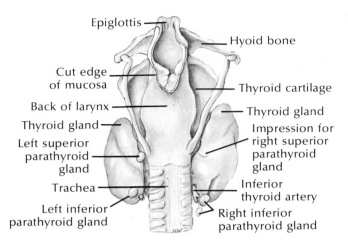

Fig. 8-9. Thyroid and parathyroid glands, posterior view. The specimen is that of a child with an asymmetric larynx. The mucosa and perichondrium have been removed except around the aditus. The right inferior parathyroid gland is double in this case.

portant in determing this formation. The secretion of the parathyroids, parathormone, plays a role along with vitamin D in the calcium balance of the body by strongly stimulating bone resorption, thus releasing calcium and phosphate into the circulation. To have bone growth or remodeling, it is necessary to have this calcium-phosphate product; without it, calcification does not take place normally.

In hypoparathyroidism the most striking manifestation is tetany, an uncontrolled twitching of the muscles of the body. This is caused by a lowering of the calcium ion concentration of the fluids of the body to the point at which the nervous system becomes hyperirritable. Treatment to raise the blood calcium will correct the condition.

Hyperparathyroidism results in an increased blood calcium concentration and, consequently, lethargy and lassitude. As a result of the high blood calcium, relatively huge quantities of calcium salts are excreted in the urine. The individual cannot be kept in a positive calcium balance, and there is a progressive decalcification of the bones, caused by increased bone resorption. Usually such a condition is associated with an adenoma, or tumor, of one of the parathyroid glands, the removal of which tends to relieve the condition.

SUPRARENAL GLANDS

Anatomy. A suprarenal, or adrenal, gland fits like a cap over the superior end of each kidney (see Fig. 8-1). There is a fibrous capsule, the tunica fibrosa, a cortex of glandular tissue, and an inner mass, the

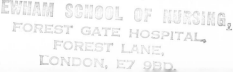

medulla, which is very vascular and composed of chromaffin tissue, so called because it stains yellow or brown when treated with dyes containing chromium salts. The cortex and medulla are functionally two endocrine glands and have different embryologic origins; the cortex is a derivative of the mesoderm of the primitive body wall, whereas the chromaffin tissue develops from the ectoderm (neural crest) in close relation to the sympathetic ganglia. Each suprarenal gland normally has three arteries, one from the inferior phrenic, one from the aorta, and one from the renal artery.

Each gland is richly supplied with nerves, forming a suprarenal plexus in the capsule. There are nerve connections with the celiac plexus and directly from the splanchnic nerves. The sympathetic nerve fibers from the above sources (1) control the blood supply to the gland and (2) stimulate release of epinephrine from the cells of the medulla. The cortex appears to receive no functional motor innervation.

Functions. The adrenal cortex is essential for life. The steroid hormones produced by the cortex can be divided into three major categories: glucocorticoids, mineral corticoids and the sex steroids, or androgens. The glucocorticoids affect metabolism of protein, fat, and glucose; the mineral corticoids control the electrolyte balances of sodium, chloride, and potassium, and the sex steroids cause masculinizing effects. Animals deprived of the adrenal cortex show a rapid decline in body weight, profound weakness, low blood pressure, low blood volume, a decline in blood sodium, and an increase in blood potassium. In man, Addison's disease, which shows many of the signs just described, is relieved by the administration of corticosteroids.

The adrenal cortex may also have an influence on the gonads. During childhood, hypertrophy of the cortex leads to precocious sexual development, and in an adult, to an excessive masculinization.

The adrenal medulla produces epinephrine, which has the same effects on the organism as does the stimulation of sympathetic nerves (thoracolumnar outflow), and may be looked upon as a mechanism to fortify the body for increased activity. Epinephrine causes an increase in the heart rate, an increase in blood pressure, an increased blood flow, and decreased activity of the gastrointestinal tract. The adrenal medulla is not essential for life.

PANCREAS

The pancreas is really a union of two organs having entirely different functions. The pancreatic tissue proper, or exocrine pancreas, is associated with and will be discussed with the digestive system (see Figs. 12-17 and 12-18). The islands of Langerhans, or endocrine pancreas, are collections of four types of cells, A, B, C, and D, which secrete two major hormones, glucagon and insulin. The product of the C cells has not been determined; the D cells probably secrete gastrin, although both may simply be variants of the A or B cells. The A cells secrete glucagon, the physiologic role of which is not clear. A review of its properties, however, suggests that glucagon may (1) stimulate insulin release and (2) increase the peripheral availability and utilization of glucose. Insulin secreted by the B cells is concerned with carbohydrate metabolism. In the usual histologic preparation the islands appear as spheroidal masses of pale staining cells arranged in the form of anastomosing cords. Interspersed between and in intimate contact with the cells making up the cords are numerous blood vessels, an arrangement that facilitates exchange of secretion between cells and vessels. The blood supply to the pancreas is derived from branches of celiac and superior mesenteric arteries, and venous return is via the portal system. Nerve fibers to the pancreas are derived from (1) the greater splanchnic, which controls vascularization of the gland, and (2) the vagus, stimulation of which causes secretion from the exocrine portion of the gland.

Insulin   In hypofunction of the islets the blood sugar rises to abnormally high levels (hyperglycemia), and as a result, glucose is excreted in the urine (glycosuria). These are the outstanding characteristics of diabetes mellitus. There seems to be an impaired ability in both the storage and the oxidation of glucose. Symptoms of diabetes include excessive urination, including night urination, thirst, dry throat, weight loss, and nocturnal cramps in the muscles of the legs and feet. Treatment, which includes diet, is aimed at keeping the blood glucose level within normal physiologic limits.

GONADS   The testes and ovaries, in addition to forming the male or female reproductive cells, secrete into the blood stream certain hormones that control the appearance of the secondary sex characteristics. Testosterone is the most important hormone secreted by the testis, and estrogen and progesterone are secreted by the ovary. Testosterone and estrogen control the appearance and development of secondary sex characteristics such as body contours, distribution of hair, voice change, and maturation of the reproductive organs. Progesterone acts mainly in the preparation of the uterus for implantation as well as on the breast for milk production.

PLACENTA   The placenta is an organ developed within the uterus during pregnancy so that the growing fetus may secure nourishment from and excrete waste material into the maternal blood stream. Throughout

272

pregnancy three placental hormones, estrogen, progesterone, and placental lactogen, are produced that act on the ovary, hypothalamus, and pituitary gland. These high levels of female hormones block ovulation during this period and also influence breast development.

The glands described in the foregoing discussions of this chapter are known to have endocrine functions. The liver is described with the digestive system, although it is known to have endocrine as well as exocrine functions. In the remaining discussions of this chapter, certain structures of the body are grouped that, at the present time, have not been proven to have any endocrine function. It is, however, convenient to describe them here.

MISCELLANEOUS STRUCTURES

The pineal body is a small cone-shaped mass of tissue, about 6 mm in length, attached by means of a hollow stalk to the roof of the third ventricle of the brain and lying on the superior colliculi. The cavity of the stalk is a recess of the third ventricle.

Pineal body

The pineal body is covered by pia mater, and fibrous septa, formed from the pia, subdivide the gland into small lobules. The most distinctive cells within the lobules are large and round, with granular cytoplasm and deeply staining nuclei.

The pineal body appears to produce a substance (melatonin) that, in conjunction with a hypothalamic substance, delays puberty until the normal time.

Associated with the plexuses of the sympathetic system and with its ganglia are tiny masses of chromaffin tissue, known as paraganglia. The development, chemical reaction, and structure of each of these tiny structures resemble those of the medulla of the suprarenal gland. They vary greatly in number; as many as 70 have been found, but usually there are not nearly this many.

Paraganglia

The most prominent are the aortic paraganglia. In the newborn child these are a pair of elongated masses of tissue nearly 12 mm in length lying in front of the abdominal aorta, near the origin of the inferior mesenteric artery. They regress during childhood and in the adult are scarcely visible.

Near the beginning of each internal carotid artery there is located a small mass of tissue containing groups of epitheliallike cells and numerous blood capillaries. The carotid branch of the glossopharyngeal nerve innervates the body. The cells of the body are very sensitive to slight changes in the amounts of oxygen and carbon dioxide in the blood and are therefore known as chemoreceptors. They are important in the reflex regulation of respiration.

Carotid and aortic bodies

273

There are similar small masses of tissue, the aortic bodies, located near the arch of the aorta and innervated by branches from the vagus nerves. These bodies are not to be confused with the aortic paraganglia.

REVIEW QUESTIONS

1. Where is the hypophysis located?
2. List and give functions for the hormones associated with the adenohypophysis.
3. What hormones are associated with the neurohypophysis?
4. Describe the thyroid gland. What are its functions?
5. What is the result of hypothyroidism in infancy? In adult life?
6. Where are the parathyroid glands located? What is their function?
7. Where are the suprarenal glands located?
8. What are the symptoms of a deficiency in adrenal cortical activity?
9. What portion of the pancreas has an endocrine function?
10. Name three secondary sex characteristics.
11. What is the essential characteristic of an endocrine gland?
12. Where is the pineal body located?
13. What is the nerve supply of the carotid body?
14. What is the function of the carotid body?
15. What is the embryonic source of the neurohypophysis and of the adenohypophysis?

CHAPTER 9

THE CIRCULATORY SYSTEM

The circulatory system consists of (1) a muscular pump, the heart, (2) a system of distributing vessels—arteries, capillaries, and veins, (3) a circulating fluid, the blood, and (4) an auxiliary system for returning fluid from the tissue spaces, the lymphatic system.

The blood is discussed in Chapter 2, and the lymphatic system is discussed in Chapter 10.

The blood is pumped from the heart through the arteries, which subdivide into smaller and smaller vessels, ending in capillaries, which form networks in all the tissues of the body except cartilage, the cornea, and outer layers of the skin. From these capillaries arise venules, which unite to form small veins; these in turn are tributaries of larger vessels, which give place to the great veins emptying into the heart.

This entire system has one continuous smooth lining, endothelium, which, together with a small amount of connective tissue, forms the tunica intima. Capillaries have only this one coat, but veins and arteries have two other coats, the tunica media, composed of smooth muscle, and the tunica adventitia, composed of connective tissue. The smooth muscle fibers of the tunica media have a circular arrangement, and in a few of the largest arteries a small number of longitudinal muscle fibers are found in the tunica adventitia. The amount of fibrous and elastic tissue varies, the arteries having more elastic tissue than the veins; in the first portions of the aorta and pulmonary arteries there is a great deal of elastic tissue and almost no smooth muscle. In a cross section of any artery and its accompanying veins (Fig. 9-2), the arterial

275

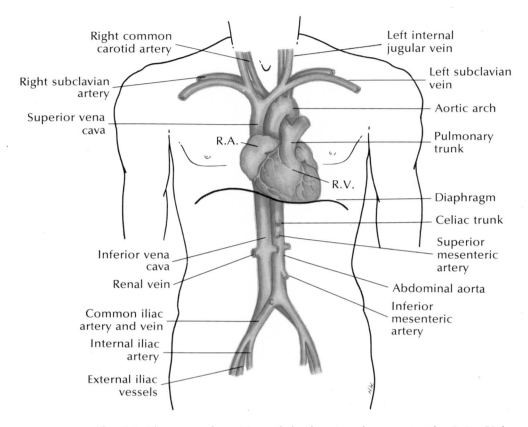

Fig. 9-1. The general position of the heart and great vessels. *R.A.*, Right atrium; *R.V.*, right ventricle.

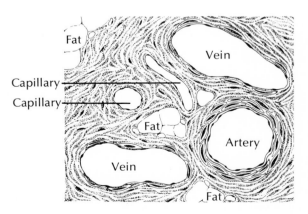

Fig. 9-2. Cross section of small artery, accompanying veins, and capillaries.

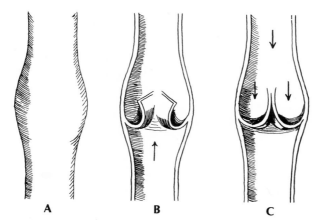

Fig. 9-3. Vein valves. **A,** External view showing dilatation at site of valve. **B,** Vein opened and valves opened. **C,** Valves closed to prevent backflow of blood.

wall is thicker and stronger, and the lumen remains round; the veins collapse when empty, and the lumen almost disappears.

In veins, which carry blood against the force of gravity, folds of the endothelium or tunica intima, called valves, are placed to allow blood to flow freely towards the heart. The valves come together and occlude the vessel when the blood tends to flow away from the heart (Fig. 9-3). Valves, therefore, are commonest in the lower extremity and are absent in the veins of the head and neck, the venae cavae, and the pulmonary and portal systems. Valves are not present in arteries.

Arteries with their accompanying veins usually run along the flexor side of a limb where they are well protected from injury and where there is little stretch on the vessels during movement. An artery is usually more deeply placed than its accompanying veins and lymphatic channels.

Arteries are well supplied with fine nerve fibers received from nearby nerve trunks. These fibers form extensive plexuses about the arteries and contain sensory fibers as well as vasomotor sympathetic fibers. The larger blood vessels have within their walls smaller vessels to nourish the tunics; these are known as vasa vasorum (vessels of vessels).

The blood carries oxygen and dissolved food material to the cells of the body and carries waste material from the tissues to the excretory organs of the body, namely, to the lungs, the kidneys, and the skin (Fig. 9-4).

277

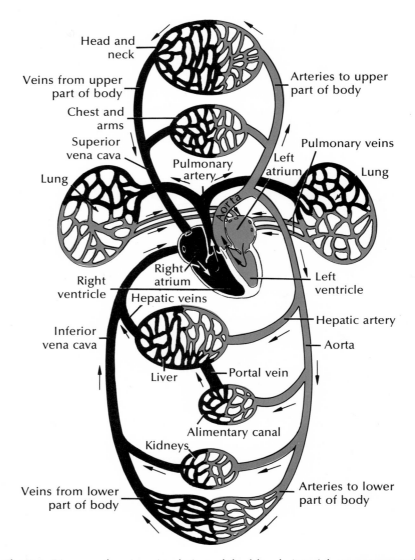

Fig. 9-4. Diagram showing circulation of the blood. Arterial, or oxygenated, blood is shown in red; venous blood is shown in black. (From Schottelius, B. A., and Schottelius, D. D.: Textbook of physiology, ed. 17, St. Louis, 1973, The C. V. Mosby Co.)

278

Blood vessels are subdivided into the following three groups:
1. The pulmonary system, which carries blood to and from the lungs
2. The portal system, which carries blood from the spleen, stomach, and intestines to the liver
3. The general or systemic system, which carries blood to and from the heart for the rest of the body

HEART

The heart is a four-chambered muscular organ completely divided into right and left portions by a septum. In each half there is an upper chamber, the atrium, which receives blood from the veins and a lower chamber, the ventricle, which pumps blood out into the arteries. There is an opening leading from the atrium to the ventricle supplied with valves that prevent blood from flowing back into the atrium when the ventricle contracts. There are valves performing a similar function at the outlet of each ventricle into the artery.

The heart, enclosed by pericardium, lies in the lower part of the mediastinum posterior to the sternum, between the lungs, above the middle portion of the diaphragm, and anterior to the esophagus and the thoracic portion of the aorta.

The base of the heart is formed largely by the left atrium. The left pulmonary veins enter the left atrium on its left border. On the right border the superior and inferior venae cavae enter the right atrium,

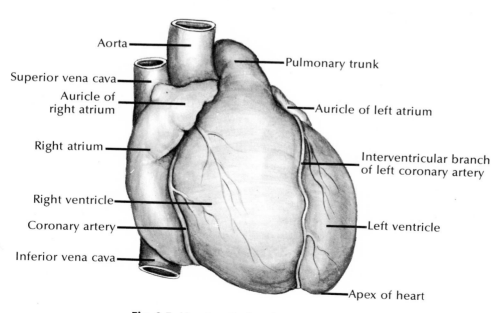

Fig. 9-5. Heart, anterior view.

279

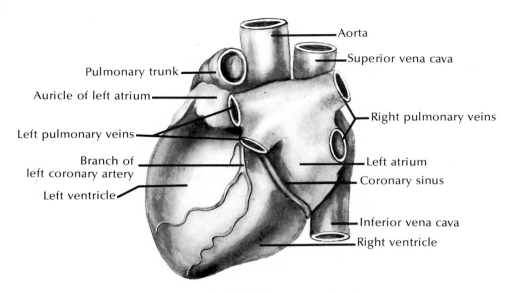

Aorta

Superior vena cava

Pulmonary trunk

Auricle of left atrium

Right pulmonary veins

Left pulmonary veins

Branch of
left coronary artery

Left atrium

Coronary sinus

Left ventricle

Inferior vena cava

Right ventricle

Fig. 9-6. Heart, posterior view.

and the right pulmonary veins pass transversely behind the right atrium to enter the left atrium.

The right border of the heart, formed by the right atrium, lies closely parallel to the right margin of the sternum from the level of the third to the sixth costal cartilage.

The inferior border of the heart extends from the level of the junction of the sixth right costal cartilage with the sternum to the fifth left intercostal space, about 7.5 cm from the sternum. This border is formed mostly by the right ventricle, but on the extreme left, the left ventricle enters into its composition at the apex of the heart.

The left border extends from the apex obliquely upward to the junction of the left third costal cartilage and the sternum. It is formed mainly by the left ventricle but at its upper end by a small part of the left atrium also.

In short, in thickset persons the heart lies more horizontally on the diaphragm, and its apex is a little higher and more to the left than in slender, tall persons.

Chambers of heart   The right atrium receives venous blood (blood, poor in oxygen and rich in carbon dioxide, returning from all parts of the body) from the venae cavae and from the walls of the heart itself by way of the coronary sinus. The opening from the right atrium into the right ventricle is called the tricuspid orifice because the valve has three cusps.

280

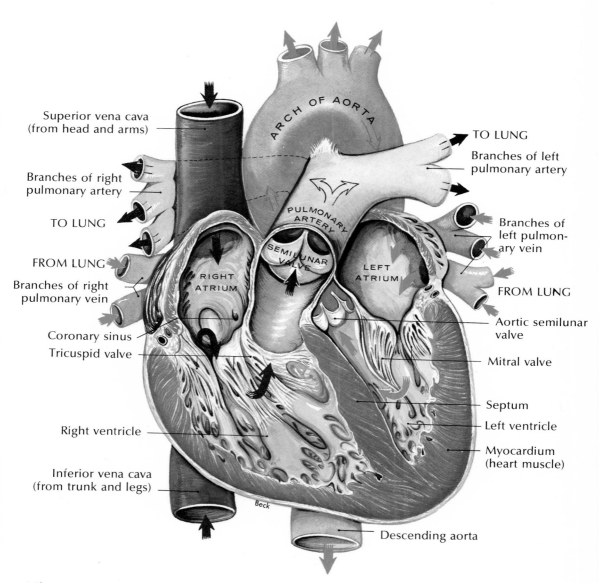

Fig. 9-7. Frontal section of the heart showing the four chambers, valves, openings, and major vessels. Arrows indicate direction of blood flow. Black arrows represent unoxygenated blood and red arrows oxygenated blood. The two branches of the right pulmonary vein extend from the right lung behind the heart to enter the left atrium. (From Anthony, C. P., and Kolthoff, N. J.: Textbook of anatomy and physiology, ed. 8, St. Louis, 1971, The C. V. Mosby Co.)

The walls of the right atrium are relatively thin and smooth except in front where the muscles are arranged in columns to form pectinate bundles. The outer side of the atrium has an outpouching called the auricle because of its earlike shape.

The left atrium receives oxygenated blood from the lungs by way of the four pulmonary veins. The left atrioventricular valve is called the mitral valve and has only two cusps. There are pectinate muscles in the wall, and there is an auricular appendage on the lateral side.

In the wall separating the two atria is a small oval depression, the fossa ovalis, marking the site of an opening between the two atria, which closed at birth.

The right ventricle has much thicker walls than the atria. It receives venous blood from the right atrium and pumps it through the pulmonary trunk into the lungs. The opening into the artery is guarded by a valve having three cusps. The musculature of the ventricle is arranged in projecting muscle columns, called trabeculae carneae.

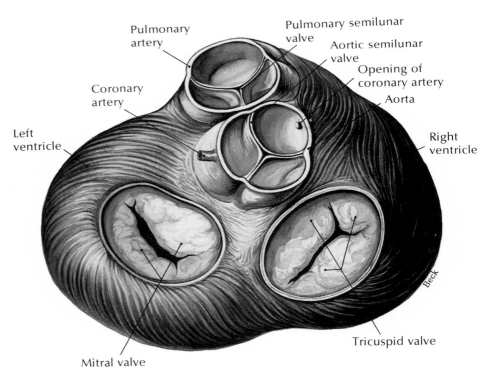

Fig. 9-8. The valves of the heart, superior view. The atria are removed to show the mitral tricuspid valves. (From Anthony, C. P., and Kolthoff, N. J.: Textbook of anatomy and physiology, ed. 8, St. Louis, 1971, The C. V. Mosby Co.)

Other muscle bundles form cone-shaped masses, called papillary muscles. From the apex of each papillary muscle a strong, white band, chorda tendinea, extends to the edge of the tricuspid valve. One of the trabeculae carneae stretches across the lower part of the cavity of the right ventricle and is known as the moderator band.

The left ventricle has even thicker walls than the right ventricle. It receives oxygenated blood from the left atrium and sends it through the aorta to all parts of the body. The aortic opening has a valve of three cusps similar to the one for the pulmonary trunk. The ventricular wall is provided with trabeculae (columnae) carneae. The papillary muscles of the left ventricle are larger than those of the right and connect with the edges of the mitral valve by means of the chordae tendineae.

The valves between the right ventricle and the pulmonary trunk and between the left ventricle and the aorta are three simple semilunar flaps attached at their outer border to the wall of the vessel. They are composed of endothelium, with some strengthening bands of fibrous tissue. Each ventricular valve is a fold of endothelium, but the free margin is irregular and attached to the chordae tendineae. In contractions of the ventricle the chordae tendineae keep the valves from turning inside out. The action is very similar to that of the cords of a parachute. The right atrioventricular orifice will admit three fingers, and the left, two.

In the septum between the two halves of the heart is a bundle of pale muscle fibers that partakes somewhat of the nature of nerve tissue and is the conducting system of the heart. It begins as a small node in the lower part of the posterior wall of the right atrium, near the opening of the superior vena cava; this node is known as the sinoatrial, or sinuatrial, node (SA node). The atrioventricular node (AV node) is located in the interatrial wall of the right atrium, just above the opening of the coronary sinus. From the AV node arises the atrioventricular bundle (bundle of Kent or bundle of His), which runs anteriorly in the atrial septum and then into the ventricular septum, where it divides into right and left branches, which break up into many fine strands beneath the endocardium and pass to the muscle bundles of the ventricles. This final network is also called the Purkinje system. In summary, the conducting system of the heart consists of the sinoatrial node, the atrioventricular node, the atrioventricular bundle with two branches, and the final network beneath the endocardium, or inner lining, of the ventricles (Fig. 9-9).

The intrinsic beat of the heart (72 per minute in a normal adult), beginning in the embryo prior to external nervous control, can operate without outside influence. This factor is utilized in heart transplants,

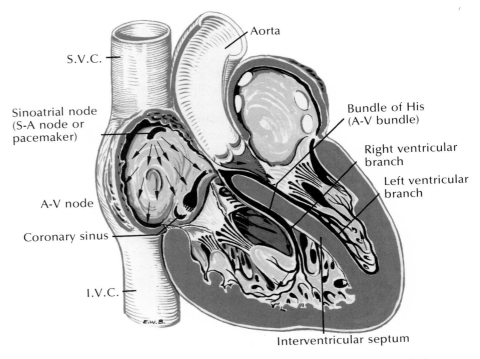

Fig. 9-9. Illustration showing intrinsic nervous mechanism of the mammalian heart. (From Schottelius, B. A., and Schottelius, D. D.: Textbook of physiology, ed. 17, St. Louis, 1973, The C. V. Mosby Co.)

in which all external nerves are severed. Once a transplanted heart is in place, an electric shock will initiate the intrinsic system. Although the external nerve supply is the major modifying influence on heart rate, cardiac responses to increased physiologic demand appear to be quite adequately controlled by other factors such as hormonal mechanisms.

Nerve fibers pass to the heart from the vagus nerves (cranial autonomic outflow) and from the upper thoracic nerves (thoracolumbar autonomic outflow). Sensory nerve fibers accompany the thoracic branches, and since the first and second thoracic nerves also receive sensory fibers from the inner side of the arm, patients with heart disease (angina pectoris or coronary thrombosis) often complain of severe pain in the inner side of the left arm when the actual source of pain is in the heart, a condition known as referred pain.

The postnatal circulation of blood through the heart may be summarized in the following manner. Venous blood received from the venae cavae into the right atrium passes through the tricuspid orifice into the right ventricle, which in turn pumps the blood through the pulmonary orifice into the pulmonary trunk and thus to the lungs. Oxygenated blood is received from the lungs into the left atrium through the pulmonary veins and passes through the mitral orifice into the left ventricle, which pumps it into the aorta and so to all parts of the body.

In the fetus, the placenta acts as an organ of nourishment, excretion, and respiration. Fetal blood passes to the placenta by way of the umbilical arteries, which are branches of the internal iliac (hypogastric) arteries. Oxygenated blood returns to the fetus by way of the umbilical vein. When this blood reaches the liver, most of it is shunted around this organ by means of the ductus venosus and empties into the inferior vena cava and on into the right atrium.

Entering the right atrium are two major streams of blood. Oxygenated blood from the inferior vena cava enters the right atrium, and although some enters the right ventricle, the majority is directed through the foramen ovale into the left atrium. The oxygenated blood then passes into the left ventricle and on into the aorta to be supplied to both oxygen-demanding as well as rapidly growing regions such as the brain, heart, and upper limbs. Deoxygenated blood returning via the superior vena cava enters the right atrium and is directed almost exclusively into the right ventricle. It then passes into the pulmonary trunk, but since the lungs are nonfunctional, the majority of the deoxygenated blood is shunted via the ductus arteriosus into the arch of the aorta distal to the branches to the head and upper limbs. The descending aorta in the embryo therefore carries blood with only a medium level of oxygen saturation (Figs. 9-10 and 9-11).

Important changes occur in the circulation pattern at birth. Placental circulation ceases causing a drop of pressure in the inferior vena cava and the right atrium. Aeration of the lungs is associated with a marked increase in pulmonary flow and a dramatic rise in pressure in the left atrium above that of the right. The increased left atrial pressure forces the valve of the foramen ovale to close. Initially this is only a functional closure that can be overcome by an increase in right atrial pressure. With time, however, the closing is anatomical, caused by a proliferation of endothelial and fibrous tissue, and the foramen eventually is represented by the fossa ovale, a thin oval area on the atrial septum. The umbilical arteries eventually become the lateral umbilical ligaments, two fibrous bands lying beneath the anterior parietal peritoneum and passing from the umbilicus into the true pelvis (see Fig. 9-20). The umbilical vein becomes the ligamentum teres hepatis, or round ligament of the liver, passing as a cord from the umbilicus, within the falciform ligament of the liver, to the

285

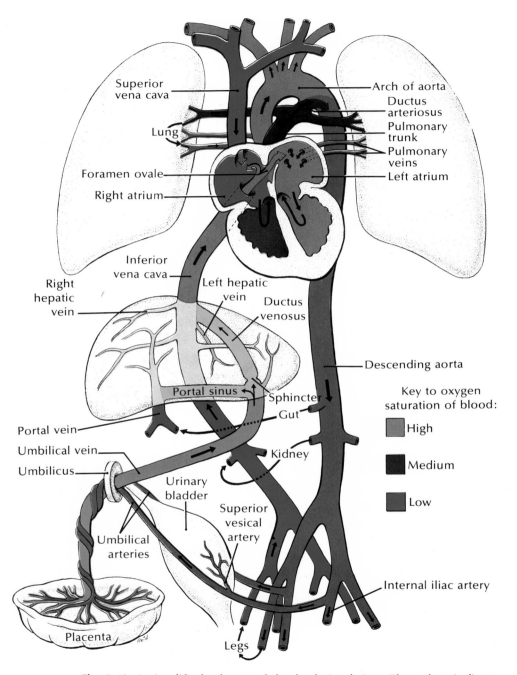

Superior
vena cava

Arch of aorta

Ductus
arteriosus

Pulmonary
trunk

Lung

Pulmonary
veins

Foramen ovale

Left atrium

Right atrium

Inferior
vena cava

Left hepatic
vein

Right
hepatic
vein

Ductus
venosus

Descending aorta

Portal sinus

Sphincter

Gut

Key to oxygen
saturation of blood:

High

Portal vein

Umbilical vein

Kidney

Medium

Umbilicus

Low

Urinary
bladder

Superior
vesical
artery

Umbilical
arteries

Internal iliac artery

Placenta

Legs

Fig. 9-10. A simplified scheme of the fetal circulation. The colors indicate
the oxygen saturation of the blood and the arrows show the course of the
fetal circulation. The organs are not drawn to scale. (From Moore, K.: The
developing human, Philadelphia, 1973, W. B. Saunders Company.)

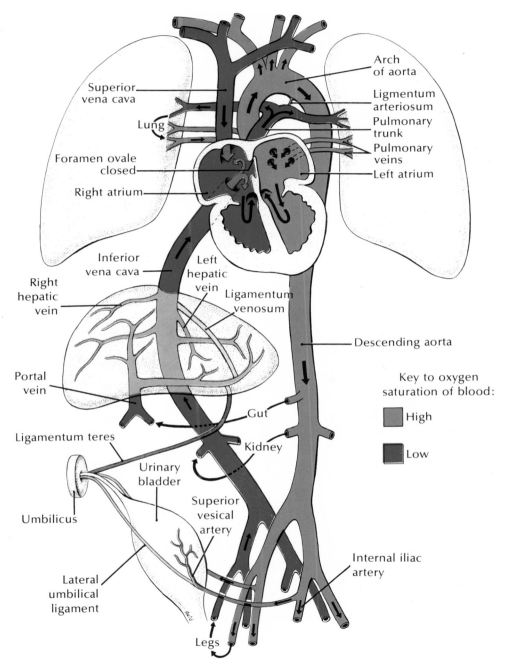

Fig. 9-11. A simplified representation of the circulation after birth. The adult derivatives of the fetal vessels and structures that become nonfunctional at birth are also shown. The arrows indicate the course of the neonatal circulation. The organs are not drawn to scale. (From Moore, K.: The developing human, Philadelphia, 1973, W. B. Saunders Company.)

287

porta hepatis. The ductus venosus and the ductus arteriosus become fibrous cords.

In health the heart is roughly proportionate to the size of a person and is often said to be as large as the clenched fist. Average measurements for the adult heart are 12.5 cm in length, 9 cm in breadth, and 6 cm in thickness.

Skeleton of heart

The heart has a fibrocartilaginous skeleton that surrounds and gives insertion to the valves. The myocardial fibers also originate from and insert into this skeleton. Hence, upon contraction, the heart is literally "wrung out," an effective means of propelling blood through and out of the heart chambers.

Pericardium

The pericardium is a sac that surrounds the heart. It lies in the middle mediastinum posterior to the sternum. The pericardium has a serous lining like that of the pleura; the parietal layer lines the pericardial sac; the visceral layer covers the heart itself.

The visceral layer continues over the beginnings of the great vessels to merge into the parietal layer at the base of the heart.

Enveloping the parietal serous membrane is a tough, fibrous coat, called the fibrous pericardium. This dense coat prevents overdistension of the heart, and by fibrous connections to the sternum and central tendon of the diaphragm, anchors the heart to the mediastinum.

Clinical considerations

Heart sounds. The heart sounds are produced by the shutting of two sets of valves causing a sound commonly described as lub-dub or thump-bump. The first sound is caused by the closing of the inlet valves, the right and left atrioventricular valves, and the second by the closing of the outlet or semilunar valves. The inlet valves open and shut at about the same time as do the outlet valves. When the ventricles fill with blood the inlet valves shut coinciding with ventricular emptying, or systole. The second sound is heard at the beginning of ventricular filling, or diastole. Auscultation of heart sounds is performed over the major valve area; however, sounds are transmitted in the direction of blood flow, resulting in a shift in location of the valve areas from the site of topographic projection (Fig. 9-12). Abnormal sounds or noises, the so-called heart murmurs, may or may not indicate a disease state. A diseased or narrowed valve, such as occurs following rheumatic fever, will cause increased velocity and turbulence in the blood flow with a coinciding murmur.

Congenital heart defects. Hereditary or environmental factors, often in conjunction, cause approximately 1 of every 1000 babies to be born with some form of heart defect. With the aid of new surgical tech-

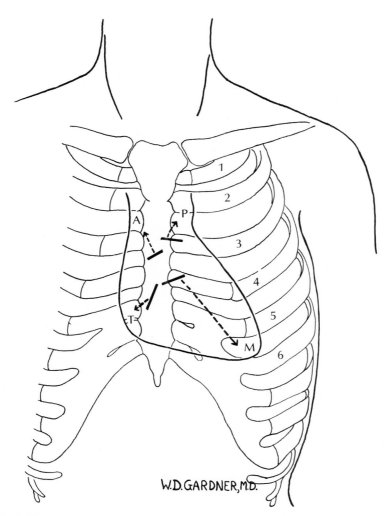

Fig. 9-12. Projection of the cardiac outline and the valve areas to the chest wall. *A*, Aortic valve clinical or auscultatory area; *P*, pulmonary valve clinical or auscultatory area; *T*, tricuspid valve clinical or auscultatory area; *M*, mitral valve clinical or auscultatory area. Solid bars connected to the clinical areas by arrows represent the actual anatomic locations. Numbers indicate rib levels. (From Gardner, W. D.: Diagnostic anatomy, St. Louis, The C. V. Mosby Co.)

niques many of these are now repairable. Blue baby, a term familiar to many, refers to a child born with a defect that allows various amounts of incoming venous blood to pass directly through the heart and into the body again without being oxygenated in the lungs. Common causes are a patent foramen ovale or ductus arteriosus (Figs. 9-10 and 9-11).

ARTERIES
Pulmonary trunk

The single artery arising from the right ventricle is called the pulmonary trunk to distinguish it from its two branches, the right and left pulmonary arteries. The pulmonary trunk arises from the upper left portion of the right ventricle on the anterior aspect of the heart, curves superiorly and then posteriorly, passing to the left of the ascending aorta to divide about 5 cm from its origin into right and left branches. The right branch passes posterior to the ascending aorta and the superior vena cava, enters the hilus of the right lung, and subdivides into branches for the lobes. The left branch of the pulmonary trunk passes into the hilus of the left lung.

Thoracic aorta and
branches

The aorta arises from the base of the left ventricle. At its origin it lies to the right of and behind the pulmonary trunk. The ascending part of the aorta passes upward in front of the right branch of the pulmonary trunk. The aortic arch curves over this vessel to occupy a position to the left of the vertebral column. The aorta then descends through the posterior part of the mediastinum and passes behind the diaphragm into the abdomen.

At its origin the ascending aorta has a dilated portion, and the three semilunar valves that guard the orifice form three secondary aortic sinuses (the sinuses of Valsalva). The two coronary arteries that supply the heart arise from two of the aortic sinuses. The right coronary arises from the right aortic sinus and has several branches: the anterior ventricular, right atrial, right marginal, and posterior interventricular. The left coronary arises from the left aortic sinus and has anterior interventricular, left atrial, and circumflex branches. The two interventricular branches anastomose with each other at the apex of the heart, and the circumflex branch of the left coronary anastomoses with the terminal part of the right coronary to form an arterial ring around the base of the ventricles.

Three branches originate from the arch of the aorta:
1. Brachiocephalic trunk (innominate)
2. Left common carotid
3. Left subclavian

The brachiocephalic trunk subdivides to form the right subclavian and right common carotid arteries. The subclavian artery supplies the upper extremity and gives one important branch, the vertebral artery, to the brain.

Each common carotid artery passes up into the neck beside the trachea and divides into the external and internal carotid arteries. The carotid sinus is a dilatation of the terminal portion of the common carotid and of the beginning of the internal carotid. Its walls are quite elastic, and the sensory nerve endings from this region passing to the glossopharyngeal nerve are part of the blood pressure and respiratory regulating mechanisms.

The external carotid supplies the structures of the neck, face, mouth, jaws, and scalp. Its branches are the superior thyroid, lingual, facial (external maxillary), occipital, posterior auricular, ascending pharyngeal, superficial temporal, and (internal) maxillary arteries. Frequently the facial and lingual arise from a common linguofacial trunk. The middle meningeal artery is a branch of the maxillary artery

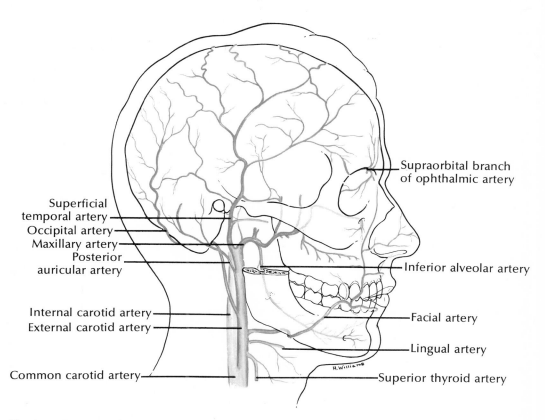

Fig. 9-13. Arteries of the face. Deeper vessels are shown in paler color than superficial vessels.

291

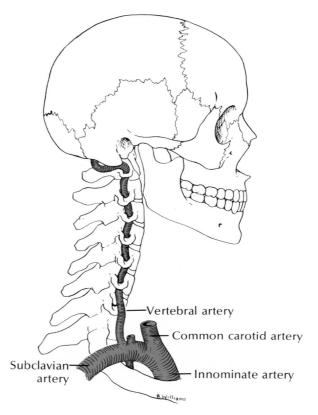

Fig. 9-14. Location of the vertebral artery. (From Anthony, C. P., and Kolthoff, N. J.: Textbook of anatomy and physiology, ed. 8, St. Louis, 1971, The C. V. Mosby Co.)

and plays an important role in the blood supply of the meninges of the brain. Other branches of the maxillary artery supply the nasal cavity and palate.

The internal carotid, having no branches in the neck, enters the middle cranial fossa through the carotid canal, where it helps to form the arterial circle at the base of the brain. The vertebral arteries pass up through the lateral foramina of the cervical vertebrae and through the foramen magnum into the cranial cavity (Figs. 9-14 and 9-15). On the undersurface of the brain stem the two vertebral arteries unite to form the basilar artery, which continues into the middle cranial fossa. By means of anastomotic branches the two internal carotids and the basilar artery form an arterial circle at the base of the brain (circle of Willis). From these vessels arise the arteries supplying the brain. The anterior and middle cerebral arteries are branches of the internal

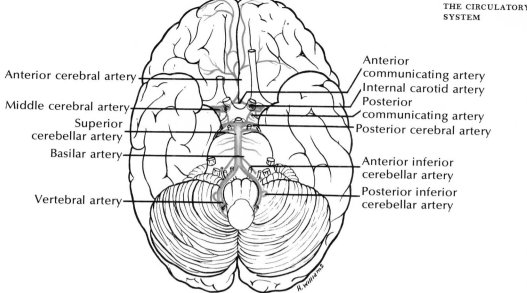

Fig. 9-15. Arteries of base of brain. (Male, 45 years of age.)

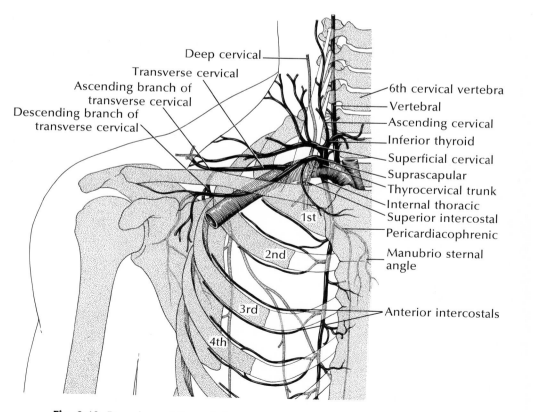

Fig. 9-16. Branches of the subclavian artery.

293

carotid; the posterior cerebral artery is a branch of the basilar. The ophthalmic artery, supplying the eyeball and forehead, also comes from the internal carotid. The various cerebellar arteries arise from the vertebral or basilar artery.

The subclavian artery, having given origin to the vertebral artery, supplies branches to the shoulder, chest wall, and neck. These branches are the thyrocervical trunk, the transverse cervical artery, the suprascapular artery, the internal thoracic (internal mammary) artery, and the costocervical trunk (Fig. 9-16). The continuation of the subclavian artery into the armpit is called the axillary artery, which in turn continues into the upper arm as the brachial artery. The axillary artery has six branches that supply the region of the shoulder joint: the supreme thoracic, thoracoacromial, lateral thoracic, subscapular, and anterior and posterior humeral circumflex arteries (Figs. 9-17 and 9-18). The brachial artery has muscular branches and also gives off the profunda artery of the arm and the superior and inferior ulnar collateral arteries. At the elbow the brachial artery divides into the radial and ulnar arteries, which pass down, one on each side of

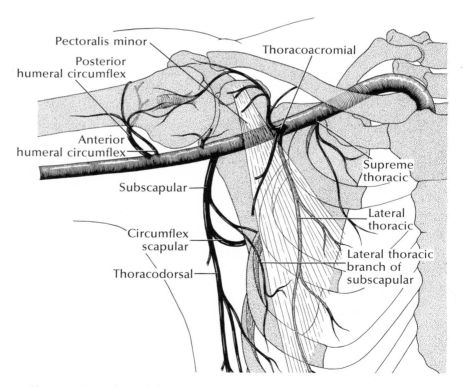

Fig. 9-17. Branches of the axillary artery.

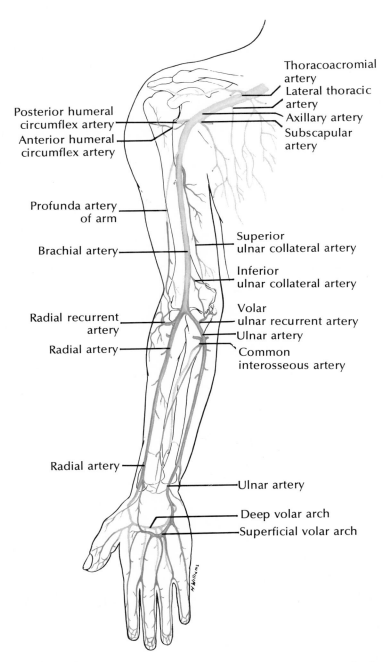

Posterior humeral
circumflex artery

Anterior humeral
circumflex artery

Thoracoacromial
artery

Lateral thoracic
artery

Axillary artery

Subscapular
artery

Profunda artery
of arm

Brachial artery

Superior
ulnar collateral artery

Inferior
ulnar collateral artery

Radial recurrent
artery

Radial artery

Volar
ulnar recurrent artery

Ulnar artery

Common
interosseous artery

Radial artery

Ulnar artery

Deep volar arch

Superficial volar arch

Fig. 9-18. Arteries of upper extremity, anterior view. Deeper vessels shown
in paler color than superficial vessels.

295

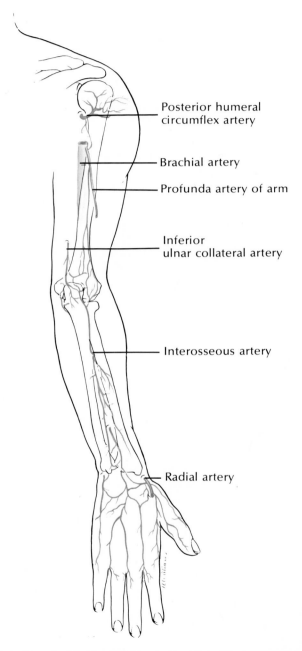

Posterior humeral
circumflex artery

Brachial artery

Profunda artery of arm

Inferior
ulnar collateral artery

Interosseous artery

Radial artery

Fig. 9-19. Arteries of upper extremity, posterior view. Deeper vessels are
shown in paler color than superficial vessels.

the forearm, giving off muscular and interosseous branches. In the palm the ulnar and radial arteries form two palmar arches, a superficial and a deep, which give off numerous branches to the hand and fingers. The extensive anastomosis of the palmar arteries makes it difficult to control arterial hemorrhage of the hand, and often each end of a cut vessel must be tied. The pulse is usually palpated at the inferior end of the radial artery where it lies just under the skin on the front of the radius (Fig. 9-18).

An anastomosis is, in an anatomical sense, a connecting channel between blood vessels. Three types of anastomosis are found in the body, arterial, venous, or arteriovenous. **Anastomosis**

Arterial anastomoses are connections between two or more arteries or their branches. They are particularly evident around joints and in vital organs such as the brain. An exception to this is the blood supply via coronary arteries to the walls of the heart. The coronary arteries are peculiar in that each branch follows its own course to some area of the heart having few if any connections with nearby branches. If one of the coronary arteries or its branches are obstructed either by a deposition of foreign tissue, such as a mass of fat forming on the inside of the arterial wall, a condition known as atherosclerosis, or by a blood clot, the cardiac muscle that depends on the occluded coronary vessel will die and be replaced by a connective tissue scar. Some people have more coronary connections than others, and as the percentage of collateral channels increases, the incidence of death from coronary disease decreases.

The arterial circle around the base of the brain (the circle of Willis) exemplifies further the importance of arterial anastomosis (Fig. 9-15). Brain tissue receives its blood supply from the two internal carotids and the two vertebral arteries. In the circle of Willis these vessels or their branches are united by communicating channels. If, for example, the right internal carotid is occluded, blood will flow from the vertebrals and the left internal carotid via the communicating channels, bypassing the occlusion and thereby maintaining blood supply to the region.

An example of the importance of arterial anastomosis around a joint can be seen when occlusion occurs in the axillary artery. Branches of the subclavian, namely, the transverse cervical and suprascapular, supply the medial or vertebral border of the scapula, the supraspinous and infraspinous fossae and associated musculature, respectively. Intercostal vessels, branches of the thoracic aorta and the internal thoracic artery, also supply the serratus anterior, which inserts into the vertebral border of the scapula. Collateral, or communi-

297

cating, arterial channels from these vessels join with branches from the subscapular and subscapular circumflex arteries, which arise from the axillary. As long as the occlusion is proximal to the subscapular artery and distal to the branches of the subclavian involved in the anastomosis, blood will flow backwards via the subscapular to the axillary and into the upper limb (Figs. 9-16 and 9-17).

The descending portion of the thoracic aorta supplies branches to the chest wall, the esophagus, the bronchi, and the mediastinum. There are usually nine pairs of intercostal arteries for the nine lower intercostal spaces. There are also intercostal branches from the internal thoracic artery, and the first and second intercostal spaces are supplied from the costocervical trunk.

Abdominal aorta and branches

The abdominal aorta supplies both visceral and parietal branches. The visceral branches include the following:

1. One suprarenal artery to each suprarenal gland
2. One renal artery to each kidney
3. One spermatic artery to each ovary (or testis)
4. A single median celiac trunk dividing into three main branches, namely, hepatic, splenic, and left gastric (see Fig. 10-10)
5. A single median superior mesenteric artery that supplies many branches to the small intestine and the proximal half of the large intestine (see Fig. 10-11)
6. A single median inferior mesenteric artery that supplies branches to the distal half of the large intestine (see Fig. 10-11)

The parietal branches go to the diaphragm (inferior phrenic artery) and to the dorsal abdominal wall (lumbar arteries).

There are anastomoses in the region of the pancreas between branches of the celiac and superior mesenteric arteries, and branches from superior and inferior mesenteric arteries going to the colon anastomose with each other in the mesocolon. The three main branches of the celiac trunk have large anastomotic connections with each other around the stomach.

The abdominal aorta divides into the common iliac arteries in front of the fourth lumbar vertebra. Each common iliac artery in turn divides into the internal iliac (hypogastric) and the external iliac arteries (Fig. 9-20).

The internal iliac artery supplies the structures lying within the walls of the pelvis, the buttocks, and the genitalia. It has an anterior and a posterior division, and its branches are quite variable. Usually from the posterior division arise the iliolumbar, lateral sacral, and superior gluteal arteries. From the anterior division arise the obturator, inferior gluteal, internal pudendal, inferior vesical, middle hemor-

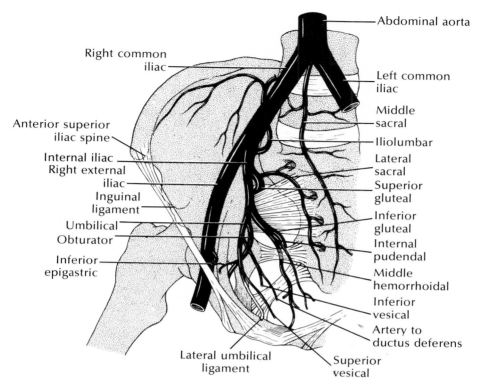

Right common iliac

Anterior superior iliac spine

Internal iliac
Right external iliac
Inguinal ligament
Umbilical
Obturator
Inferior epigastric

Abdominal aorta

Left common iliac

Middle sacral

Iliolumbar

Lateral sacral

Superior gluteal

Inferior gluteal

Internal pudendal

Middle hemorrhoidal

Inferior vesical

Artery to ductus deferens

Lateral umbilical ligament

Superior vesical

Fig. 9-20. The branches of the right internal iliac (hypogastric) artery.

rhoidal (rectal), and superior vesical (remains of the umbilical artery of the fetus) arteries. In women the uterine and vaginal arteries also arise from the anterior division.

A more detailed description of the arterial supply is given with the discussion of the individual visceral organs.

The main blood supply of the lower extremity is the external iliac artery, which becomes the femoral in the thigh and the popliteal behind the knee, beyond which it subdivides into the anterior and posterior tibial arteries, which pass down the anterior and posterior aspects of the leg (Figs. 9-21 and 9-22). The posterior tibial passes around the medial malleolus into the sole of the foot where it subdivides into medial and lateral plantar branches. The posterior tibial artery can be palpated just below and behind the medial malleolus. The anterior tibial artery passes down the front of the leg on the lateral side of the tibia to the dorsum of the foot where it is called the dorsalis pedis. The terminal branches of the anterior and posterior tibial arteries anastomose to form arterial arches in the sole of the foot, from which vessels pass to the toes.

299

Table 13. Main arteries

Name	Chief branches	Area supplied
Ascending aorta	Coronary	Heart
Aortic arch	Brachiocephalic Left subclavian Left common carotid	
Brachiocephalic	Right subclavian Right common carotid	Head and neck
Common carotid	Internal carotid External carotid	Brain Neck and face
Subclavian	Vertebral Internal thoracic Thyrocervical trunk Axillary	Brain Chest Neck Upper extremity
Axillary	Thoracoacromial trunk Subscapular Brachial	Shoulder Arm
Brachial	Profunda brachii Radial ⟩ Ulnar	Arm Forearm and hand
Abdominal aorta	Celiac trunk Superior mesenteric Inferior mesenteric Renal Spermatic Common iliac	 Small intestine Large intestine Kidney Testis or ovary
Celiac	Hepatic Left gastric Splenic	Liver Stomach Spleen
Common iliac	Internal iliac External iliac	Pelvic region
External iliac	Inferior epigastric Femoral	Lower abdominal wall Lower extremity
Femoral	Profunda femoris Popliteal	Thigh
Popliteal	Anterior tibial ⟩ Posterior tibial	Leg and foot

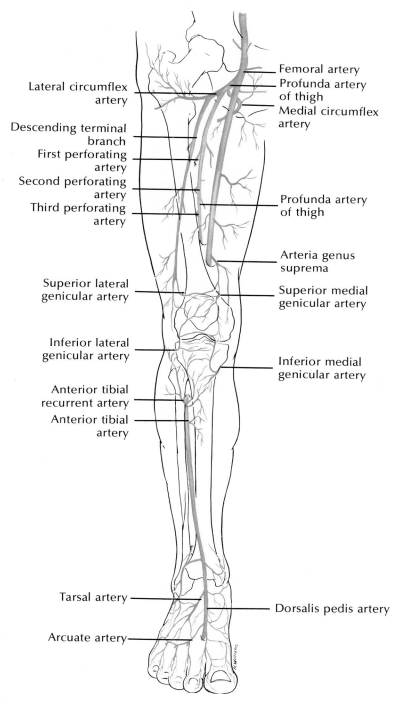

Lateral circumflex
artery

Descending terminal
branch
First perforating
artery
Second perforating
artery
Third perforating
artery

Superior lateral
genicular artery

Inferior lateral
genicular artery

Anterior tibial
recurrent artery
Anterior tibial
artery

Tarsal artery

Arcuate artery

Femoral artery
Profunda artery
of thigh
Medial circumflex
artery

Profunda artery
of thigh

Arteria genus
suprema

Superior medial
genicular artery

Inferior medial
genicular artery

Dorsalis pedis artery

Fig. 9-21. Arteries of lower extremity, anterior view. Deeper vessels are
shown in paler color than superficial vessels.

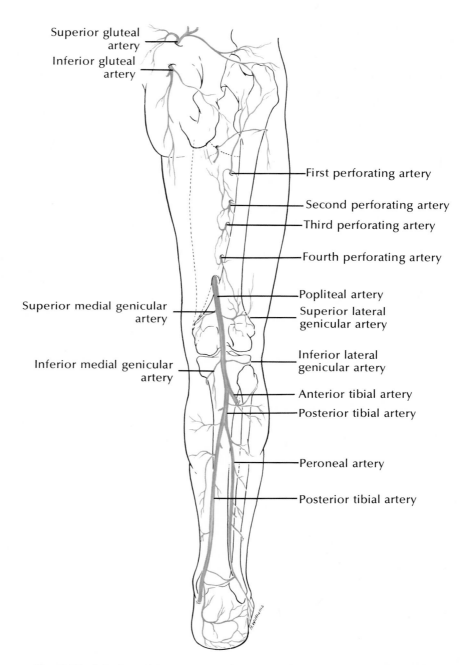

Superior gluteal
artery

Inferior gluteal
artery

First perforating artery

Second perforating artery

Third perforating artery

Fourth perforating artery

Popliteal artery

Superior lateral
genicular artery

Superior medial genicular
artery

Inferior lateral
genicular artery

Inferior medial genicular
artery

Anterior tibial artery

Posterior tibial artery

Peroneal artery

Posterior tibial artery

Fig. 9-22. Arteries of lower extremity, posterior view. Deeper vessels are
shown in paler color than superficial vessels. The adductor magnus muscle
is dotted in to show relation to perforating arteries.

302

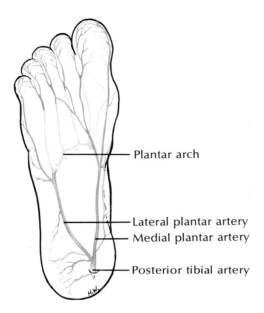

— Plantar arch

— Lateral plantar artery
— Medial plantar artery

— Posterior tibial artery

Fig. 9-23. Arteries of sole of foot. Deeper vessels are shown in paler color than superficial vessels.

The obturator artery supplies branches to the muscles in the medial portion of the thigh and a branch to the hip joint.

The external iliac artery has the following branches: inferior epigastric and deep circumflex iliac. The femoral artery, in addition to numerous muscular branches, has the superficial circumflex iliac, superficial epigastric, superficial and deep external pudendal arteries, the profunda artery of the thigh, and the highest artery of the knee. The popliteal gives off five genicular branches that enter into an anastomosis at about the knee joint.

Within each extremity there are numerous anastomosing branches about each joint. If the main blood channel is blocked off, the distal portion of the limb is able to receive nourishment by blood flowing through these communicating channels, which in time become large enough to permit normal functioning of the part. The main anastomoses about the hip, knee, ankle, shoulder, elbow, and wrist joints are shown in the colored drawings of the arteries.

In the foregoing description of the arteries reference has been made to counting the pulse by palpating various peripheral vessels. For convenience this information will be summarized here. It is customary to take the pulse by palpating the radial artery at the wrist, but if this is impractical, the pulse may be obtained by palpating the 303 superficial temporal artery anterior to the ear, the common carotid artery along the anterior border of the sternocleidomastoid muscle, the facial artery along the lower border of the mandible about halfway between the angle and symphysis, the brachial artery along the medial edge of the biceps brachii muscle, the femoral artery in the groin, the posterior tibial artery behind the medial malleolus, or the dorsalis pedis artery on the dorsum of the foot.

VEINS

Venous anastomoses are generally more numerous, irregular, and larger than arterial anastomoses. Communications between deep and superficial veins, especially in the lower limbs, are clinically important, since these channels are involved in the formation of varicosities. Communications are common between systemic veins; however, anastomosis between portal and systemic systems occurs only at limited sites, such as the end of the esophagus and lower end of the rectum, around the umbilicus, and on the posterior abdominal wall.

The very large arteries and those for the viscera usually have but one accompanying vein, but the remaining arteries usually have two companion veins with the same name as the artery they accompany. The veins from the inferior extremities and abdomen empty into the inferior vena cava; those of the head, neck, upper extremities, and chest wall empty into the superior vena cava. The coronary sinus returns blood from the heart. From each lung there are two pulmonary veins that empty into the left atrium.

Certain veins and venous sinuses and systems require special mention. These are the superficial veins of the head and extremities, the azygos vein, the venous sinuses of the cranium, the portal vein, and the vertebral venous system.

The pattern of superficial veins is extremely variable from person to person, and indeed there are marked differences on the right and left sides of the same person. The following descriptions define the usual formation.

Superficial veins

The superficial veins of the face and scalp are abundant and anastomose freely. They tend to converge at a common meeting point below the ear by two main channels: the posterior auricular and the retromandibular veins. These form the external jugular vein, which passes downward over the sternocleidomastoid muscle to the base of the neck where it empties into the junction of the internal jugular and the subclavian veins.

The superficial veins of the upper extremity begin in the dorsal and palmar venous arches of the hand. These arches at the wrist tend to form two main channels, a cephalic vein and a basilic vein.

304

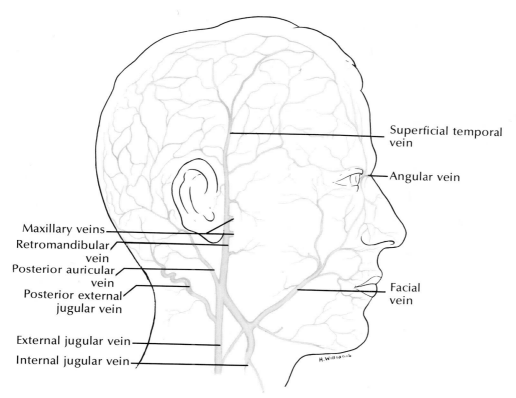

Fig. 9-24. Superficial veins of the face and neck.

The cephalic vein passes up the lateral side of the forearm and upper arm, emptying into the axillary vein just below the clavicle. Occasionally it passes over the clavicle to empty into the external jugular vein.

The basilic vein passes up the medial side of the forearm and upper arm, ultimately joining the axillary vein. There are several connecting veins in the forearm. In front of the elbow there is usually a prominent vessel, called the median cubital vein, which connects the basilic and cephalic veins. This is the vessel of choice for venipuncture and blood transfusions.

The superficial veins of the lower extremity begin at the ends of the dorsal venous arch on the foot. The great saphenous vein (long saphenous) springs from the arch at the front on the inner side of the ankle. It passes up the medial side of the leg and thigh and empties into the femoral vein just below the inguinal ligament. The small saphenous (short saphenous) vein begins on the lateral side of the

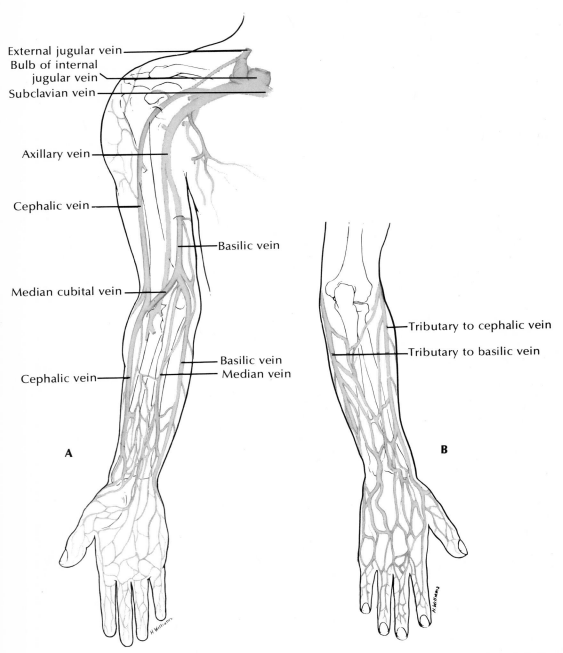

External jugular vein

Bulb of internal
jugular vein

Subclavian vein

Axillary vein

Cephalic vein

Basilic vein

Median cubital vein

Tributary to cephalic vein

Tributary to basilic vein

Basilic vein
Median vein

Cephalic vein

A

B

Fig. 9-25. A, Superficial veins of upper extremity, anterior view. An occasional connection between cephalic vein and external jugular vein is shown in dotted lines. **B,** Superficial veins of forearm, posterior view.

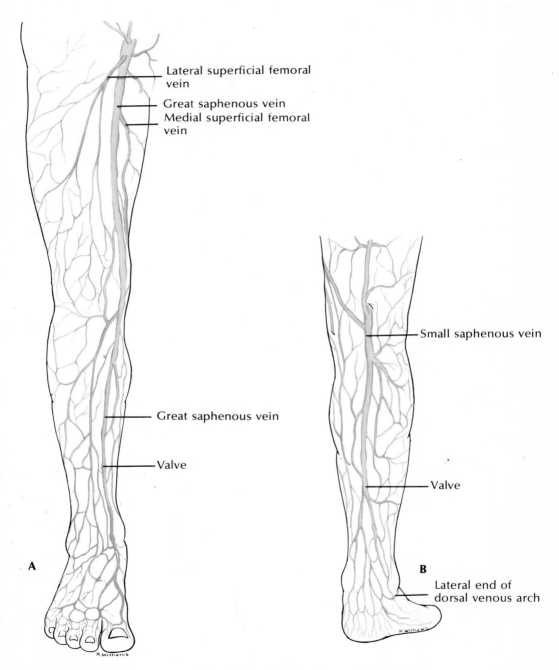

Fig. 9-26. A, Great saphenous vein and tributaries. **B,** Small saphenous vein
and tributaries.

307

ankle, passes up the back of the leg, and empties into the popliteal vein behind the knee. Venous valves that break up the column of blood into segments are common in the saphenous veins, forming small expansions in the course of the vessel. Valves are also found in other veins but are less numerous.

Azygos veins

The azygos vein arises in the right posterior abdominal wall at the level of the first or second lumbar vertebra, passes upward on the right side of the vertebral column behind the diaphragm to the right of the aorta, and empties into the terminal part of the superior vena cava. In the abdomen it receives blood from the right lumbar veins, and usually there is an anastomosis with the right renal vein, the right common iliac vein, and the inferior vena cava. In the thorax it receives blood from the accessory azygos veins. On the left side in the posterior abdominal wall the hemiazygos vein passes upward through the left crus of the diaphragm, crosses anterior to the vertebral column, and empties into the azygos vein. The accessory hemiazygos drains blood

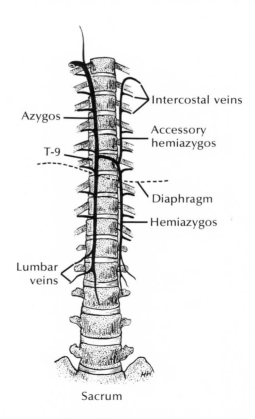

Fig. 9-27. Azygos veins.

from the upper intercostal spaces on the left into the azygos or the hemiazygos vein. The azygos veins drain blood from the lumbar area, from the chest wall, from the bronchial veins, and from the mediastinum and serve as an intermediate blood channel between the superior and inferior venae cavae (Fig. 9-27).

The portal vein receives blood from the large and small intestines, stomach, spleen, and pancreas and conveys the absorbed food material to the liver. Within the liver, portal blood is distributed by venous capillaries to the hepatic vein, which in turn joins the inferior vena cava. The pattern of formation of the portal system varies; however, the splenic and superior mesenteric veins commonly unite behind the neck of the pancreas to form the single portal vein. The inferior mesenteric may join the splenic or may empty into the junction of splenic and superior mesenteric. Another tributary of the portal is the left gastric, which drains the lesser curvature of the stomach and lower portion of the esophagus.

Portal vein

Obstruction of the portal vein in or near the liver, as in hepatic cirrhosis, causes portal hypertension, a serious condition. Since valves in the portal vein are rudimentary, portal blood diverted form the liver, leads to backflow into and dilation of the tributaries of the portal vein and especially of the anastomotic channels that exist between the portal and caval systems. Although such channels are numerous, they are also typically small; therefore, portal hypertension leads to marked enlargement and tortuosity. Superiorly, blood backflows via the left gastric into esophageal veins, which are tributaries of the azygos. The esophageal veins located in the submucosa of the esophagus dilate from the increased pressure, creating the danger of spontaneous or mechanical rupture into the lumen of the esophagus. Inferiorly the superior rectal, a branch of the inferior mesenteric, and the inferior rectal, a branch of the caval system, anastomose in the submucosa of the anal canal. Increased pressure in the superior or inferior rectal veins causes dilation and bulging of the varicosities into the anal canal resulting in a condition known as hemorrhoids (Fig. 9-28).

Within the spinal canal is a rich plexus of thin-walled veins without valves. These veins form anterior and posterior venous sinuses extending the entire length of the canal. They communicate freely with each other about the spinal cord; they have connections above with the blood sinuses within the cranium; they receive branches from the veins of the trunk by way of connecting channels that pass through the intervertebral foramina; they have connections with the veins that drain the pelvic viscera.

Vertebral venous system

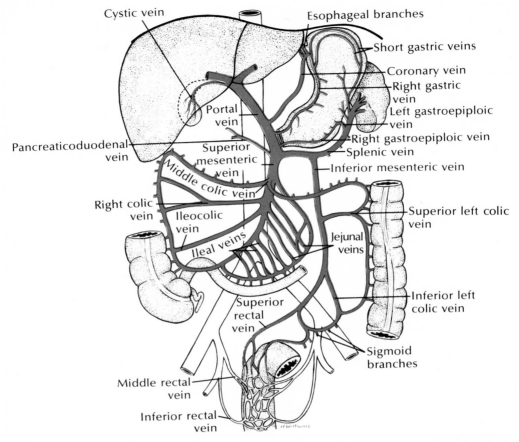

Fig. 9-28. Portal vein and tributaries. Note the anastomosis with inferior esophageal veins and with inferior hemorrhoidal veins of the systemic circulation.

When the pressure within the thorax and abdomen is increased, less blood flows toward the heart in the venae cavae, and there is a tendency for a retrograde flow of blood into the vertebral venous plexuses. This is a path by which infections and metastatic tumors may find their way into the brain and bones without going through the portal, systemic, or pulmonary circuits.

Clinical considerations

Varicose veins. A vein is said to be varicose when its diameter is enlarged and its course is tortuous. Neither the circulatory nor the anatomical factors leading to the development of varicosities are clearly understood. Often stressed is the concept that incompetent valves in the saphenous system leads to increased venous pressure; however,

310

it is not certain whether the incompetence of the valves precedes or is the result of the varicosities. Any factor that leads to pooling of blood in the saphenous system will aid in the formation of varicose veins. Hereditary factors have been implicated, and this factor assumes importance when women consider using the pill as a method of birth control. Hormones, specifically estrogen and progesterone, in the pill tend to cause loosening of the venous walls; therefore, a hereditary predisposition toward varicosities will be augmented by use of the pill. Occupations in which an individual stands relatively still for long periods of time tend to cause pooling or slowing of the circulation, a condition that also tends to increase the incidence of varicose veins.

Danger area of the face. The facial vein, the chief drainage route for the face, starting at the angle of the eye as the angular vein, communicates with the supraorbital as well as the ophthalmic vein (Fig. 9-30). The ophthalmic vein drains directly into the cavernous sinus, a large venous sinus located lateral to the sella turcica of the sphenoid bone. Since the veins of the head and face are without valves, blood can flow in either direction. Infections of the face may cause dissemination of septic material into the facial vein, causing thrombosis. If normal flow in the facial vein is blocked, infection, if not treated, may travel via the facial to ophthalmic to cavernous sinus, with the imminent danger of meningitis occurring.

CRANIUM
Venous sinuses
within the cranium

These sinuses are found between the layers of the dura mater and receive blood from the brain. The superior sagittal sinus begins near the crista galli in the anterior cranial fossa and passes posteriorly in the superior margin of the falx cerebri. When the sinus reaches the level of the internal occipital protuberance, it usually turns to the right, forming the right transverse sinus, which passes around the wall of the posterior cranial fossa and becomes the right internal jugular vein in the jugular foramen.

The inferior sagittal sinus begins near the crista galli but passes posteriorly in the free inferior margin of the falx cerebri. Immediately behind the corpus callosum it is joined by the great cerebral vein (the vein of Galen) from the cerebral hemispheres. In this manner the straight sinus is formed. The straight sinus passes posteriorly in the line of union of the falx cerebri with the tentorium cerebelli, as far as the internal occipital protuberance. At this point it becomes the left transverse sinus, which is continued into the left internal jugular vein. At the internal occipital protuberance there is frequently a communication between the right and left transverse sinuses, called the confluence of sinuses. The distal portion of each transverse sinus is fre-

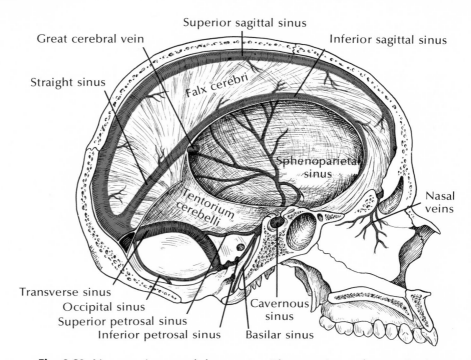

Great cerebral vein

Superior sagittal sinus

Inferior sagittal sinus

Straight sinus

Falx cerebri

Sphenoparietal sinus

Nasal veins

Tentorium cerebelli

Transverse sinus

Occipital sinus

Superior petrosal sinus

Inferior petrosal sinus

Cavernous sinus

Basilar sinus

Fig. 9-29. Venous sinuses of dura mater. The anterior and posterior intercavernous sinuses are not labeled, but their cut edges are shown on the
anterior and posterior walls of the sella turcica. The connection between
the nasal veins and the beginning of the superior sagittal sinus is not always
demonstrable.

quently called the sigmoid sinus, and the transverse sinuses are also
known as lateral sinuses.

There are several other smaller venous sinuses in the base of the
skull. The cavernous sinuses together with the anterior and posterior
intercavernous sinuses from a circular sinus about the sella turcica.
The superior and inferior petrosal sinuses are lodged along the petrous
portion of the temporal bone. The sphenoparietal sinuses are found
along the edge of the small wings of the sphenoid. The occipital sinus
is found posterior to the foramen magnum, and the basilar sinus is
found anterior to the foramen magnum. These sinuses all drain eventually into the internal jugular veins. The petrosal sinuses connect the
cavernous sinuses with the sigmoid sinuses. The occipital and basilar
sinuses connect with each other on either side of the foramen magnum and with the vertebral venous system. Through the emissary
foramina the blood sinuses within the cranium communicate with the
veins of scalp and face and with the diploic veins; these communica-

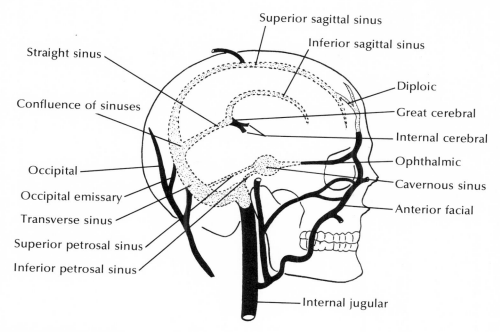

Fig. 9-30. The dural venous sinuses, the internal jugular vein, and some diploic and emissary veins. (From DiDio, L. J. A.: Synopsis of anatomy, St. Louis, 1970, The C. V. Mosby Co.)

tions form one possible pathway for the passage of infections into the cranial cavity.

In addition to the great cerebral vein, a number of superficial cerebral veins empty directly into the superior longitudinal sinus; veins from the cerebellum, pons, and medulla drain into the various venous sinuses in the base of the skull.

After early childhood the brain case is a closed box of bone. Within this rigid box is the brain, which is very delicate and sensitive to alterations in intracranial blood pressure. Also the brain is a most active organ requiring a constant and abundant supply of arterial blood. Four large arteries (two vertebral and two internal carotid) bring blood into the cranial cavity. These arteries enter into the formation of the arterial circle at the base of the brain. If this anastomotic circle is adequate in all its parts, it is possible, if one of the arteries is blocked, for blood to be shunted through the circle to the endangered area of the brain, and the entire brain continues to function normally. The venous sinuses anastomose freely with each other, and there are connections

**Intracranial blood
pressure**

313

through emissary vessels with veins outside the cranial cavity. At all times it is necessary that the amount of blood within the cranial cavity be maintained at a constant level; the volume of arterial blood entering must be equal to the amount of venous blood leaving. If there is a sudden lowering of the blood pressure, the individual faints; if the intracranial pressure increases, the individual eventually becomes unconscious. If the cerebral cortex is deprived of arterial blood for more than a few minutes, irreparable damage results.

REVIEW QUESTIONS

1. What are the differences between an artery, a vein, and a capillary?
2. Name the four main chambers of the human heart.
3. What structures form the borders of the heart?
4. Name the main parts of the conducting system of the heart.
5. Trace a drop of blood through the pulmonary blood system, starting at the right atrium.
6. Trace a drop of blood from the inferior vena cava to the aorta.
7. Discuss heart sounds.
8. List five places in the body where the pulse may be taken.
9. Describe the great saphenous vein.
10. List the venous sinuses of the dura mater.
11. Describe briefly the arterial supply of each of the following: the upper extremity, the lower extremity, and the brain.
12. What is the function of the heart?
13. Describe the coronary circulation.
14. Where is the carotid sinus? What is its nerve supply?
15. What is the nerve supply of the heart?
16. Describe briefly the circulation of blood in the fetus.
17. The portal vein carries blood from what organs?
18. Discuss arterial anastomoses around the base of the brain and the shoulder girdle.

CHAPTER 10

THE LYMPHATIC SYSTEM

The lymphatic system begins in meshes of connective tissues as closed capillaries that anastomose to form rich plexuses, or networks. These capillaries unite to form the first collecting trunks, or afferent vessels, that go to regional lymph nodes. A node is an encapsulated mass of lymphocytes. Within the node the collecting trunks break up into capillaries and are reunited into efferent trunks. The terminal collecting trunks empty into the subclavian veins. The entire lymphatic system acts as a secondary system for the return of fluid and particulate matter from peripheral tissues and organs to the superior vena cava.

A lymph nodule, or follicle, is a small, nonencapsulated mass of lymphocytes in a mesh of reticular tissue. Each lymph node contains several nodules. Also, lymph nodules occurring singly or in groups are found beneath the epithelium of mucous membranes, particularly of the respiratory and digestive tracts. The tonsils are aggregates of lymph nodules and are described in the discussion of the pharynx. The lymph nodules of the small intestine are described in the discussion of that organ.

The capillary walls of the lymphatic system have only a very thin endothelial layer, which makes them permeable to substances of greater molecular size than those that can pass through the thicker endothelial wall of a blood capillary. The collecting trunks have, in addition, a covering of connective tissue containing scattered smooth muscle and elastic fibers. A collecting trunk has a wall similar to that of a vein but possesses many more valves. The shape of lymphatic vessels varies with the structures through which they pass. In muscles,

such as those in the diaphragm, the lumen in cross section looks like a
mere slit, but in loose connective tissue the lumen is widely dilated.
Lymphatics course almost exclusively through the structures of the
connnective tissue type; they are found on the surface of an organ and
deep within it. There is very little anastomosis between the superficial and deep lymphatics of any structure. Collecting trunks tend
to be grouped in the vicinity of blood vessels and lie superficial to
and not deeper than those vessels, a fact of much significance in surgery.

Unlike circulation in the circulatory system, in which blood
is propelled by contraction of the heart, circulation in the lymph
system is controlled as follows:

1. Contraction of adjacent muscles that compresses the lymphatic
   vessels and moves the lymph in a direction determined by the
   valves
2. Pulsation of nearby vascular channels with resultant pressure,
   especially on deep lymphatic vessels
3. Respiration and the resulting relatively low pressure in the
   subclavian veins where the lymph trunks terminate
4. Contraction of smooth muscle in the walls of the larger
   lymphatic vessels

A lymph node has a capsule of white fibrous connective tissue,

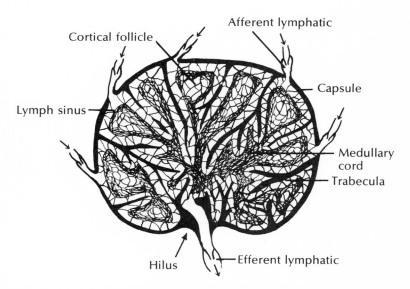

Fig. 10-1. A lymph node. This is a diagram showing the connective tissue
framework of a node; the fine mesh represents reticular tissue; the lymphocytes have been omitted.

with trabeculae extending inward and partially subdividing the substance of the node into lobules and forming the structural framework. Dense masses of lymphocytes in reticular tissue form the follicles of the cortex beneath the capsule. The central portion or medulla contains cords of lymphocytes in reticular tissue. At the hilus where the blood vessels of the node enter and leave and where the efferent lymphatic trunk arises, the medulla reaches the surface, and there is no cortex. The afferent lymphatic vessels, of which there are usually several for each node, pierce the capsule separately. The lymph sinuses are spaces beneath the capsule and around the trabeculae, extending inward along the follicles and cords of cells. The lymph enters the node from the afferent vessels, filters through the sinuses, and leaves at the hilus through the efferent vessel. Lymph nodes have several functions. They act as a center for production of lymphocytes; they act as a phagocytic organ in which lymph is purified, and they act as a site of antibody formation in immunologic reactions.

Lymph nodes vary markedly in shape, color, size, consistency, and number. Though lymph nodes are present throughout life, they are characteristically frequent, large, and obvious in childhood. They increase in size and regress according to the subjection to, or freedom of tissues from, bacterial invasion or tumor growth. The lymph nodes that drain the air passages become black because they receive and deposit particles of dust brought to them by way of the lymphatics of the lungs. Other lymph nodes, such as those of the abdomen, remain pink throughout life. In persons suffering from long-continued illness, such as chronic tuberculosis, the lymph nodes are large, firm, and apparently more numerous. In acute infections they are swollen and tender and may break down into abscesses.

Lymphatics not only drain lymph back into the blood stream from the tissue spaces, but also the lacteals, or the lymph capillaries in the villi of the small intestine, absorb products of fat digestion and empty them into the blood stream by way of the thoracic duct.

There are no lymph nodes or lymphatics within the cranium. The superficial nodes are arranged in a ring that lies along the lower border of the mandible, about the ear, and at the junction of neck and head. The deep nodes lie along the deeper blood vessels of the neck. There are numerous lymphatics connecting the nodes of the superficial ring and others passing from superficial to deep nodes. There are also many channels draining lymph from the tonsillar masses of the pharynx. The lymphatic masses of the air passages together with the various lymph nodes constitute very important barriers to infections of the mouth and upper air passages.

**LYMPHATICS OF
HEAD AND NECK**

317

I. Superficial nodes
  A. Occipital group at the back of the head
  B. Retroauricular (mastoid) group over the mastoid process be-
     hind the ear
  C. Parotid group (anterior auricular) in and about the parotid
     gland

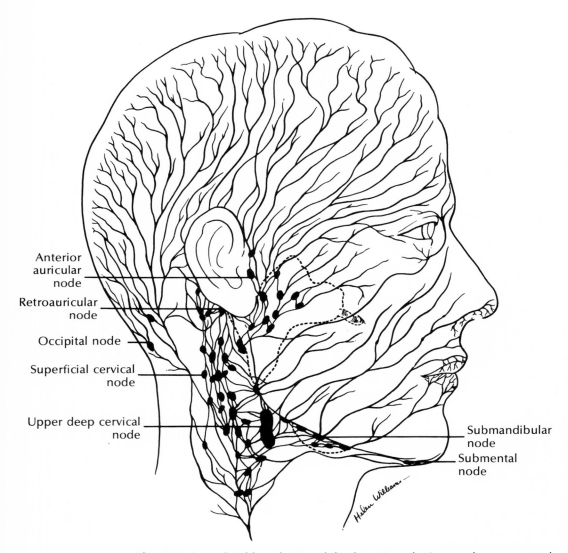

Anterior
auricular
node

Retroauricular
node

Occipital node

Superficial cervical
node

Upper deep cervical
node

Submandibular
node

Submental
node

Fig. 10-2. Superficial lymphatics of the face. Lymphatic vessels represented
by black lines. In life they are actually moniliform. Parotid and submandibular salivary glands are indicated by dotted lines to show their relation to
lymph nodes. (After Sappey.)

318

    D. Submandibular (submaxillary) group below and parallel to the mandible

    E. Submental group beneath the chin

 II. Deep nodes

    A. Retropharyngeal nodes between the pharynx and the vertebral column

    B. Deep cervical chain along the internal jugular vein

    C. Supraclavicular group along the subclavian artery

The lymphatics of the scalp form a rich plexus and unite into three sets of collecting trunks on each side: a frontal group ending in the anterior auricular nodes, a parietal group draining into the retroauricular nodes, and an occipital group going to the occipital nodes. Lymphatic channels pass from these nodes into deep cervical nodes.

The lymphatics of the lips, eyelids, cheeks, gums, and skin of the nose drain to nearby nodes and thence into cervical nodes (Fig. 10-2).

Lymphatics of the nasal cavity, air sinuses, and pharynx drain into cervical and retropharyngeal nodes. At the angle of the jaw is a submandibular node that becomes enlarged and tender in infections of the tonsillar region. This must not be mistaken for the tonsil itself. The retropharyngeal nodes are likely to become very large in infections of the nose and throat. In young children they may become so large as to push the posterior wall of the pharynx far forward. If pus forms, a retropharyngeal abscess results.

The lymphatics of the tongue drain from the tip to the submental nodes, from the sides to the submandibular nodes, and from the back and deeper portions to the deep cervical nodes.

In the axillary nodes nearly all the superficial and deep lymphatics of the upper limb meet. There are, however, a few scattered nodes in other parts of the arm that lie on the course of collecting trunks.

LYMPHATICS OF UPPER EXTREMITY

The epitrochlear node, usually single, lies on the deep fascia about 3.5 cm proximal to the medial epicondyle of the humerus. Into this node drain some of the superficial collecting trunks on the medial (ulnar) side of the hand and the ring and little fingers. The efferent vessels accompany the basilic vein and pierce the deep fascia in the middle part of the upper arm to empty into the deep lymphatics that accompany the axillary vessels.

The axillary nodes drain not only the upper extremity but also the thoracic and abdominal wall, down to the level of the umbilicus. The axillary nodes are embedded in the axilla and are subdivided in the following manner:

Axillary nodes

    1. The humeral, or lateral chain, in close relation to the axillary

319

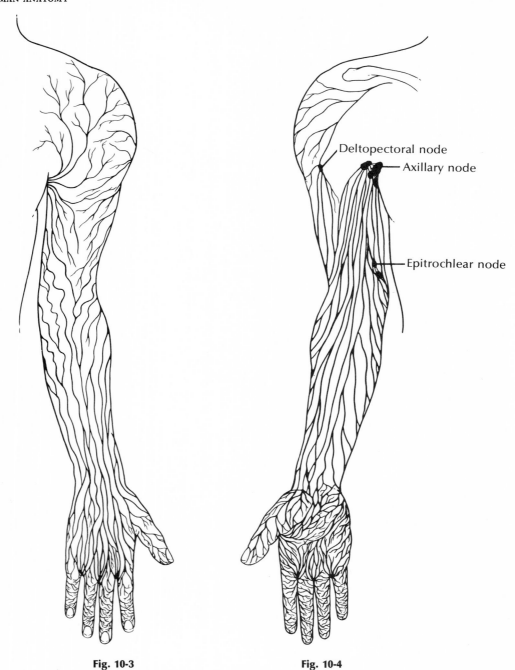

Deltopectoral node

Axillary node

Epitrochlear node

Fig. 10-3   **Fig. 10-4**

Fig. 10-3. Superficial lymphatics of upper extremity, posterior view. (After Sappey.)
Fig. 10-4. Superficial lymphatics of upper extremity, anterior view. (After Sappey.)

vein, receives nearly all the lymphatics of the upper limb.

2. The thoracic, pectoral, or medial chain, lying along the lateral thoracic artery, drains particularly the anterior chest wall and breast.

3. The subscapular, or posterior chain, lying along the subscapular vessels, drains the scapular region and the lower part of the neck.

4. An infraclavicular, or anterior group, lying along the upper border of the pectoralis minor, receives mainly efferent vessels from the other axillary groups.

5. A central group in the apex of the axilla receives efferent vessels from the other groups.

The superficial lymphatic network reaches its maximum development on the palmar surface of the fingers and is much less rich on the dorsum. These networks give rise to collecting trunklets that converge toward the sides of the fingers and run over the dorsum of the hand in the interdigital spaces, forming numerous anastomoses.

The trunklets from the medial and lateral sides and from the distal portion of the palm drain into the network on the dorsum of the hand; those from the central portion of the palm drain by a single trunk, formed beneath the superficial palmar fascia and passing laterally around the side of the hand to the dorsum. The trunklets from the central proximal part of the palm drain into collecting trunks on the volar aspect of the forearm.

From the course of the lymphatics it is easy to understand why spreading infections from fingers and from most of the palm cause early swelling and redness of the dorsum of the hand even though the source of the infection is on the palmar aspect.

As the collecting trunks pass up the forearm, they merge with each other, thus diminishing their total number. In the forearm there are about 30, but in the upper arm, 15 to 18 (Sappey).

On the ventral (anterior) aspect of the forearm are three groups of collecting trunks: the medial and lateral groups coursing along the respective borders and the middle group accompanying the median vein. The trunks on the dorsum are more tortuous, especially near the elbow. In the upper arm the three anterior groups course in parallel lines, with frequent intercommunications, to empty into the humeral chain of nodes. The innermost trunks may be interrupted by the epitrochlear node and follow the deep lymphatics of the arm; the outermost trunk may drain to nodes in the deltopectoral triangle an area located between the clavicular portions of the deltoid and pectoralis major muscles.

321

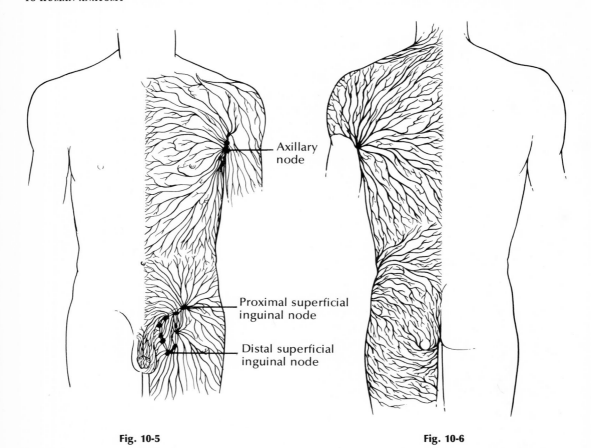

Axillary
node

Proximal superficial
inguinal node

Distal superficial
inguinal node

Fig. 10-5

Fig. 10-6

Fig. 10-5. Superficial lymphatics of trunk, anterior view. (After Sappey.)
Fig. 10-6. Superficial lymphatics of trunk, posterior view. (After Sappey.)

The deep lymphatics accompany the brachial artery and its branches. There are radial, ulnar, and interosseous trunks arising in the neighborhood of the peripheral distribution of the vessels that they accompany. They terminate in the humeral trunk along the brachial artery.

Mammary gland

The lymphatics of the breast are extremely numerous. A knowledge of the main channels, however, is of particular importance because carcinomas of the breast may metastasize, or spread, along these vessels.

Deep and subcutaneous vessels communicate in the subareolar plexus, and from the plexus, two major trunks arise that pass laterally and superiorly to the anterior pectoral group of axillary nodes.

322

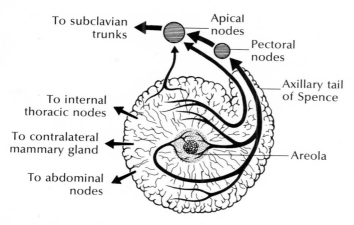

To subclavian trunks

Apical nodes

Pectoral nodes

Axillary tail of Spence

To internal thoracic nodes

To contralateral mammary gland

Areola

To abdominal nodes

Fig. 10-7. Lymph drainage from left breast. (Modified from Gardner, E., Gray, D. J., and O'Rahilly, R.: Anatomy, Philadelphia, 1969, W. B. Saunders Company.)

There also may be lymphatics passing directly to the apical group of axillary nodes but rarely to nodes along the axillary artery.

In addition to the chief drainage of the breast, there are some vessels from the medial part of the breast that join the nodes along the internal thoracic artery. Communications also exist across the midline between the lymphatic plexuses of the two breasts, and lymphatics from the lower medial aspect of the mammary gland may occasionally join abdominal nodes in the region of the diaphragm. Thus, metastasis may occasionally occur to the opposite side or to the abdomen.

The lymphatics of the lower extremity terminate in the inguinal lymph nodes, which are subdivided into a superficial and a deep group.

LYMPHATICS OF LOWER EXTREMITY

1. The superficial inguinal nodes are found in the subcutaneous tissue about the medial end of the inguinal ligament. There is a proximal group that lies parallel to the ligament and a distal group that lies parallel to the great saphenous vein. The nodes vary greatly in number and size. Their afferent vessels originate in the leg, perineum, scrotum or labia, skin of penis or clitoris, anus, and wall of the trunk up to the level of the umbilicus. The efferent vessels end in deep inguinal nodes and thence to the nodes along the external and common iliac arteries.

2. Deep inguinal nodes are few in number and lie around the femoral artery as it enters the thigh.

323

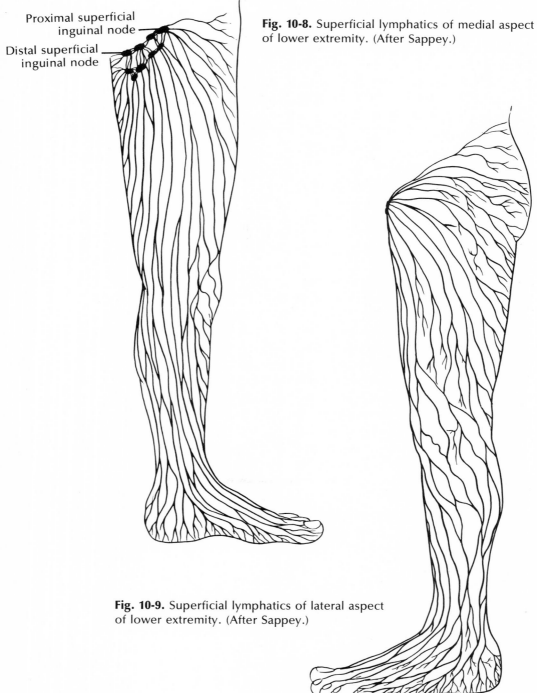

Proximal superficial
inguinal node

Distal superficial
inguinal node

Fig. 10-8. Superficial lymphatics of medial aspect
of lower extremity. (After Sappey.)

Fig. 10-9. Superficial lymphatics of lateral aspect
of lower extremity. (After Sappey.)

324

Posterior to the knee and lying close to the popliteal vein are several small nodes to which afferent vessels come from the lateral side of the calf of the leg above the small saphenous vein, from the collecting trunks accompanying posterior tibial and peroneal arteries, from the knee joint, and from the anterior tibial lymph node. Most of the efferent lymphatics drain into the deep inguinal nodes.

The superficial lymphatic network gives rise to three groups of collecting trunks. Those accompanying the great saphenous vein drain the region of the first, second, and third toes and the medial portion of the foot. They ascend in parallel lines to the inguinal nodes. The collecting trunks of the lateral aspect of the foot pass upward and forward to empty into the collecting channels accompanying the great saphenous vein. Some collecting trunks from the lateral aspect of the foot and from the heel accompany the small saphenous vein to the knee and empty into the most superficial popliteal node. Collecting trunks from the lateral gluteal region pass around the outer side of the thigh to reach the superior lateral superficial inguinal nodes. From the inner third of the buttock and anal region the collecting trunks pass medially around the thigh to the lower superficial inguinal nodes.

The deep lymphatics accompany the main blood vessels, namely, the pedal and anterior tibial vessels and the plantar and posterior tibial vessels. They communicate with the popliteal nodes and then course along the femoral vessels. Accessory lymphatics from the obturator and gluteal vessels join the femoral collecting trunks and terminate in the deep inguinal or internal iliac (hypogastric) nodes. Deep and superficial lymphatics are independent, though generally they do communicate with each other through popliteal and superficial inguinal nodes.

The superficial lymphatics of the scrotum, skin, and prepuce of the penis, the labia majora, and the coverings of the clitoris and skin of anal region and buttocks, together with those of the abdominal wall up to the umbilicus, drain to the superficial inguinal lymph nodes.

Afferent vessels of the deep inguinal lymph nodes are those from the superficial nodes, lymphatics accompanying the femoral vessels, and lymphatics from the glans of the penis or clitoris.

The lymphatic drainage of the skin and subcutaneous tissue has been given in considerable detail because of its importance in the spread of infections. It explains the apprehension of a surgeon when he sees red streaks of inflammation on a forearm and upper arm produced by infections spreading along the collecting trunks. The disappearance of these red streaks under treatment means that the infection is being localized to the original site.

325

**LYMPHATICS OF
PELVIS**

The lymph nodes lying within the cavity of the pelvis are more or less artificially grouped in accordance with their location along the blood vessels.

1. External iliac lymph nodes are scattered along the course of the vessels and receive lymph from the inguinal nodes and some from the anterior abdominal wall.
2. Internal iliac (hypogastric) lymph nodes lie in relation to the internal iliac artery and its branches and receive lymph from the pelvic viscera and some also from the perineum and buttocks.
3. The common iliac lymph nodes are in reality an upward extension of the internal and external iliac chains and above are continued as the aortic nodes of the abdominal cavity.

It is simpler to look upon the internal iliac group as the nodes of the cavity of the pelvis and upon the external and common iliac groups as the nodes of the brim.

In general the lymphatics of a viscus are distributed in a superficial network beneath the capsule and in a series of deep channels within the substance. These channels drain toward the hilus, or site where the chief blood vessels enter and leave.

The lymphatics of the pelvic organs usually drain along the accompanying blood vessels. The nodes of the brim (external and common iliac nodes) receive the efferent vessels of the nodes of the cavity (internal iliac) and, in addition, numerous direct efferents from the pelvic organs. Also, efferent vessels from the upper part of the rectum, the upper part of the uterus, and the uterine tube and ovary (in the male, the testis) pass directly into aortic nodes of the abdominal cavity.

**LYMPHATICS OF
ABDOMEN**

The nodes situated within the upper abdominal cavity may, for purposes of description, be subdivided into numerous groups, but the subdivision is artificial and there are many intercommunications.

1. Aortic lymph nodes are most numerous on the left side of the aorta, between the origin of the left renal artery and the beginning of the left common iliac artery. This group becomes continuous with the nodes lying above the inferior mesenteric artery. Above the level of the renal arteries the aortic group is difficult to distinguish from the celiac and superior mesenteric groups. There are some small nodes, the lateral lumbar lymph nodes, scattered along the parietal branches of the aorta to the dorsal abdominal wall.
2. Inferior mesenteric lymph nodes are subdivided into groups lying along the branches of the artery.
3. Superior mesenteric lymph nodes have a less regular distribu-

tion than those of the inferior mesenteric group but are very numerous. The nodes scattered within the mesentery are said to number between 100 and 200.

4. Celiac lymph nodes are arranged about the celiac trunk and its branches. Most of the celiac nodes are situated along the upper edge of the pancreas, but some are located within the lesser and greater omenta.

The lymphatics of the stomach pass by means of three streams to the celiac nodes: from the fundus and upper part of the gastric tube to nodes on the left side, from the lower portion of the gastric tube to nodes just above the pancreas, and from the pyloric canal to the lower

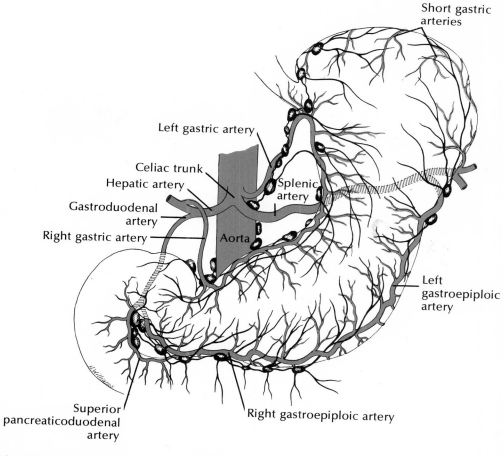

Fig. 10-10. Arterial supply and lymphatic drainage of the stomach. (After Cutler and Zollinger.)

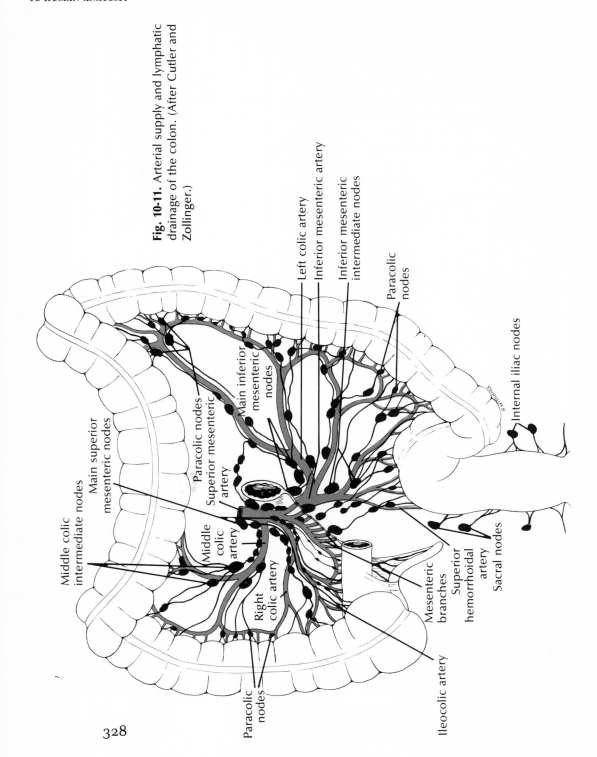

Fig. 10-11. Arterial supply and lymphatic drainage of the colon. (After Cutler and Zollinger.)

celiac nodes on the right side. These streams intermingle and boundaries of drainage are not clear cut.

The lymphatics of the small intestine drain into nodes lying in the mesentery. The lymph is usually relayed through several nodes before reaching the main nodes of the superior mesenteric group.

The lymphatics from the proximal portion of the large intestine drain to the superior mesenteric group of nodes and from the distal portion to the inferior mesenteric group.

The lymphatics of the pancreas drain to adjacent nodes.

The lymphatics of the gallbladder and of most of the liver drain to the celiac group, but the collecting vessels from the surface next to the diaphragm and the anterior abdominal wall drain upward to nodes in the thoracic cavity.

The lymphatics of the spleen drain lymph to nodes in the left portion of the celiac group.

Lymphatics of the kidneys are not numerous and drain to nearby aortic nodes.

Lymphatics of the suprarenal glands go mainly to aortic and celiac nodes but some pass upward to thoracic nodes.

Lymphatics of the testes and ovaries drain into abdominal nodes close to the cisterna chyli.

The lymph nodes of the thorax are divided into several small superficial groups and a large bronchial group. The superficial group includes the following:

LYMPHATICS OF THORAX

1. Sternal nodes lying just behind the sternum and receiving afferents from the thoracic wall and diaphragm
2. Intercostal nodes found in the intercostal spaces and draining lymph from the chest wall
3. Anterior mediastinal nodes, which receive afferent vessels from the liver, diaphragm, and mediastinum
4. Posterior mediastinal nodes, which receive afferents from the diaphragm, mediastinum, and esophagus

The bronchial group includes all the nodes associated with the distal portion of the trachea and bronchi and is subdivided into the following groups:

1. Tracheobronchial nodes situated in the angle between trachea and bronchus on either side
2. Intertracheobronchial nodes placed below the trachea in the angle between the bronchi
3. Bronchopulmonary nodes located in the hilus of each lung
4. Pulmonary nodes lying within the substance of the lung, usually in the angle between two bronchial branches

329

The lymphatics of the lungs and visceral pleura drain through the pulmonary and bronchopulmonary nodes to the nodes about the trachea.

The lymphatics of the heart drain to the tracheobronchial nodes.

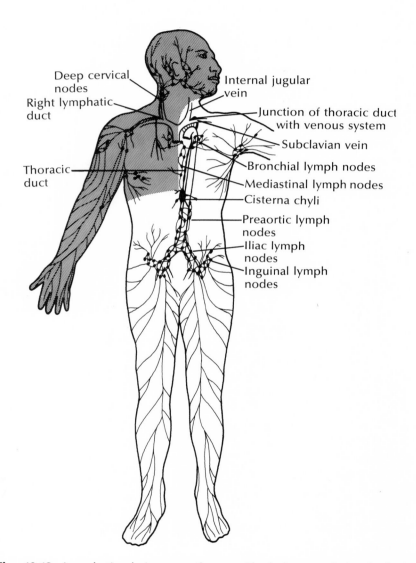

Fig. 10-12. Lymphatic drainage pathways. Shaded area of the body is drained via the right lymphatic duct, which is formed by the union of three vessels: the right jugular trunk, the right subclavian trunk, and the right bronchomediastinal trunk. Lymph from the remainder of the body enters the venous system by way of the thoracic duct.

The lymphatics of the abdomen and legs unite to form a single channel, the thoracic duct, which commences as a dilated sac, the cisterna chyli, at the upper border of the second lumbar vertebra and terminates at the junction of the left internal jugular and sub-clavian veins. The left jugular, subclavian, and bronchomediastinal collecting trunks usually empty into the terminal part of the thoracic duct but may empty separately into the vein. On the right side these three collecting trunks usually empty singly into the junction of the right internal jugular and subclavian veins, and there is no common right lymphatic duct (Fig. 10-12).

Terminal collecting trunks

The thoracic duct runs superiorly in front of the bodies of the vertebrae, through the aortic orifice of the diaphragm and behind the esophagus, crossing from the right side to the left of the vertebral column at the lower border of the body of the sixth thoracic vertebra. It curves upward to the left above the subclavian artery to its termina-tion. It may, and frequently does, empty by several openings.

The spleen is a lymphatic organ lying beneath the left dome of the diaphragm. It lies lateral to the left kidney and superior and poste-rior to the cardiac portion of the stomach and the splenic flexure of the colon.

SPLEEN

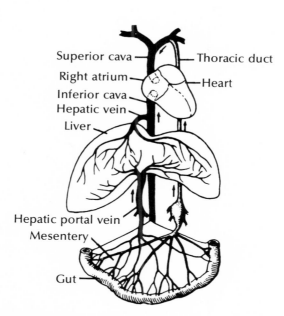

Superior cava — — Thoracic duct

Right atrium —

Inferior cava — — Heart

Hepatic vein —

Liver —

Hepatic portal vein

Mesentery

Gut

Fig. 10-13. Diagram of thoracic duct and portal system. (After Wieman; from Jackson, D. E.: Experimental pharmacology and materia medica, ed. 2, St. Louis, The C. V. Mosby Co.)

331

In formalin-embalmed bodies the spleen has definite borders and impressions upon its surface produced by the molding contact with adjacent viscera. The diaphragmatic surface is convex, but the undersurface has three concave areas due to contact with the stomach, kidney, and splenic flexure.

The spleen is much like a large lymph node, but the capsule is thicker and the trabeculae are larger. The supporting tissue contains more elastic fibers and a few smooth muscle cells. Therefore the spleen, in contrast to a lymph node, may be distended or contracted. During life it is soft and elastic and varies in size with

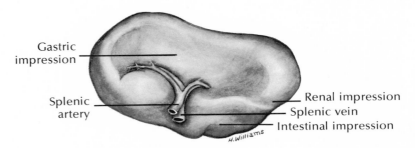

Gastric impression

Splenic artery

Renal impression

Splenic vein

Intestinal impression

Fig. 10-14. Medial aspect of the spleen.

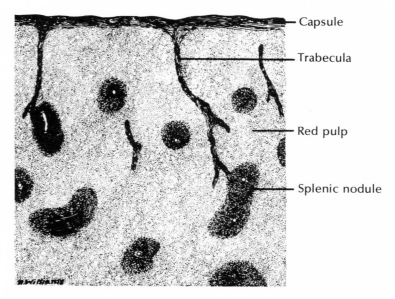

Capsule

Trabecula

Red pulp

Splenic nodule

332   **Fig. 10-15.** Section of human spleen.

the blood flow. It becomes larger and softer in acute infections, and in certain diseases such as malaria and leukemia, it becomes permanently enlarged and firmer than normal.

The splenic artery, a branch of the celiac, enters the organ at the hilus. The splenic vein drains into the portal circulation. Nerves pass to the spleen from the celiac ganglion. The Latin name for spleen is *lien,* and the splenic artery and vein are sometimes called the lienal artery and vein.

The spleen has a peritoneal covering, the tunica serosa. Beneath this is the tunica propria, or capsule, a strong fibroelastic covering containing some smooth muscle. Trabeculae pass inward from the tunica propria to divide the central portion of the organ into lobules. The lobules contain masses of lymphatic cells arranged about a central arteriole. Each of these masses is a splenic nodule. The larger nodules are visible to the naked eye as small dots. The splenic nodules compose the white pulp of the spleen. The diffuse masses about the nodules form the red pulp. The red pulp contains lymphocytes, reticuloendothelial cells, and all the cells found in circulating blood. There is a fine mesh of reticular tissue in both the red and the white pulp.

The spleen has various functions. It produces lymphocytes. It acts as a storehouse for red cells and aids in altering the relation between the amount of blood plasma and cells with varying needs of the body. The reticuloendothelial cells destroy worn-out red cells. It produces new blood cells during infancy and childhood.

THYMUS

The thymus is a two-lobed structure lying posterior to the upper part of the sternum and anterior to the beginning of the aorta and pulmonary trunk. It is relatively large at birth but begins to shrink at about the age of puberty, and in an adult it is usually represented by a small mass of connective tissue and fat. At any given age there may be great variation in size. The organ is pink in early life and becomes yellowish-pink with age. It has a fibrous capsule from which septa pass into the substance of the organ, separating it into primary and secondary lobules. The lobules contain lymphatic nodules.

Branches of the internal thoracic artery supply the thymus, and nerve filaments come from the vagus and upper thoracic segments of the cord.

There is increasing evidence that the thymus plays a very important role in enabling the body to produce mechanisms against infection, that is, in developing immunity. This appears to be true particularly in infancy. Minute amounts of thymic secretion stimulate other lymphoid organs, such as the spleen, to produce lymphocytes.

REVIEW QUESTIONS

1. What is the general function of the lymphatic system?
2. Give a brief description of a lymph node.
3. Describe briefly the lymphatic drainage of the scalp.
4. The axillary lymph nodes drain lymph from what areas of the body?
5. The inguinal lymph nodes drain lymph from what areas of the body?
6. Where does the thoracic duct begin? Where does it terminate?
7. Where is the spleen located?
8. Give three functions of the spleen.
9. Where is the thymus located?
10. Where do the lymphatics of the stomach drain?
11. Describe lymphatic drainage from the breast.

CHAPTER 11

THE RESPIRATORY SYSTEM

The organs of breathing consist of a series of air passages including the nasal chambers, pharynx, larynx, trachea, and bronchi
and the lungs to which these passages lead. The mouth serves as a secondary respiratory passage if the nasal passages are blocked. The
pharynx is a pathway used by both the digestive and respiratory
systems (Fig. 11-1).

The external nose is roughly triangular in shape. The upper angle is **NOSE**
called the root, and the portion containing the external openings, or
nostrils, is called the base. The lateral wall of each external opening is
called the ala of the nose. The tip of the nose is the apex, and the bridge
of the nose is that bony portion between the root and the apex. The
root, dorsum, and upper portion of the sides of the nose are bony, but
the lower and more prominent part is formed by several cartilages. The
nasal cavity is subdivided into two portions by the nasal septum, the
posterior part of which is formed from the vomer and vertical plate of
the ethmoid; the anterior part is composed of cartilage (Fig. 11-2).

Attached to the lateral wall of the nasal cavity are three scroll-like
processes of bone, the nasal conchae or turbinates. The inferior concha
is a separate bone articulating with the maxilla, but the superior and
middle conchae are portions of the ethmoid.

Each turbinate is covered by mucous membrane; that covering the
inferior turbinate is thick and soft, giving a rounded, bulbous appearance to the posterior end, that covering the middle turbinate is less
thick, and that covering the superior turbinate is thin and firm.

The lining of the nose just within the nostrils is stratified squamous

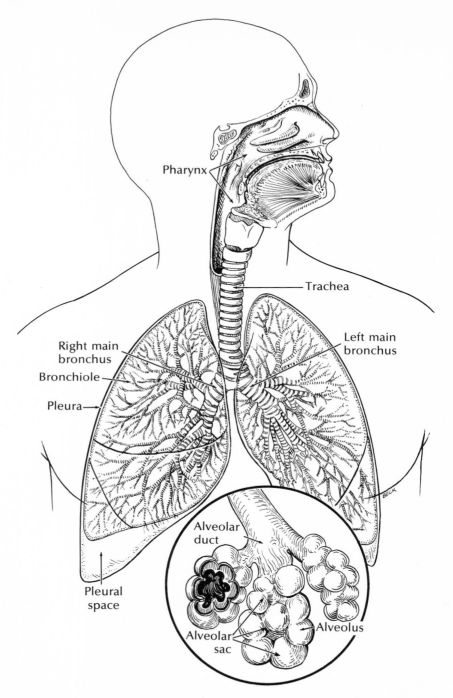

Pharynx

Trachea

Right main
bronchus

Left main
bronchus

Bronchiole

Pleura

Alveolar
duct

Pleural
space

Alveolus

Alveolar
sac

Fig. 11-1. The pharynx, trachea, and lungs. The inset shows the grapelike
alveolar sacs, in which the interchange of oxygen and carbon dioxide takes
place through the thin walls of the alveoli. Capillaries (not shown) surround
the alveoli. (From Anthony, C. P., and Kolthoff, N. J.: Textbook of anatomy
and physiology, ed. 8, St. Louis, 1971, The C. V. Mosby Co.)

336

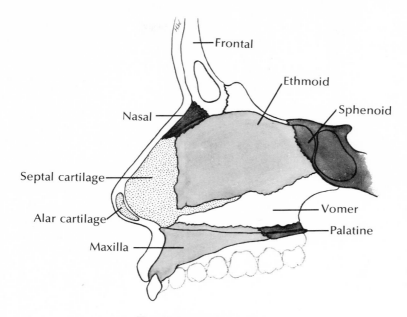

Fig. 11-2. Nasal septum.

epithelium, but this soon changes to pseudostratified, ciliated, columnar epithelium lying upon a dense layer of connective tissue, the tunica
propria. Within the tunica propria are branched tubuloalveolar mucus-
producing glands. A small portion of the mucosa covering the medial surface of the superior concha and the nearby surface of the
septum contains the olfactory cells specialized for the registration
of odors.

The nasal mucosa is richly supplied with blood vessels, particularly that over the inferior concha. Most of the blood vessels are terminal
branches of the maxillary artery, but the external portion of the nose
receives small arterial branches from the facial artery, and the upper
portion of each nasal cavity receives branches from the ophthalmic
artery. The veins drain into the facial veins, into a plexus of veins
about the pterygoid muscles, and also into the blood sinuses of the
dura mater of the brain.

The turbinates, especially the inferior, act as radiators for warming
and moistening the inhaled air. Just inside the nostrils are many hairs
that act as a sieve to remove dust particles from the air, thus protecting
the air passages leading to the lungs.

The conchae subdivide the nasal cavity into several parts. The inferior meatus lies below the inferior concha and is the chief air passage;
the middle meatus, which is closed in front, lies between the middle

337

and inferior conchae; the superior meatus lies between the superior and middle conchae; the sphenoethmoid recess lies superior and posterior to the superior concha. The superior meatus serves as an air trap to hold the air relatively motionless, thus facilitating the sense of smell. Air sinuses, described in detail in the next discussion of this chapter, open into it, as into the middle meatus. The nasolacrimal duct empties into the inferior meatus (Fig. 11-4).

The hard palate, which also serves as the floor of the nasal cavity, is formed by the palatine process of the maxilla and the horizontal palatal process of the palatine bone.

The roof of the nasal cavity is formed mainly by the cribriform plate of the ethmoid.

The nasal cavity communicates with the upper portion of the pharynx through two posterior openings, called the choanae or posterior nares.

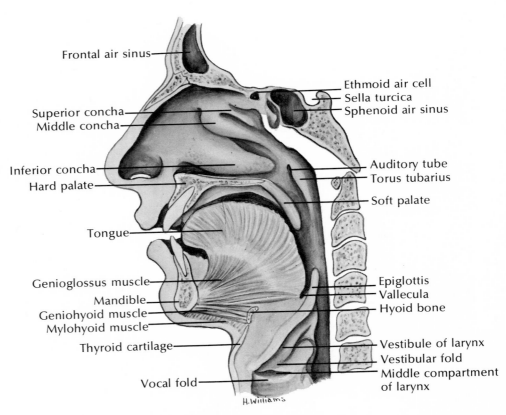

Fig. 11-3. Sagittal section of face and neck.

The air sinuses connected with the nose are the frontal, ethmoid, sphenoid, maxillary, and indirectly, the mastoid sinuses (see Plate X, Trans-vision). Those connected directly with the nose are called collectively the paranasal air sinuses. Each is lined with mucous membrane continuous with that of the nose (Fig. 11-4).

The frontal air sinuses, located in the frontal bone superior to the orbits, are generally two in number, varying greatly in size and shape; they may be partially subdivided by extra septa and are usually not symmetrical. The frontal air sinus empties into the middle meatus.

The ethmoid air sinuses form a labyrinth of small irregular spaces within each lateral mass of ethmoid bone. These vary greatly in size and number, but are usually divided into three groups: a posterior group that empties into the superior meatus, and the anterior and middle groups both of which usually empty into the middle meatus.

The sphenoid air sinuses are located in the body of the sphenoid bone. They are usually two in number, separated by a septum. The sphenoid sinus empties into the sphenoethmoid recess. Occasionally the sphenoid sinuses are completely absent.

The maxillary sinuses are found one on each side inferior to the orbit within the body of the maxilla. Each empties into the middle meatus, behind the opening of the frontal sinus (Fig. 11-5).

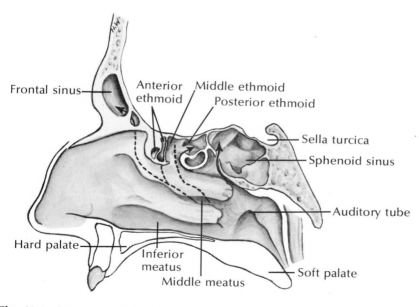

Fig. 11-4. Openings of air sinuses. Arrows indicate the openings from the nasal passages into the sinuses. (Male, 57 years of age.)

339

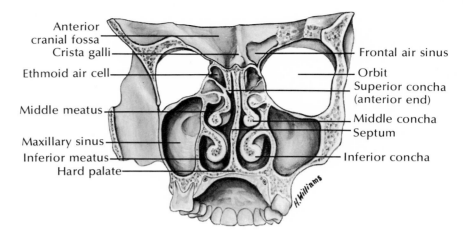

Anterior cranial fossa
Crista galli
Ethmoid air cell
Middle meatus
Maxillary sinus
Inferior meatus
Hard palate

Frontal air sinus
Orbit
Superior concha (anterior end)
Middle concha
Septum
Inferior concha

Fig. 11-5. Vertical section through the nose. Plane of the section passes slightly obliquely through the left first molar tooth and behind the second right premolar tooth. Posterior wall of right frontal sinus removed.

The mastoid air cells open into the middle ear, which is connected with the nasopharynx by way of the auditory tube. All the air sinuses therefore open into the nose, or nasopharynx.

The ophthalmic division of the trigeminal nerve carries sensory fibers from the frontal, ethmoid, and sphenoid sinuses; the maxillary division carries those from the maxillary sinus; and the glossopharyngeal nerve carries those from the mastoid air cells.

Since the opening of an air sinus usually lies above the level of its floor, drainage is impeded if excess fluid is secreted. Furthermore, the openings during life are quite small and, in an acute cold, frequently become obstructed by the swelling of the mucous membrane. Infection within a sinus is known as sinusitis.

PHARYNX

During respiration the pharynx serves as a passageway for air from the nose to the larynx. The pharynx is discussed in Chapter 12.

LARYNX

The larynx is often called the voice box, thus stressing its secondary function. If the larynx is removed surgically, the patient cannot sing and the spoken voice loses much of its flexibility and quality, becoming harsh and monotonous. However, the patient can usually be trained to speak quite adequately. The primary functions of the larynx are to regulate the flow of air into and out of the trachea and to prevent any foreign object from entering the trachea.

340   The larynx lies in the midline of the neck anterior to the fourth,

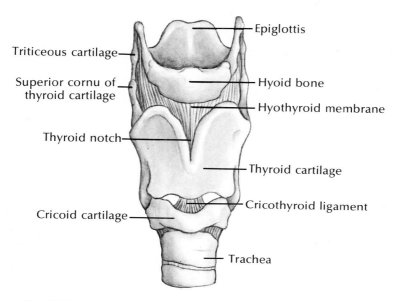

Triticeous cartilage—

Superior cornu of
thyroid cartilage—

Thyroid notch—

Cricoid cartilage—

—Epiglottis

—Hyoid bone

—Hyothyroid membrane

—Thyroid cartilage

—Cricothyroid ligament

—Trachea

Fig. 11-6. Anterior aspect of larynx. (Male, 64 years of age.)

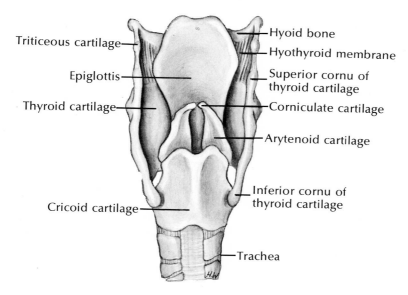

Triticeous cartilage—

Epiglottis—

Thyroid cartilage—

Cricoid cartilage—

—Hyoid bone

—Hyothyroid membrane

—Superior cornu of
thyroid cartilage

—Corniculate cartilage

—Arytenoid cartilage

—Inferior cornu of
thyroid cartilage

—Trachea

Fig. 11-7. Posterior aspect of larynx. (Male, 64 years of age.)   341

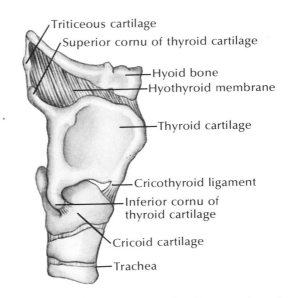

Triticeous cartilage
Superior cornu of thyroid cartilage
Hyoid bone
Hyothyroid membrane
Thyroid cartilage
Cricothyroid ligament
Inferior cornu of thyroid cartilage
Cricoid cartilage
Trachea

Fig. 11-8. Right lateral view of larynx. (Male, 64 years of age.)

fifth, and sixth cervical vertebrae. Behind it lies the lower part of the pharynx leading to the esophagus. The great vessels of the neck and vagus nerve lie on each side. Anteriorly, two layers of muscles arise on the sternum and are inserted into the front of the laryngeal wall (sternohyoid and sternothyroid muscles). The sternocleidomastoid muscle is the prominent muscular mass on each side of the larynx. The larynx is a hollow box lined with mucous membrane. Its walls are formed by several cartilages bound together by elastic membranes.

Cartilages of larynx   There are three single cartilages (thyroid, cricoid, and epiglottis) and three paired cartilages (arytenoid, corniculate, and cuneiform).

The thyroid is the largest of these cartilages. It forms the anterior part of the larynx and is shaped somewhat like the covers of an open book, with the back of the book forming the prominent projection in the neck (Adam's apple). The cricoid cartilage is shaped like a signet ring, with the signet part posterior and the band anterior. The epiglottis is a leaflike cartilage. Its stem is directed inferiorly to attach to the thyroid cartilage in the midline between the two leaves. Its upper broad portion projects superiorly behind the base of the tongue.

The arytenoid cartilages are two small pyramid-shaped masses crowning the signet part of the cricoid at the back of the larynx. The corniculate cartilages are two tiny cones, one placed on the apex of each arytenoid cartilage. The cuneiform cartilages, not always present,

342

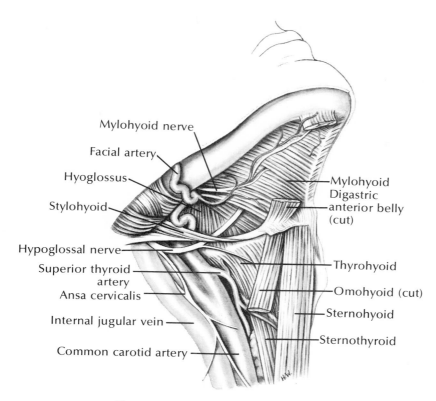

Fig. 11-9. Extrinsic muscles of larynx.

are two tiny rods placed in the mucous membrane fold joining the epiglottis to the arytenoids.

The thyrohyoid membrane fills the interval between the hyoid bone and upper margin of the thyroid cartilage.

The elastic cone, or cricothyroid membrane, is attached to the lower border of the thyroid and arytenoid cartilages superiorly and to the cricoid cartilage inferiorly, completing the wall of the larynx anteriorly and laterally. The thickened central portion of the membrane is known as the cricothyroid ligament. The upper portion of this membrane, attached to the arytenoid posteriorly and to the thyroid anteriorly, forms the vocal ligament underlying each vocal fold.

The laryngeal cavity is subdivided into three parts by two pairs of mucous membrane folds in the lateral wall, the upper pair being the vestibular folds, or false cords, and the lower pair the vocal folds, or true cords. The portion of the larynx above the vestibular folds is called the vestibule of the larynx. The aryepiglottic folds of mucous

Cavity of larynx

343

membrane, extending from the epiglottis anteriorly to the arytenoid cartilages posteriorly, separate the vestibule from the piriform recess (food gutter) of the pharynx on each side. The epiglottis separates the vestibule from the valleculae, which are a pair of depressions between the base of the tongue and the epiglottis. The middle compartment (ventricle) of the larynx is quite small and lies between the vestibular and vocal folds. The lowest compartment of the larynx lies inferior to the vocal folds and is continuous with the trachea.

The mucous membrane of the larynx is closely adherent to the epiglottis and to the vocal folds. Over the upper surface of the epiglottis and the vocal folds there is stratified squamous epithelium; elsewhere the mucous membrane is loosely attached, has pseudostratafied, ciliated columnar epithelium, and may become enormously swollen, preventing the passage of air. A surgeon must then insert a tube through the larynx to open up a passageway (intubation) or make an external opening into the trachea (tracheotomy) to preserve life.

Muscles of larynx

The numerous muscles associated with the larynx are divided into an extrinsic group and an intrinsic group. The extrinsic group includes all muscles attached to the larynx and to the hyoid bone, which is functionally a portion of the larynx (Fig. 11-10).

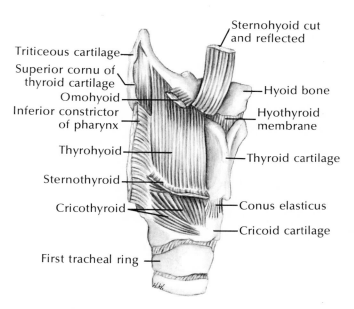

Triticeous cartilage

Superior cornu of thyroid cartilage

Omohyoid

Inferior constrictor of pharynx

Thyrohyoid

Sternothyroid

Cricothyroid

First tracheal ring

Sternohyoid cut and reflected

Hyoid bone

Hyothyroid membrane

Thyroid cartilage

Conus elasticus

Cricoid cartilage

Fig. 11-10. Extrinsic muscles of the larynx. This is a right oblique view of the structures. (Male, 65 years of age.)

Anterior to the larynx are placed the sternohyoid, sternothyroid, thyrohyoid, and omohyoid muscles (see Fig. 5-3). The sternohyoid is a thin, straplike muscle that originates from the upper edge of the manubrium of the sternum and passes upward to be inserted into the front of the hyoid bone. The sternothyroid is also a thin, flat muscle that arises from the upper edge of the sternum. It lies beneath (deeper than) the sternohyoid muscle and is inserted into the anterior surface of the thyroid cartilage. The thyrohyoid muscle arises just above the insertion of the sternothyroid muscle and is inserted into the lower edge of the hyoid bone. The omohyoid is another ribbonlike muscle composed of two muscular bellies and an intermediate tendinous part. The inferior belly arises from the superior border of the scapula and the superior belly is inserted into the lower margin of the hyoid, lateral to the attachment of the sternohyoid muscle. There is a strong band of deep cervical fascia holding the intermediate tendon close to the posterior surface of the clavicle.

Superior to the larynx are the digastric, stylohyoid, mylohyoid, and geniohyoid muscles. The digastric has two muscular bellies and a middle tendinous portion. The posterior belly arises from the mastoid bone and passes inferiorly and anteriorly toward the hyoid bone. The intermediate tendon has a fibrous attachment to the body of the hyoid, and then the anterior belly of the muscle continues superiorly and anteriorly to be inserted into the lower edge of the mandible near the midline. The stylohyoid arises from the styloid process of the temporal bone and passes inferiorly beside the posterior belly of the digastric muscle to be inserted into the body of the hyoid bone. The mylohyoid arises from the mylohyoid line of the mandible and is inserted partly into the body of the hyoid bone and partly into a fibrous band extending from the middle of the hyoid to the symphysis of the mandible. This muscle helps to form the floor of the mouth (see Fig. 5-3). The geniohyoid is associated with the mylohyoid in forming the floor of the mouth.

The muscles just described have a varied nerve supply. The posterior belly of the digastric and the stylohyoid are supplied from the facial nerve, the anterior belly of the digastric and the mylohyoid from the motor portion of the trigeminal, and the remaining muscles are innervated from branches of first, second, and third cervical nerves (ansa cervicalis).

The extrinsic muscles of the larynx alter its position in speaking and in swallowing. If you place your finger on the larynx and swallow, it is obvious that the entire larynx moves superiorly and anteriorly. At the completion of swallowing, the larynx moves in the reverse direction.

345

The intrinsic muscles of the larynx alter the shape of the various portions of the larynx itself (Figs. 11-11 and 11-12). It is not necessary to learn the attachments of this very complex group, but the more important functions should be known (Fig. 11-13).

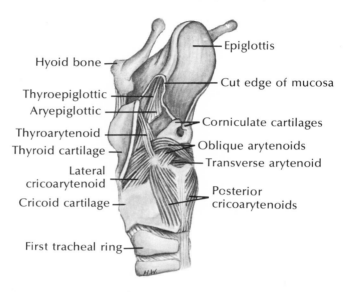

Fig. 11-11. Intrinsic muscles of the larynx, left oblique view. (Male, 65 years of age.)

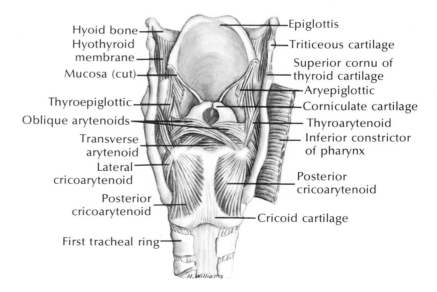

Fig. 11-12. Intrinsic muscles of the larynx, posterior view. (Male, 65 years of age.)

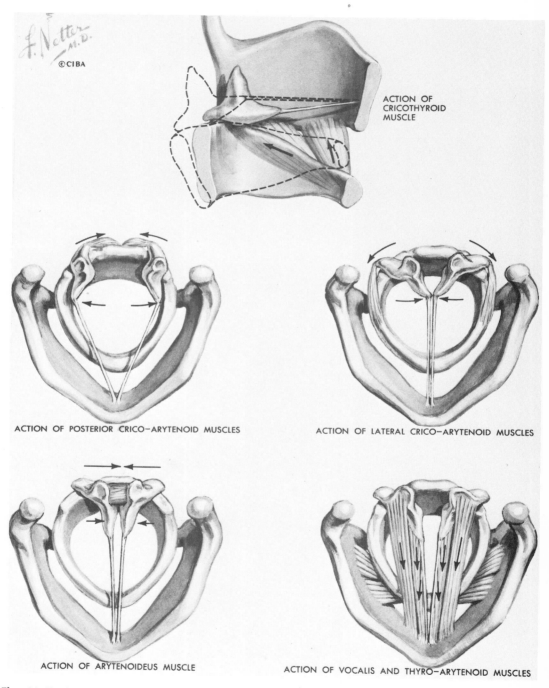

ACTION OF
CRICOTHYROID
MUSCLE

ACTION OF POSTERIOR CRICO–ARYTENOID MUSCLES

ACTION OF LATERAL CRICO–ARYTENOID MUSCLES

ACTION OF ARYTENOIDEUS MUSCLE

ACTION OF VOCALIS AND THYRO–ARYTENOID MUSCLES

Fig. 11-13. Action of intrinsic laryngeal muscles. (From DeWeese, D. D., and Saunders, W. H.: Textbook of otolaryngology, ed. 4, St. Louis, 1973, The C. V. Mosby Co.)

The aryepiglottic muscles lying within the aryepiglottic folds and the transverse and oblique arytenoids placed between the arytenoid cartilages act as a sphincter of the laryngeal inlet. During the process of swallowing, these muscles close the vestibule and thus prevent food from entering the larynx. The epiglottis does not fold back as a lid to the laryngeal opening, but it does tend to divert liquids to either side. The ventricular muscle lying within the vestibular fold acts as an accessory sphincter closing the middle compartment of the larynx. The cricothyroids are said to tense the vocal folds, whereas the vocal muscles and thyroarytenoids relax them. The lateral and posterior cricoarytenoids alter the position of the vocal folds, the lateral cri-

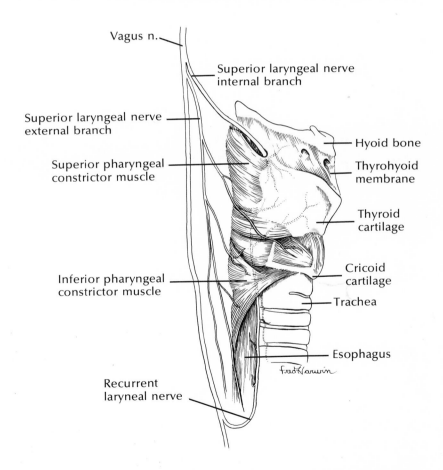

Fig. 11-14. Laryngeal nerve supply. The lowermost relationships of recurrent nerves vary on the left and the right and are not drawn. (From DeWeese, D. D., and Saunders, W. H.: Textbook of otolaryngology, ed. 4, St. Louis, 1973, The C. V. Mosby Co.)

coarytenoids drawing them together and the posterior cricoarytenoids separating them.

The ability to alter the position of the vocal folds is of great physiologic importance. The interval between the vocal folds is never more than a few millimeters and is the narrowest part of the air passages. In speaking we vary this width and thus regulate the rate of air flow from the lungs. When a person holds his breath, he does it mainly by contraction of the lateral cricoarytenoid muscles, which pull the vocal folds together and close the opening completely. The posterior cricoarytenoid muscles are the only muscles that have the opposite action; in persons in whom these muscles are paralyzed, the opening between the vocal folds becomes permanently and dangerously narrowed. The action of separation of the vocal folds, or abduction, is so vital that it has led some anatomists to regard the posterior cricoarytenoid muscles as the most important striate muscles in the body (Fig. 11-13).

All the intrinsic muscles of the larynx are supplied by the recurrent laryngeal nerve except the cricothyroid, which is supplied by the external laryngeal branch of the superior laryngeal nerve. The internal laryngeal branch of the superior laryngeal nerve carries the sensory fibers for the mucosa of the larynx superior to the vocal folds. The mucosa of the inferior compartment of the larynx receives sensory innervation through the recurrent laryngeal nerve (Fig. 11-14).

The larynx is larger in men than in women, the difference becoming particularly noticeable at puberty. It is associated with the "change of voice" characteristic of boys at that time.

TRACHEA

The trachea, or windpipe, extends from the level of the inferior border of the sixth cervical vertebra to the superior border of the fifth thoracic vertebra, where it divides into two main bronchi. In the neck the isthmus of the thyroid gland lies in front, and the lobes of the thyroid gland lie on each side of the trachea. Within the thorax the trachea lies in the posterior part of the mediastinum, behind the heart and great vessels. Posterior to the trachea is the esophagus, and posterior to that again are the bodies of the vertebrae. In the groove between the trachea and esophagus the recurrent laryngeal nerve passes superiorly to the larynx.

In the lower part of the neck, inferior to the isthmus of the thyroid gland, the anterior surface of the trachea is covered only by fascia and skin.

The trachea is kept permanently patent by a series of cartilaginous bands. These bands only partially encircle the trachea, for the posterior part is missing. The back of the trachea is therefore flat and com-

349

posed of fibromuscular tissue. The walls between the cartilaginous rings are quite elastic, enabling the trachea to adjust itself to various positions of the body. The mucous membrane lining the trachea is continuous with that of the larynx superiorly and is continued inferiorly into the bronchi. It has pseudostratified, ciliated columnar epithelium.

In infancy and early childhood the tracheal cartilages are soft; they stiffen in the later years of childhood.

BRONCHI

The bronchi, which connect the trachea with the lungs, have incomplete rings and plaques of cartilage in their walls to keep them open. The left bronchus is smaller than the right and passes more directly laterally, whereas the right continues almost vertically. For this reason foreign bodies that get into the trachea almost always lodge in the right bronchus or in one of its branches. All the branches of the left bronchus are given off below the left pulmonary artery, but the right bronchus just below its origin gives off a branch above the right pulmonary artery. This branch is called the eparterial bronchus.

There are usually two left bronchial arteries arising from the aorta, and one right bronchial artery that may arise from the aorta or from an intercostal branch or from a left bronchial artery. The bronchial arteries accompany the bronchi and carry oxygenated blood to the bronchi, the pleura, and some mediastinal structures.

THORACIC CAVITY

Before discussing the lungs it is best to describe the thoracic cavity and its subdivisions. The trachea, esophagus, and blood vessels are enclosed by fascia. On either side there is a fanshaped layer of fascia (Sibson's fascia) attached medially to the cervical vertebrae and laterally to the inner edge of the first rib. This layer of fascia forms the superior limit of each half of the thoracic cavity and seals the cavity off from the root of the neck. Inferiorly, the thoracic cavity is separated from the abdominal cavity by a sheet of muscle, called the diaphragm.

The thoracic cavity lodges the two pleural cavities, each containing a lung. The pleural cavities are completely separated from each other by the mediastinum, or connective tissue, in which the heart lies. In addition to containing the heart, the mediastinum contains the pericardium surrounding the heart, the pulmonary trunk and arteries, the thoracic aorta and its branches, the trachea and part of the bronchi, the esophagus, the vagus nerves, the phrenic nerves, the thoracic duct, many lymph nodes and lymph vessels, and the thymus or its fibrous remainder.

350   Each pleural cavity has a lining of serous membrane, the pleura,

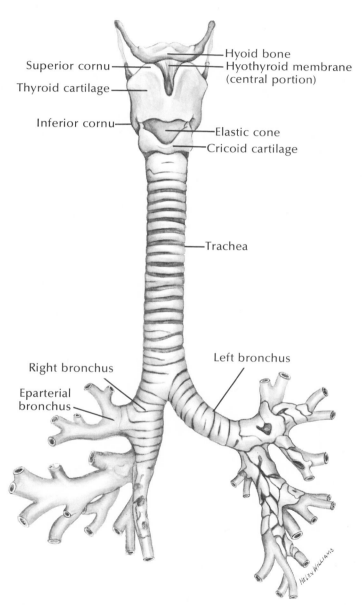

Fig. 11-15. Larynx and trachea, anterior view. Cartilage plaques omitted
from branches of right bronchus.

that completely covers its inner surface. This serous membrane is reflected at the root of the lung. The layer lining the chest wall is called the parietal pleura, and the layer over the lung is called the visceral pleura.

The parietal pleura is well supplied with sensory nerve endings. These give rise to the sensations of pain in pleurisy. In empyema, pus

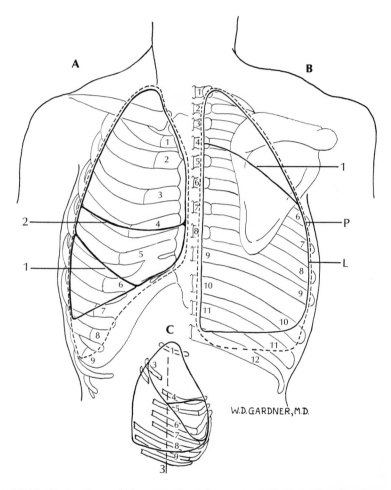

W.D. GARDNER, M.D.

Fig. 11-16. Projection of the margins, fissures, and pleural reflections of the right lung to the chest wall. **A,** Anterior surface of the lung and chest wall: *1,* primary fissure of the right lung; *2,* secondary fissure of the right lung. **B,** Posterior surface of the lung and chest wall: *1,* primary fissure of the right lung; *P,* line of pleural reflection (broken line); *L,* margin of the lung (solid line). **C,** Lateral surface of the lung and chest wall: *3,* midaxillary line. All numbers within a drawing refer to the rib number. (From Gardner, W. D.: Diagnostic anatomy, St. Louis, The C. V. Mosby Co.)

collects between the two layers of pleura and occasionally between lobes of a lung. In pleural effusions, fluid collects between the visceral and parietal pleurae. In operating to withdraw fluid, a surgeon passes a hollow needle through the chest wall and through the parietal pleura.

Posteriorly, the parietal pleura is reflected from the inner surface of the ribs to the sides of the mediastinum in a straight line parallel

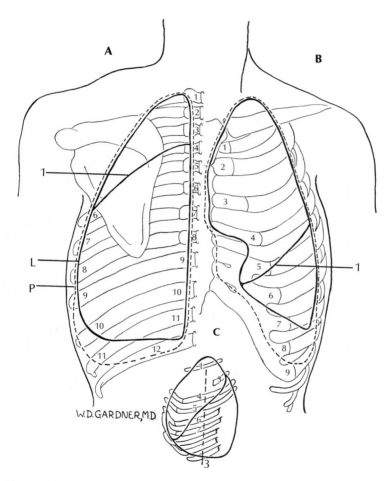

Fig. 11-17. Projection of the margins, fissures, and pleural reflections of the left lung to the chest wall. **A,** Posterior surface of the lung and chest wall: *1,* primary fissure of the left lung; *L,* margin of the lung (solid line); *P,* line of pleural reflection (broken line). **B,** Anterior surface of the lung and chest wall: *1,* primary fissure of the left lung. **C,** Lateral surface of the lung and chest wall: *3,* midaxillary line. All numbers within a drawing refer to the rib number. (From Gardner, W. D.: Diagnostic anatomy, St. Louis, The C. V. Mosby Co.)

353

and close to the vertebral column from the first to the twelfth thoracic vertebrae.

Anteriorly, on the right, the pleura is reflected from the costal surface to the mediastinal surface along a line extending from the root of the neck down the middle of the sternum to the level of the junction of the sixth costal cartilage. On the left the line is like that of the right, down to the level of the fourth costal cartilage where it deviates from the midline, being pushed aside by the heart. In this roughly triangular space behind the left half of the sternum the parietal pericardium is in contact with the anterior chest wall. The extent of this triangular area is extremely variable. If the pericardial sac is distended, it pushes the pleural sac still farther to the left, and then, if great care is used, fluid may be aspirated from the pericardial cavity.

At the line of attachment of the diaphragm to the body wall the pleura is reflected from the inner surface of the thorax onto the superior surface of the diaphragm. Since this line of reflection marks the lowest limit to which the fully distended lung can descend, its position should be kept in mind. On the left the line starts anteriorly at the junction of the sixth costal cartilage with the sternum; it passes almost horizontally around the chest, crossing, successively, the obliquely directed seventh rib at the junction with its costal cartilage, the eighth rib in the midclavicular line, the tenth rib in the midaxillary line, and the junction of the twelfth rib with the last thoracic vertebra. On the right the line of reflection follows the cartilage of the seventh rib, crosses the eighth rib at the midclavicular line, and from there on pursues a course identical with that of the left (Figs. 11-16 and 11-17).

LUNGS In a healthy adult the lung is spongy in consistency throughout and practically fills its pleural cavity. It is attached to the mediastinum on its medial aspect by the reflection of pleura and by the pulmonary vessels and bronchi that enter the substance of the lung. Normally the parietal pleura is nowhere adherent to the visceral pleura. The color of the lung of a baby is pink, because of contained blood, but in an adult this color is masked by a mottled blue-gray color produced by particles of dust and soot permanently incorporated in its tissue. The lung of a baby who has not breathed is solid and sinks in water. After birth, respiration causes the lung to become spongy and filled with air, so that it no longer sinks in water. Complete opening of the air spaces of the lung is not attained until two or three weeks after birth.

The apex of the lung is the blunt, rounded, superior end that projects up into the base of the neck above the first rib. The base of the lung is concave and rests on the diaphragm. The hilus is a wedge-shaped area on the medial surface where the great vessels and bronchi

354

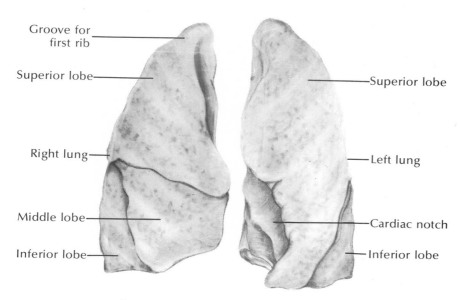

Groove for first rib

Superior lobe

Right lung

Middle lobe

Inferior lobe

Superior lobe

Left lung

Cardiac notch

Inferior lobe

Fig. 11-18. Anterior surface of lungs.

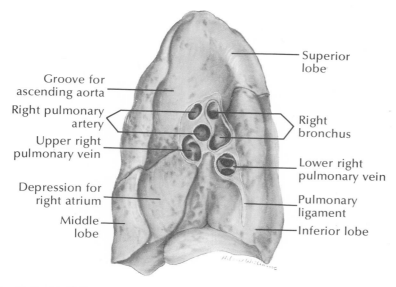

Superior lobe

Groove for ascending aorta

Right pulmonary artery

Upper right pulmonary vein

Depression for right atrium

Middle lobe

Right bronchus

Lower right pulmonary vein

Pulmonary ligament

Inferior lobe

Fig. 11-19. Medial surface of the right lung. Same lung as seen in Fig. 11-18.   355

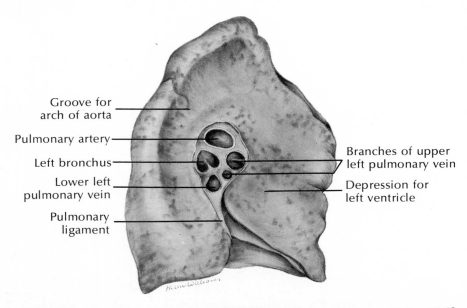

Groove for
arch of aorta

Pulmonary artery

Left bronchus

Lower left
pulmonary vein

Pulmonary
ligament

Branches of upper
left pulmonary vein

Depression for
left ventricle

Fig. 11-20. Medial surface of the left lung. Same lung as seen in Fig. 11-18.

enter the lung substance. These structures grouped together are called the root of the lung, each composed of one pulmonary artery, two pulmonary veins, nerves, lymphatics, bronchial vessels, and a main bronchus. The parietal pleura is reflected over these vessels onto the surface of the lung where it becomes the visceral pleura. The reflection extends inferiorly for some distance below the hilus to form the pulmonary ligament.

The left lung has two lobes, an upper and a lower lobe. The right lung has three lobes, an upper, middle, and lower lobe. The right upper and middle lobes correspond to the left upper lobe. The right lung is shorter, wider, and slightly larger than the left. The lower medial portion of the left lung presents a hollowed area occupied by the heart.

Each pulmonary lobe may be divided into several segments based upon the branching of the bronchial tree. The regions of the lungs aerated by tertiary (third order) bronchi are designated broncho-pulmonary segments, of which there are considered to be ten and nine in the right and left lungs, respectively (Boyden). Pulmonary and small systemic arteries also divide and run close to the bronchi, whereas pulmonary veins run at some distance from the air passages. The third-order arterial branches are intrasegmental, whereas the corresponding third-order veins are intersegmental. The veins, therefore, outline or form a "venous fence" around each broncho-

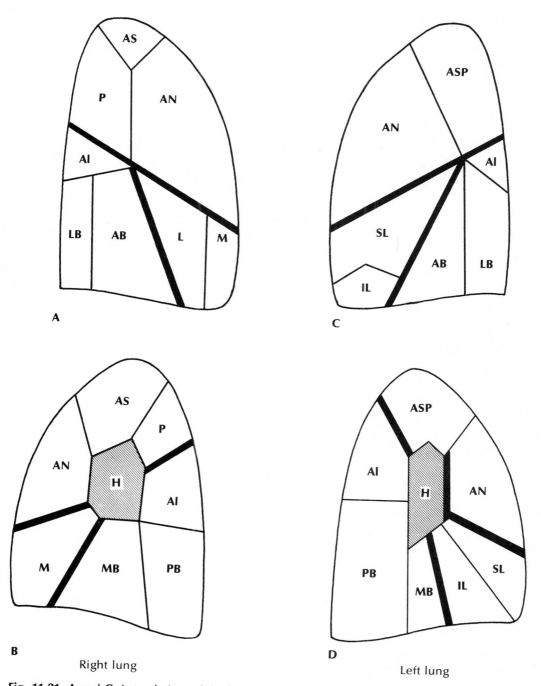

Fig. 11-21. A and **C,** Lateral view of the lungs. **B** and **D,** Medial view of the lungs. The limits of the bronchopulmonary segments are shown. **A** and **B,** Right lung. **C** and **D,** Left lung. The thick lines indicate the limits between lobes. *H,* Pulmonary hilus. (From DiDio, L. J. A.: Synopsis of anatomy, St. Louis, 1970, The C. V. Mosby Co.)

Right lung

Left lung

pulmonary segment. A disease condition may be limited to one or more segments. Therefore, it is possible for a surgeon using the veins as an intersegmental guide to resect only the diseased segments, leaving the rest of a pulmonary lobe intact. The bronchopulmonary segments are listed as follows and are illustrated in Fig. 11-21.

	Right lung	*Left lung*
Superior lobe	Apical (AS)	Apicoposterior (ASP)
	Posterior (P)	
	Anterior (AN)	Anterior (AN)
Middle lobe	Lateral (L)	Superior lingular (SL)
	Medial (M)	Inferior lingular (IL)
Inferior lobe	Apical (AI)	Apical (AI)
	Medial basal (MB)	Medial basal (MB)
	Anterior basal (AB)	Anterior basal (AB)
	Lateral basal (LB)	Lateral basal (LB)
	Posterior basal (PB)	Posterior basal (PB)

As the bronchi pass into the substance of the lung, they subdivide into smaller and smaller tubes, the smallest being known as bronchioles. These in turn end in small ducts having many outpocketings, or alveoli (see Fig. 11-1). The larger subdivisions of the primary bronchi have an inner lining of pseudostratified columnar epithelium. Beneath this is a layer of smooth muscle and a layer of connective tissue and cartilage plaques. As the air passages become smaller, the epithelium gradually changes, the cilia are lost, and the cells become flatter until finally they become squamous in the alveolar ducts. The cartilage plaques entirely disappear in the smaller bronchi, and the smooth muscle fibers cease in the alveolar ducts.

There is a very rich capillary network about the alveoli. Respiration occurs by an interchange of gases through the walls of alveolus and capillary.

A pulmonary lobule is considered to be the primary unit of the lung. It consists of the final bronchiole (respiratory bronchiole), the associated alveolar ducts and alveoli, capillaries, and nerve fibers.

The nerves to the lung come from the vagus (cranial autonomic outflow) and the upper thoracic segments of the cord (thoracolumbar autonomic outflow).

In certain parts of the air passages, the surface epithelium possesses cilia. These cilia beat in such a manner as to cause the mucus on the surface to flow toward the pharynx. In the nasal cavity this is a posterior flow, and in the lower respiratory passages it is a superior flow. Small particles of dust and carbon (smoke) are carried by the mucus into the pharynx. Here, the mucus may be swallowed or expectorated.

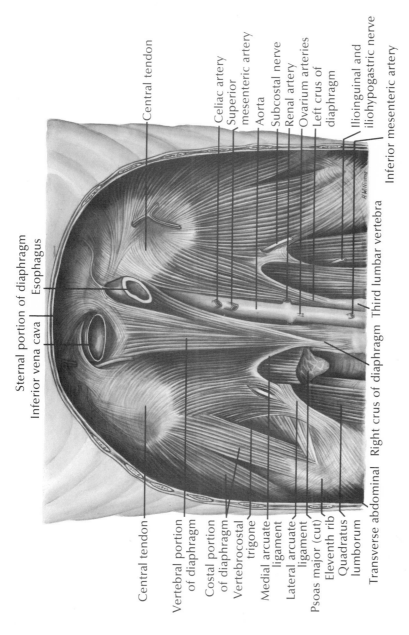

Sternal portion of diaphragm
Inferior vena cava
Esophagus

Central tendon

Celiac artery
Superior mesenteric artery
Aorta
Subcostal nerve
Renal artery
Ovarium arteries
Left crus of diaphragm
Ilioinguinal and iliohypogastric nerve
Inferior mesenteric artery

Central tendon
Vertebral portion of diaphragm
Costal portion of diaphragm
Vertebrocostal trigone
Medial arcuate ligament
Lateral arcuate ligament
Psoas major (cut)
Eleventh rib
Quadratus lumborum
Transverse abdominal
Right crus of diaphragm
Third lumbar vertebra

Fig. 11-22. Abdominal surface of the diaphragm. (Female, 31 years of age.)

359

MUSCLES OF RESPIRATION

The muscles used in breathing include the diaphragm, a large number of small muscles between the ribs, and certain accessory muscles that are attached superiorly to the upper ribs and others that are attached inferiorly to the xiphoid and lower ribs (Fig. 11-22).

The diaphragm is a muscular septum placed between the thoracic and abdominal cavities. It arises by a series of muscular bands from the posterior aspect of the xiphoid, from the inner surface of the lower six costal cartilages, from the anterior surface of the lumbar vertebrae, and from the fascia covering the deep muscles of the back. The central portion is tendinous, and the various muscle bundles are inserted into the central tendon.

The diaphragm presents domes that are concave below and convex above, the dome on the right rising to a higher level than the one on the left. The liver lies inferior to the right dome and the stomach inferior to the left. The heart rests on the superior surface of the diaphragm between the two domes.

The superior surface is covered on each side by parietal pleura and in the central portion by parietal pericardium. Most of the inferior surface is covered by parietal peritoneum.

Numerous structures pass through the diaphragm, namely, the inferior vena cava, the esophagus, the vagal trunks, and several small arteries. The aorta and thoracic duct pass through an arch at the back of the muscle and not through its substance, and the azygos vein passes behind the diaphragm, just to the right of the aorta.

The small muscles attached to the ribs include the following:

1. Eleven sets of intercostal muscles are present on each side. An external intercostal muscle arises from the lower border of a rib; its fibers pass inferiorly and anteriorly to be inserted into the upper edge of the rib below, and it is analogous to the external oblique abdominal muscle. An internal intercostal muscle arises from the lower border of a rib; its fibers pass inferiorly and posteriorly to be inserted into the rib below, and it is analogous to an internal oblique abdominal muscle. An innermost intercostal muscle also arises from the lower border of a rib; its fibers pass inferiorly and posteriorly to be inserted into the rib below, and it is analogous to the transverse abdominal muscle.

2. The subcostal muscles are similar to the innermost intercostals but are found only in the lower chest. They are not attached to adjacent ribs but pass over more than one rib between origin and insertion.

3. The transverse thoracic muscle arises from the deep surface of the sternum and passes out to an insertion into the costal cartilages.

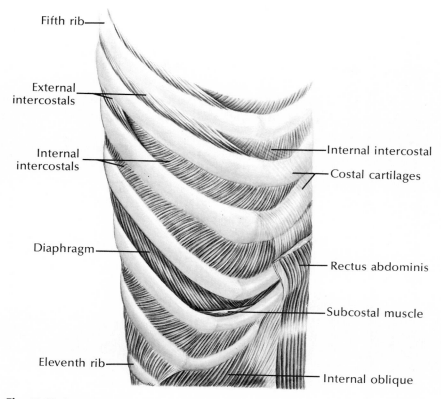

Fifth rib

External intercostals

Internal intercostals

Diaphragm

Eleventh rib

Internal intercostal

Costal cartilages

Rectus abdominis

Subcostal muscle

Internal oblique

Fig. 11-23. Intercostal muscles of the right chest wall. (Male, 57 years of age.)

4. Twelve pairs of levator costarum muscles arise from the transverse processes of the last cervical and upper 11 thoracic vertebrae and attach to the rib below.

In the neck are three scalene muscles that arise from the tubercles of the transverse processes of cervical vertebrae. The anterior scalene is inserted into the first rib anterior to the subclavian artery. The middle scalene is inserted into the first rib posterior to the subclavian artery. The posterior scalene is inserted into the lateral side of the second rib.

In inhalation of air, the size of the pleural cavity is increased in three directions. Expansion of the chest wall lowers the intrathoracic pressure, and air enters from the outside through the air passages into the lungs.

The vertical length of the pleural cavity is increased by contraction of the diaphragm. The muscular bands pull on the central tendon from every side, flattening out the diaphragm and pushing the abdomi-

361

nal viscera inferiorly and anteriorly. The muscles of the abdominal wall control and limit this visceral movement.

The ribs are so articulated with the vertebral column that they tend to rotate out and up with inhalation. Thus the size of the chest is increased from side to side and from anterior to posterior. The first rib is raised and fixed by contraction of the scalene muscles. The small muscles attached to the ribs likewise contract in series from above downward.

The abdominal muscles, particularly the rectus abdominis, anchor the sternum so that raising of the ribs must result in a more horizontal position of the obliquely placed costal cartilages. This increases the expansibility of the chest.

In exhalation the respiratory muscles relax. The weight of the thoracic cage, the elasticity of the costal cartilages, the inherent elasticity of the lungs, and the tone of the abdominal muscles that push the abdominal viscera and diaphragm superiorly all cause air to be forced out of the lungs.

The diaphragm, composed of voluntary skeletal muscle, is innervated by the phrenic nerves, which arise from the third, fourth, and fifth cervical spinal cord segments. The intercostal muscles are innervated by branches of the first through eleventh thoracic spinal nerves. The respiratory motoneurons in both phrenic and intercostal nerves are found in the ventral horn of the corresponding spinal cord segments. The phrenic nerves carry sensory fibers from the central portion of the diaphragm, above and below; sensory fibers from the peripheral portion of the diaphragm are found in the lower intercostal nerves.

Respiration is subject to a considerable degree of voluntary control, which can be demonstrated by the holding of ones breath. The ability to hold ones breath, however, also demonstrates the reflex type of control that normally allows one to breathe without conscious voluntary effort.

There are a number of sensory receptors that can alter respiration. These include stretch receptors, located within the lungs and respiratory muscles, and chemoreceptors, the carotid and aortic bodies. The carotid body is located at the bifurcation of the common carotid artery, and the aortic body lies between the arch of the aorta and the pulmonary artery. Stretch receptors from the lungs pass to the brain stem via the vagus nerve, those from the respiratory muscles pass to the brain stem in the appropriate spinal nerves, and afferents from the chemoreceptors are carried with the glossopharyngeal and vagus nerves.

362 The chemoreceptors receive a rich arterial supply, and the afferent

fibers from the carotid and aortic bodies appear to respond to a lowered pH in the blood associated with a decrease in arterial oxygen tension and an increase in arterial carbon dioxide tension.

Reflexes, spinal and brain stem as well as many others, interact to produce normal rate, depth, and pattern of respiration.

REVIEW QUESTIONS

1. What organs are included in the respiratory system?
2. Describe the inferior turbinate.
3. Name the air sinuses of the skull. Where is each located? Where does each empty?
4. Name the cartilages of the larynx. Which are paired and which are unpaired?
5. What is the nerve supply of the intrinsic muscles of the larynx?
6. Give a brief description of the trachea.
7. What structures form the walls of the thoracic cavity?
8. How do the lungs of an adult differ from those of a newborn child?
9. List the muscles of respiration.
10. Describe the diaphragm.
11. Describe the mechanical processes involved in inspiration and expiration.
12. What are the functions of the nasal cavity?
13. What are the functions of the larynx?
14. What are the components of a pulmonary lobule?
15. What is the function of the posterior cricoarytenoid muscle?
16. Discuss bronchopulmonary segments.

CHAPTER 12

THE DIGESTIVE SYSTEM

The digestive, or alimentary, canal is a hollow tube with associated glands running from oral cavity to anus. Although modified in its various parts, the canal consists throughout of four coats, or layers: mucosa, submucosa, muscularis, and adventitia, or serosa (Fig. 12-1). The function of the system is to break down ingested foods into simpler substances, thereby enhancing absorption or excretion. It is interesting to note that while food is inside the gastrointestinal tract, it is in reality outside the body, since there are no membranes to be transversed in its passage through the digestive tract. The digestive, or alimentary, canal has the following subdivisions: mouth, pharynx, esophagus, stomach, and small and large intestine.

MOUTH   The mouth is bounded on each side by the cheeks, superiorly by the hard and soft palates and inferiorly by a muscular sheet attached to the mandible. Anteriorly the mouth is closed by the lips, and posteriorly it opens into the pharynx. The mouth contains the teeth and tongue. The ducts of the salivary glands empty into the mouth.

The vestibule of the mouth is the space between the teeth and the mucous membrane of the cheeks and lips. The main cavity of the mouth lies within the dental arches, inferior to the palate.

The lips have a layer of skin on the outer side that is continuous with the mucous membrane covering the lip margins and extending into the mouth. Beneath this outer layer are bands of muscle and connective tissue. These various muscles of expression were discussed in Chapter 5. The lips are richly supplied with blood vessels, lymphatics, and sensory nerves.

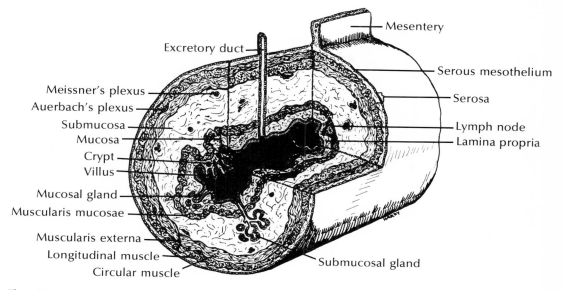

Fig. 12-1. Stereogram of general plan of gastrointestinal tract. (From Bevelander, G., and Ramaley, J. A.: Essentials of histology, ed. 7, St. Louis, 1974, The C. V. Mosby Co.)

Like the lips, the cheeks have skin on the outer surface, mucous membrane on the inner surface, and muscles and connective tissue between the two surfaces. The buccinator, the most important muscle of the cheek, helps to keep the cheeks pressed firmly against the teeth, thereby acting as an accessory muscle of mastication.

The hard palate, formed from portions of the maxillary and palatine bones, separates the mouth from the nasal cavity. The undersurface is covered by a thick layer of mucoperiosteum, so called because the mucous membrane is firmly adherent to the periosteum covering the bone.

Mucous glands are found throughout the mouth but are particularly abundant in certain areas. Beneath the mucous membrane of the lips is an almost continuous layer of small compound alveolar glands (racemose) that empty into the vestibule of the mouth. On the back of the hard palate and on the oral surface of the soft palate there are also very numerous glands.

The soft palate is attached posteriorly to the hard palate and to the sides of the mouth. It is a muscular fold covered superiorly and inferiorly by mucous membrane. In mastication it hugs the back of the tongue, shutting off the mouth from the pharynx and allowing air to flow freely into the larynx. When one swallows, the soft palate is raised,

365

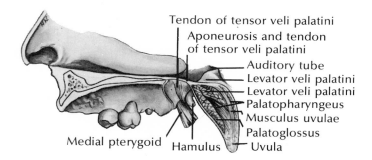

Tendon of tensor veli palatini
Aponeurosis and tendon
of tensor veli palatini
Auditory tube
Levator veli palatini
Levator veli palatini
Palatopharyngeus
Musculus uvulae
Palatoglossus
Uvula
Medial pterygoid
Hamulus

Fig. 12-2. Sagittal section of the soft palate. (Female, 44 years of age.)

closing off the nasopharynx and permitting food to pass downward into
the esophagus. Also, when one speaks or sings, the soft palate is
raised, shutting off the nasopharynx and thus directing the passage
of air through the mouth. The soft palate ends posteriorly in a median
free projection called the uvula (Fig. 12-2).

Laterally, the soft palate is continuous with a fold of the side wall
anterior to the palatine tonsil. This is known as the palatoglossal arch
(anterior pillar of the fauces). Posterior to the palatine tonsil there is
another fold in the side wall of the pharynx, called the palatopharyngeal arch (posterior pillar of the fauces). There are muscles within
these folds, attached superiorly to the soft palate and inferiorly to
the side of the tongue and pharynx, respectively. The palatoglossus
is the muscle of the anterior fold, and the palatopharyngeus is the
muscle of the posterior fold. The palatoglossus may be said to arise
from the dense fascia forming the midline of the soft palate. Here the
fibers are continuous with those of the muscle of the other side of the
palate. The palatopharyngeus is a similar muscle arising in the midline of the soft palate where its fibers are continuous with those of the
other side. These muscles aid the soft palate in closing off the mouth
from the pharynx during mastication. They also make a narrow opening through which the tongue must push food when one swallows.

The levator veli palatini muscle arises from the inferior surface of
the petrous portion of the temporal bone and passes inferiorly and
anteriorly into the soft palate. Some of its fibers are continuous with
those of the same muscle of the other side. In this way a sling for the
soft palate is formed, and in contraction of the muscles the soft palate
is pulled superiorly from the back of the tongue.

The tensor veli palatini arises from the undersurface of the sphenoid bone. As it passes inferiorly in the side wall of the pharynx, it becomes tendinous and is inserted into the soft palate. Its function is

somewhat uncertain, but it is thought to open the inner end of the auditory tube when one swallows.

The palatoglossus, palatopharyngeus, and levator veli palatini muscles receive their nerve supply from the pharyngeal plexus; the tensor veli palatini muscle is innervated by the motor portion of the trigeminal nerve.

The tongue is a muscular organ covered by mucous membrane continuous with the lining of the mouth. Muscle bundles pass through the substance of the tongue longitudinally, vertically, and laterally, thus making it a very mobile organ. Its function in chewing is to mix the food with saliva and to keep the mass of food pressed between the grinding surfaces of the teeth. It acts in swallowing by forcing the food back into the pharynx. It is also an organ of speech, aiding particularly in the production of consonantal sounds. Taste buds distributed over the mucous membrane of the tongue are the end organs for the reception of taste. The fibers carrying sensory impulses of taste for the anterior two thirds of the tongue pass through the chorda tympani branch of the seventh cranial nerve, and those for the posterior third through the ninth cranial nerve.

Other types of sensory impulses for the anterior portion of the tongue are transmitted through the fibers of the fifth nerve and for the posterior portion through the ninth nerve. The motor nerve of the tongue is the twelfth cranial, or hypoglossal, nerve.

The mucous membrane of the tongue has a layer of stratified squamous epithelium. On the superior surface are many projections, or papillae, that make the surface rough. Most of the papillae are filiform, or slender and threadlike, some are fungiform, or knoblike, and a few are vallate, or knoblike with a circular depression around each one.

The extrinsic muscles of the tongue include the hyoglossus, genioglossus, styloglossus, and palatoglossus. The palatoglossus has already been described in the discussion on the soft palate. The hyoglossus arises from the superior border of the hyoid bone and passes directly superiorly and anteriorly to be inserted into the side of the tongue. The genioglossus arises from the back of the symphysis of the mandible. Its fibers pass out in a fan-shaped manner and are inserted into the entire length of the tongue near the midline. The styloglossus arises from the styloid process of the temporal bone and passes inferiorly and anteriorly in the side wall of the pharynx to be inserted into the side of the tongue. Its fibers are intermingled with those of the hyoglossus and genioglossus muscles. The styloglossus pulls the tongue posteriorly and superiorly, the hyoglossus pulls the tongue inferiorly and posteriorly, and the genioglossus protrudes the tongue. The genioglossus also keeps the base of the tongue from falling back into the oral phar-

367

ynx, which would obstruct the airway from nose to larynx. The palato-glossus muscles receive motor fibers from the pharyngeal plexus. The other extrinsic muscles of the tongue receive their motor innervation from the hypoglossal nerve.

The floor of the mouth, composed of a muscular diaphragm, is covered by mucous membrane. The most important muscle of the diaphragm is the mylohyoid, which arises on each side from the mylohyoid line on the medial surface of the mandible. The two muscles meet in the midline beneath the tongue. They fill in the space between the two halves of the mandible and are attached inferiorly to the hyoid bone. The geniohyoid muscle arises from the posterior surface of the symphysis of the mandible and is inserted into the central portion of the hyoid. It lies in the midline deeper than the mylohyoid. The genioglossus muscle, which lies deeper than the geniohyoid, is one of the extrinsic muscles of the tongue. The anterior belly of the digastric muscle, which lies superficial to the mylohyoid, is described in the discussion on the extrinsic muscles of the larynx.

SALIVARY GLANDS

The salivary glands secrete saliva, a clear fluid that moistens the food and also contains an enzyme that digests cooked starch. The salivary glands are arranged in pairs: the parotid, the submandibular (submaxillary), and the sublingual glands.

The parotid gland lies in the side of the face, just anterior and inferior to the ear and on the masseter muscle. The facial nerve passes anteriorly beneath the gland and there breaks up into a number of branches. The retromandibular vein, the external carotid artery and its terminal branches, the great auricular nerve, and the auriculotemporal nerve are all in intimate relation with the medial surface of the gland. The parotid, or Stensen's, duct passes anteriorly around the edge of the masseter muscle, pierces the buccinator muscle, and empties into the

Table 14. Salivary glands

Name	Location	Site of opening of duct	Innervation*
Parotid	Anterior and inferior to the ear	Vestibule of mouth opposite upper second molar	Glossopharyngeal
Submandibular	Inferior to mylohyoid muscle	Floor of mouth near anterior end of tongue	Facial
Sublingual	In floor of mouth superior to mylohyoid muscle	Several openings in floor of mouth near midline	Facial

*Source of parasympathetic fibers. Thoracolumbar fibers from superior cervical ganglion go to blood vessels of each gland.

vestibule of the mouth at the level of the upper second molar. In a person with mumps this gland becomes swollen. Since the gland has a tonguelike process projecting between the temporomandibular joint and the mastoid process, opening the mouth compresses the swollen glandular process and causes pain. In a person with mumps the other salivary glands may also be swollen.

The submandibular salivary gland is smaller than the parotid and lies inferior to the body of the mandible about halfway between the angle and the point of the lower jaw. It rests on the undersurface (superficial surface) of the mylohyoid muscle. The submandibular, or Wharton's, duct passes through this muscle and opens into the floor of the mouth near the midline, under the anterior end of the tongue.

The sublingual salivary glands lie in the floor of the mouth on either side of the tongue, on the superior surface of the mylohyoid muscle. Each gland possesses several small ducts opening into the floor of the mouth, behind the opening of the submandibular duct.

Secretory nerve fibers for the parotid gland come from the otic ganglion (cranial autonomic outflow from the ninth cranial nerve) and from the superior cervical ganglion (thoracolumbar outflow along the blood vessels). The secretory nerve fibers for the submandibular and sublingual glands come from the submandibular ganglion (cranial autonomic outflow from the chorda tympani branch of the seventh cranial nerve) and the superior cervical ganglion (thoracolumbar outflow along the blood vessels). The sensory nerves for all the salivary glands are branches of the trigeminal nerve.

TEETH

Each tooth has a crown, the portion projecting above the gum, a neck, the constricted part at the gum line, and a root embedded in the jawbone. At the apex of the root there is an opening through which nerves and blood vessels enter the pulp cavity within the tooth.

The surface coating for the crown of the tooth is a very dense, smooth, white, translucent layer, called enamel. This layer ends at the gum line where it is slightly overlapped by the outer layer covering the root of the tooth. This outer layer, called cementum, is a layer of modified bone forming a sheath for the root. The bulk of the tooth lying beneath these two outer layers is called dentin. This is a dense, yellow-white, hard material having a striated appearance in thin sections. The tooth cavity within the dentin contains the dental pulp, which is composed of connective tissue surrounding the nerve endings and small blood vessels (Fig. 12-3).

The alveolar periosteum, or periodontal membrane, is a layer of fibrous connective tissue containing many blood vessels and sensory nerves, which fixes the root of the tooth in the alveolar process. This

369

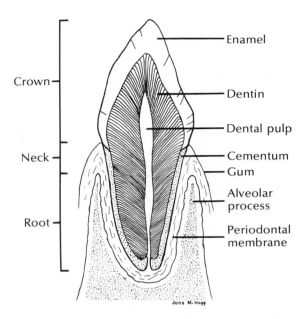

Fig. 12-3. Vertical section of an incisor tooth.

membrane is firmly attached to the cementum of the tooth and to the bone of the alveolar process.

Enamel and dentin are very rich in mineral, particularly calcium phosphate and calcium carbonate, rendering them hard and resistant to wear.

The teeth are divided into four groups:

1. *Incisors:* These are the cutting teeth, which have crowns shaped like chisels (Fig. 12-3).
2. *Canines:* These are the cuspids in which each crown terminates in a sharp point.
3. *Premolars:* These are the bicuspids in which each crown has a grinding surface with two small projections, called cusps.
4. *Molars:* These are larger teeth than the premolars and have a broad grinding surface with four cusps (see Fig. 3-22).

Each incisor and canine has one root; the premolars usually have but one root; the molars have two or three roots.

There are two successional sets of teeth, a deciduous and a permanent.

The deciduous, or milk, dentition consists of 20 teeth, 10 in each jaw. There are eight incisors, four canines, and eight molars. There are no premolars in the milk teeth. The permanent dentition consists of 32 teeth, 16 in each jaw. There are eight incisors, four canines, eight

Table 15. Time of eruption of teeth

Deciduous teeth	Months
Lower central incisors	6–8
Upper central incisors	9–12
Upper lateral incisors	12–14
Lower lateral incisors	14–15
First molars	15–16
Canines	20–24
Second molars	30–32
Permanent teeth	Years
First molars	6
Central incisors	7
Lateral incisors	8
First premolars	9–10
Second premolars	10
Canines	11
Second molars	12
Third molars	17–18

premolars, and 12 molars. The upper lateral incisors may be small or occasionally absent. Some or all of the third molars may be absent or may be present in the jaws, though they do not erupt. There is also an occasional extra incisor or a fourth molar. Table 15 gives the average time for the eruption of teeth, but there are great individual variations from this general order, and the teeth tend to erupt earlier in girls than in boys.

Roentgenograms of the jaws show that a tooth begins to calcify, that is, to form enamel and dentin, long before it erupts. The cusps of all the milk teeth are well formed at birth. The first permanent molar, or the "6-year" molar, begins to form cusps at 3 months; the second, or "12-year," molar at 3 years; and the third molar, or "wisdom tooth," at 9 years. If the teeth are to be healthy and strong, children must have ample minerals in their diet when the cusps are calcifying.

Healthy deciduous teeth are more nearly white in color than the permanent teeth, but all should be translucent. The deciduous incisors and canines are much smaller than their permanent successors. The deciduous molars are larger than their successors, the permanent premolars.

The sensory nerve supply of the upper teeth comes from branches of the maxillary division of the trigeminal nerve, and that of the teeth in the lower jaw from the mandibular division of the same nerve.

Inasmuch as the teeth are the organs of mastication, the muscles used in chewing are discussed here.

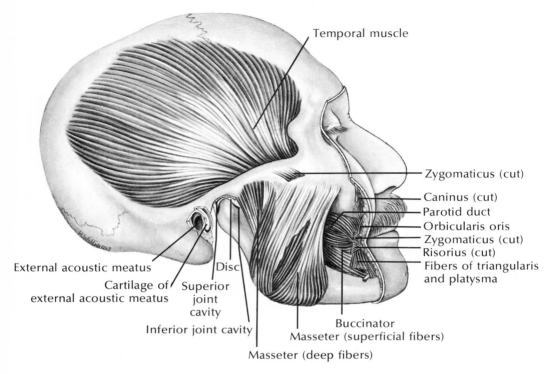

Fig. 12-4. Right temporal and masseter muscles. (Dissection by Dr. C. A. Hamann.)

MUSCLES OF MASTICATION

There are four muscles of mastication: the masseter, temporal, lateral pterygoid, and medial pterygoid muscles (Fig. 12-4). They are aided by certain accessory muscles of which the most important is the buccinator.

The masseter arises from the lower border and deep surface of the zygomatic arch and is inserted into the lateral side of the ramus, above the angle of the mandible. The temporal muscle arises from the temporal fossa on the lateral surface of the skull. It is a fan-shaped muscle. The converging fibers pass deep to the zygomatic arch to be inserted into the coronoid process of the mandible. The lateral (external) pterygoid arises from the lateral side of the lateral pterygoid lamina of the sphenoid bone and the nearby undersurface of the great wing of the sphenoid. It is inserted into the neck of the mandible. The medial (internal) pterygoid arises from the medial side of the lateral pterygoid lamina and from the nearby surface of the palatine and maxillary bones and is inserted into the medial surface of the ramus of the mandible.

372

All four are supplied from the motor part of the mandibular division of the trigeminal nerve (the masticator nerve).

The masseter, temporal, and medial pterygoid muscles close the mouth and clench the teeth. The lateral pterygoids working together protract or pull the lower jaw forward. The pterygoids on one side, working alternately with those on the other, produce lateral movements of the mandible. The posterior fibers of the temporal muscle retract or pull the jaw backward, and the anterior fibers of the temporal aid in protracting or pulling the jaw forward.

When the masticator muscles relax, the mandible drops in response to the action of gravity. When the mouth is opened wide, gravity is aided by certain muscles running from the hyoid to the mandible, namely, the anterior belly of the digastric, the geniohyoid, the mylohyoid, and the platysma muscles.

The functions of the tongue, buccinator, and orbicularis oris in mastication have already been discussed.

PHARYNX

The pharynx may be divided functionally into three parts. The superior part, or nasopharynx, lies posterior to the nose and is an air passage only. The middle part, or oropharynx, lies posterior to the mouth and serves both the respiratory and digestive tracts as a common passageway. The lower part, or laryngopharynx, lies posterior to the larynx and is a pathway for food passing into the esophagus.

The pharynx is a funnel-shaped cavity with fibromuscular walls. It is widest superiorly, beneath the skull, and gradually narrows toward its inferior end, where it becomes the esophagus. It is about 12.5 cm long and lies anterior to the cervical portion of the vertebral column. It is lined with mucous membrane that is covered with respiratory epithelium in its upper part and with stratified squamous epithelium below. A number of important muscles form the essential structure of the wall (Figs. 12-5 and 12-6).

There are three constrictors of the pharynx arranged like three cones, each fitting within the next below. The superior constrictor arises from the posterior portion of the medial pterygoid lamina, the fascia between that bone and the mandible, the mylohyoid line of the mandible, and the side of the tongue. The fibers pass around the side of the pharynx, spreading out like a fan to be attached to a fibrous band, or median raphe, in the midline posteriorly. This raphe extends from the base of the occiput downward.

The middle constrictor arises from the cornua of the hyoid bone and passes posteriorly to overlap the lower portion of the superior constrictor and to be inserted into the median raphe.

The inferior constrictor arises from the lateral side of the thyroid

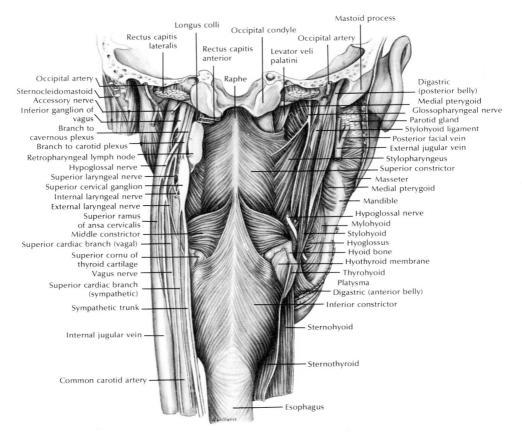

Longus colli
Rectus capitis
lateralis
Rectus capitis
anterior
Occipital condyle
Levator veli
palatini
Occipital artery
Mastoid process
Occipital artery
Raphe

Occipital artery
Sternocleidomastoid
Accessory nerve
Inferior ganglion of
vagus
Branch to
cavernous plexus
Branch to carotid plexus
Retropharyngeal lymph node
Hypoglossal nerve
Superior laryngeal nerve
Superior cervical ganglion
Internal laryngeal nerve
External laryngeal nerve
Superior ramus
of ansa cervicalis
Middle constrictor
Superior cardiac branch (vagal)
Superior cornu of
thyroid cartilage
Vagus nerve
Superior cardiac branch
(sympathetic)
Sympathetic trunk

Internal jugular vein

Common carotid artery

Digastric
(posterior belly)
Medial pterygoid
Glossopharyngeal nerve
Parotid gland
Stylohyoid ligament
Posterior facial vein
External jugular vein
Stylopharyngeus
Superior constrictor
Masseter
Medial pterygoid
Mandible
Hypoglossal nerve
Mylohyoid
Stylohyoid
Hyoglossus
Hyoid bone
Hyothyroid membrane
Thyrohyoid
Platysma
Digastric (anterior belly)
Inferior constrictor

Sternohyoid

Sternothyroid

Esophagus

Fig. 12-5. Posterior view of the pharynx. (Dissection by Dr. J. R. Nickerson.) (Male, 53 years of age.)

and cricoid cartilages. It passes posteriorly on each side like the others to be inserted into the median raphe overlapping the lower portion of the middle constrictor.

The stylopharyngeus arises from the posterior surface of the styloid process. It passes inferiorly to be inserted into the lateral wall of the pharynx between the superior and middle constrictors.

The palatopharyngeus arises in the soft palate and passes inferiorly in the palatopharyngeal arch to an insertion into the lateral wall of the pharynx between the middle and inferior contrictors. A bundle of muscle fibers that arises from the cartilage of the auditory tube and blends with the rest of the palatopharyngeus is called the salpingopharyngeus.

When one swallows, the constrictor muscles direct the passage of food inferiorly into the esophagus. The stylopharyngeus and palato-

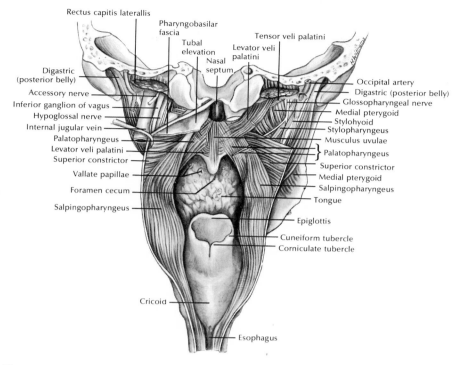

Rectus capitis laterallis
Pharyngobasilar fascia
Tubal elevation
Nasal septum
Levator veli palatini
Tensor veli palatini

Digastric (posterior belly)
Accessory nerve
Inferior ganglion of vagus
Hypoglossal nerve
Internal jugular vein
Palatopharyngeus
Levator veli palatini
Superior constrictor
Vallate papillae
Foramen cecum
Salpingopharyngeus

Occipital artery
Digastric (posterior belly)
Glossopharyngeal nerve
Medial pterygoid
Stylohyoid
Stylopharyngeus
Musculus uvulae
Palatopharyngeus
Superior constrictor
Medial pterygoid
Salpingopharyngeus
Tongue
Epiglottis
Cuneiform tubercle
Corniculate tubercle

Cricoid

Esophagus

Fig. 12-6. Interior of the pharynx, posterior view. The posterior wall has been split and each half has been reflected laterally. (Dissection by Dr. J. R. Nickerson.) (Male, 53 years of age.)

pharyngeus also take part in this action by assisting the geniohyoid, the mylohyoid, and the anterior belly of the digastric in drawing the larynx superiorly and anteriorly out of the direct line of passage of food.

Vowel sounds are produced in the pharynx, which is capable of considerable change in form by the action of its constituent muscles. Roentgenoscopic observation shows that when one enunciates the letter "a," as in father, the pharyngeal cavity is narrowed from anterior to posterior, and the soft palate is partly raised. When one says "oo" as in stool, the larynx is drawn moderately forward, and the soft palate is strongly arched. When one says "e" as in feet, the pharynx is widely dilated, the larynx is pulled anteriorly, and the soft palate is pulled sharply up and back into the nasopharynx. The increasing pull of the mylohyoid and geniohyoid muscles may be felt by pressing the finger beneath the chin and saying the vowels in order (Fig. 12-7).

The constrictors and palatopharyngeus muscles are supplied through the pharyngeal plexus; the stylopharyngeus muscle is sup-

375

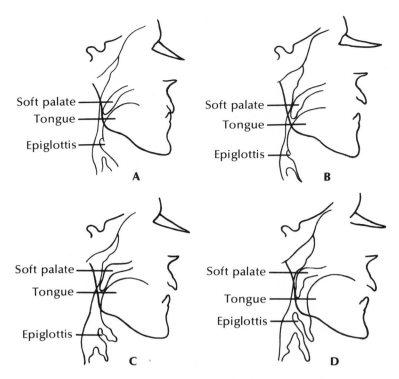

Fig. 12-7. Alterations of position of pharynx and larynx in phonation of vowels. **A,** Position in quiet respiration. **B,** Position when phonating *a* as in *father*. **C,** Position when phonating *oo* as in *stool*. **D,** Position when phonating *ee* as in *feet*. (Tracings made from roentgenograms of adult male.)

plied by the glossopharyngeal, which is also the main sensory nerve for the mucosa of the pharynx.

It is well to summarize the seven openings into the pharynx. Anteriorly and superiorly are the openings of the two choanae into the nose, inferiorly is the single opening into the mouth, still farther inferiorly is the opening into the larynx, and posterior to that is the opening into the esophagus. In the lateral wall high up on each side is the opening into the auditory tube.

TONSILS
Lying in the walls of the pharynx are masses of lymphatic tissue forming a ring about the openings into the mouth and nose. The aggregation of lymphatic tissue between the pillars of the fauces is called the tonsil. The tonsils vary greatly in size with age and with health. In a newborn infant they are quite small, but during infancy they increase in size, reaching a maximum at about the third year of age. After this they gradually diminish and should be quite small in adult life.

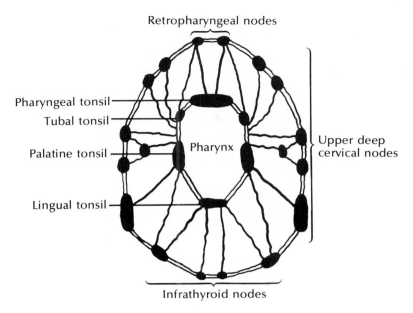

Retropharyngeal nodes

Pharyngeal tonsil

Tubal tonsil

Palatine tonsil

Pharynx

Upper deep
cervical nodes

Lingual tonsil

Infrathyroid nodes

Fig. 12-8. Lymphatic drainage of tonsils.

Like other lymphatic structures the tonsils aid in combating disease by releasing phagocytes or scavenging leukocytes to cope with bacteria on the mucosa. Therefore, they become enlarged in persons with infections and irritations of the nose and throat. If the bacteria gain the upper hand, the tonsils become inflamed. If the tonsils are chronically diseased, the surgeon removes them. In persons with nasal allergy they tend to become enlarged by accumulation of fluid (edematous swelling). The connections of the lymphatic masses of the throat with the deep and superficial lymph nodes of the neck have been discussed in Chapter 10.

Each tonsil is a mass of lymph nodules with a fine reticular tissue framework and a covering of mucous membrane. The surface is irregular because of the openings of many small pits on it. Sometimes the word tonsil is used widely to designate any of the lymphatic masses of the throat (Fig. 12-9). By this nomenclature there are the following "tonsils":

1. The palatine tonsil is a mass lying on each side in the lateral wall of the pharynx, between the palatoglossal arch and the palatopharyngeal arch. The maxillary artery and several of its branches lie just lateral to the fibrous capsule that covers the lateral surface of the tonsil. Injury to these vessels during a tonsillectomy may lead to severe hemorrhage. A quinsy is an abscess outside the fibrous capsule and is usually above the tonsil itself.

377

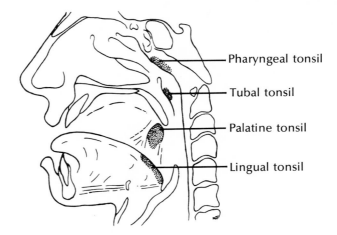

Pharyngeal tonsil

Tubal tonsil

Palatine tonsil

Lingual tonsil

Fig. 12-9. Diagram to show the location of the various tonsillar masses.

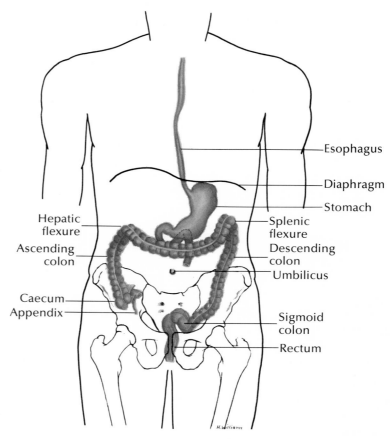

Esophagus

Diaphragm

Stomach

Hepatic
flexure

Splenic
flexure

Ascending
colon

Descending
colon

Umbilicus

Caecum

Appendix

Sigmoid
colon

Rectum

Fig. 12-10. Position of digestive organs.

2. The pharyngeal tonsil is a mass lying in the upper posterior wall of the pharynx, posterior to the choanae. This is also known as the "adenoid," and when enlarged, it produces a lobulated mass that may block the nasopharyngeal passage and the medial opening of the auditory tube.
3. The tubal tonsil is a small mass lying just posterior to the opening of the auditory tube.
4. The lingual tonsil is a lymphatic mass covering the posterior third of the tongue.

ESOPHAGUS

The esophagus, or gullet, is a muscular tube extending from the pharynx at the level of the sixth cervical vertebra, through the posterior mediastinum and diaphragm, to the cardiac orifice of the stomach. It is 25 to 30 cm long (Fig. 12-10).

The esophagus has four coverings: (1) an inner tunica mucosa with stratified squamous epithelium, (2) a tela submucosa of connective tissue, (3) a tunica muscularis composed of an inner layer of circular muscle fibers and an outer layer of longitudinally arranged muscle bands, and (4) an outer tunica adventitia of loose connective tissue blending with that in the neck and mediastinum.

The muscular coat in the upper portion is composed of striate muscle innervated through the pharyngeal plexus. Inferiorly, smooth muscle replaces the striate muscle, and this is innervated by the vagus and thoracic sympathetic nerves.

The lumen of the esophagus is stellate in outline because of the tonic contraction of its musculature. It is distended by the passage of food, but it has three relatively constricted portions, one at the upper end, a second where the esophagus passes posterior to the left bronchus, and a third where it passes through the diaphragm.

ABDOMINAL CAVITY

The abdominal cavity is that portion of the general body cavity lying inferior to the diaphragm. Anteriorly it is bounded by the muscles of the anterior abdominal wall, inferiorly by the bones of the pelvic girdle, and by the pelvic diaphragm formed by the levator ani muscles, and posteriorly by the vertebral column and by the psoas muscles and the muscles of the flanks. It is lined by a serous membrane, called the peritoneum. As in other body cavities this serous lining is reflected over the organs within the cavity. The layer lining the walls is called the parietal peritoneum, and the continuation over the organs is called the visceral peritoneum. During life the organs lie closely touching each other so that there is only a potential cavity between the parietal and visceral peritoneum.

Certain organs lying between the peritoneum and the walls of the abdominal cavity are covered only on one surface by peritoneum.

379

These are the kidneys, ureters, urinary bladder, uterus, inferior vena cava, and abdominal aorta. Such organs are called retroperitoneal organs. The pancreas and portions of the duodenum, the ascending colon, and the descending colon become retroperitoneal secondarily; that is, they had mesenteries in the embryo but lost them later. Most of the abdominal digestive tract is almost completely clothed by peritoneum. The folds of peritoneum that are reflected from the walls over the viscera are called mesenteries. Certain of these have special names. The mesentery of the small intestine is known as "the mesentery." The transverse mesocolon is the mesentery of the transverse colon. The mesoappendix is the mesentery of the appendix, and the mesovarium, the mesentery of the ovary. The mesentery of the greater curvature of the stomach is prolonged as a great fat-containing fold, the greater omentum, which hangs like an apron over the anterior aspect of the small intestine. Between the lesser curvature of the stomach and the hilus of the liver, the peritoneum continues as the lesser omentum, or gastrohepatic ligament. Other folds of the peritoneum are called ligaments; these are the gastrosplenic ligament from the stomach to spleen, the hepatoduodenal ligament from liver to duodenum, and the phrenocolic ligament from the diaphragm to the splenic flexure of the colon. In addition to acting as supporting structures, the various mesenteries serve as passageways for the arteries, veins, lymphatics, and nerves supplying the viscera to which they are attached.

STOMACH The stomach is a thick-walled tube into which the esophagus empties. A healthy, empty stomach has a thick wall and a small cavity. It is capable of great distention and may assume a great variety of shapes, depending upon its contents, the amount of tone of the muscles in its walls, and the position of the individual.

Fig. 12-11 is a tracing of the stomach of a young adult made from a roentgenogram taken while the person was standing. The stomach was visualized by means of a "barium meal." On the right is the lesser curvature extending from the cardia or esophageal opening to the pylorus or outlet. The lesser curvature is the upper or concave margin of the stomach near the liver. The lesser omentum is attached to this margin and extends toward the right to the porta hepatis of the liver. The greater curvature is the left or convex margin of the stomach. It is much longer than the lesser, and attached to it is the greater omentum. The fundus of the stomach is the dome-shaped portion superior to the cardia, lying directly beneath the left dome of the diaphragm. The body of the stomach is the midportion of the tube; its inferior end is called the pyloric portion.

380

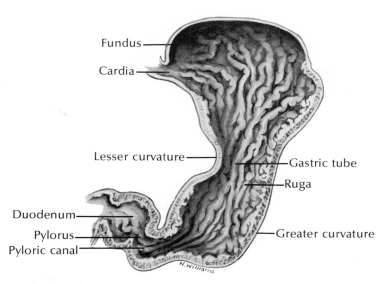

Fundus

Cardia

Lesser curvature

Gastric tube

Ruga

Duodenum

Pylorus

Pyloric canal

Greater curvature

H. Williams

Fig. 12-11. Vertical section of the stomach. Traced from a roentgenogram of adult female who had been given water containing enough barium sulfate to outline gastric walls.

The wall of the stomach has the following four coats:

1. An inner layer, called the tunica mucosa, is soft and velvety in appearance. This layer is thrown into numerous folds, or rugae, that, when the organ is contracted, run in a general longitudinal direction. As the stomach distends, the rugae lose their longitudinal disposition and ultimately disappear. The epithelium of this layer has simple columnar epithelial cells and numerous small glands that secrete mucus, enzymes, and hydrochloric acid.

2. The tela submucosa lies beneath the first layer and is composed of connective tissue.

3. The tunica muscularis has three layers of smooth muscle: an outer longitudinal layer, a middle circular layer, and a inner oblique layer.

4. The tunica serosa is composed of visceral peritoneum continuous at the greater and lesser curvatures with the peritoneum of the greater and lesser omenta.

The blood vessels of the stomach lie between the layers of the omenta along each curvature and send long branches onto the anterior and posterior surfaces. Along the lesser curvature are the left gastric artery (a branch of the celiac artery) and the right gastric branch of the hepatic artery; along the greater curvature are the left gastroepiploic branch of the splenic artery and the right gastroepiploic branch of the gastroduodenal artery of the hepatic artery. The upper portion of the greater curvature receives a few arterial branches (short gastric) directly from the splenic artery (See Fig. 10-10).

The stomach receives motor nerves from two sources, the vagus nerves and the thoracolumbar autonomic outflow. The vagal trunks, which pierce the diaphragm together with the esophagus, send many fine branches to the anterior and posterior surfaces of the stomach. The sympathetic fibers are derived from the celiac ganglion and pass to the stomach along the branches of the celiac artery. There is an intrinsic nerve plexus containing some ganglion cells in the tela submucosa, and a similar nerve plexus exists in the tunica muscularis between the layers of smooth muscle.

There are sensory nerve fibers from the stomach, and the conscious impressions arising from stimulation of these nerves are a good example of the indefiniteness of visceral sensation. We are well aware of the great discomfort of nausea, but we cannot localize the site of the sensation nor describe it accurately. The "gnawing" sensation of a gastric

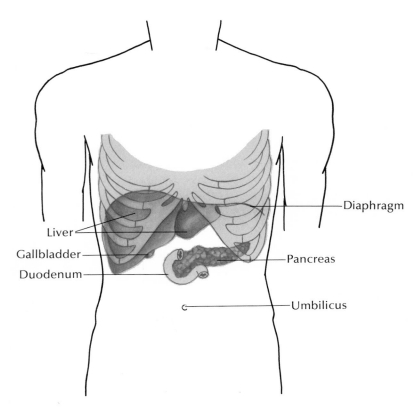

Fig. 12-12. The position of liver and pancreas.

ulcer is another example. Fibers carrying the sensation of pain travel with the sympathetic pathway, and those carrying the sensations of nausea and hunger travel with the vagus nerves.

The liver is the largest gland in the body. It secretes bile and also receives digested carbohydrates and protein from the intestine by way of the portal vein. It fills the right upper portion of the abdominal cavity from the undersurface of the diaphragm to below the costal margin. There is an extension to the left where it lies beneath the left dome of the diaphragm and above the cardia of the stomach. The inferior vena cava is embedded in a deep groove on the posterior surface of the liver. The visceral peritoneum covering the liver is reflected in certain places from the surface of the liver to join the parietal peritoneum, thus forming several ligaments. On the anterior surface is the falciform ligament, extending to the anterior abdominal wall as far inferiorly as the umbilicus; above are the right and left triangular ligaments and the coronary ligament attaching the liver to the diaphragm (Fig. 12-13). The round ligament is a round fibrous cord embedded within the free border of the falciform ligament and extending from the umbilicus to the porta hepatis. This ligament is the remains of the left umbilical vein, a blood vessel that before birth carried blood from the placenta to the liver and inferior vena cava. The inferior surface of the liver has a deep fissure, the porta hepatis, where the portal vein and hepatic artery

LIVER

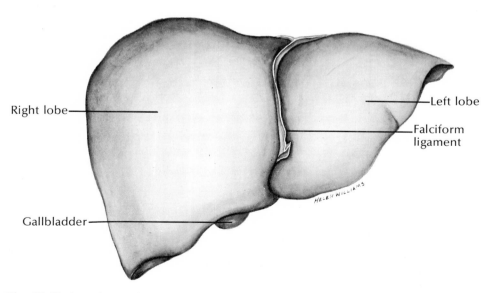

Right lobe

Left lobe

Falciform ligament

Gallbladder

Fig. 12-13. Anterior surface of the liver.

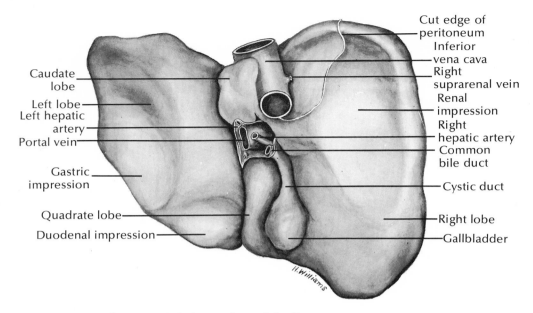

Caudate lobe

Left lobe
Left hepatic artery
Portal vein

Gastric impression

Quadrate lobe
Duodenal impression

Cut edge of peritoneum
Inferior vena cava
Right suprarenal vein
Renal impression
Right hepatic artery
Common bile duct

Cystic duct

Right lobe
Gallbladder

Fig. 12-14. Inferior surface of the liver.

pass into the liver and the hepatic ducts leave (Fig. 12-14). The right border of the lesser omentum is attached to the porta hepatis; the portal vein, hepatic artery, and bile ducts lie within the two layers of this omentum. The free border of the lesser omentum forms the epiploic foramen (foramen of Winslow), which opens into the omental bursa, a recess of the general peritoneal cavity.

The liver has four lobes:
1. The right lobe lies beneath the right dome of the diaphragm.
2. The left lobe lies beneath the left dome and is much smaller than the right.
3. The quadrate lobe is a quadrilateral area on the inferior surface of the liver lying anterior to the porta hepatis and between the gallbladder and the fossa for the round ligament.
4. The caudate lobe is another quadrilateral area on the posterior aspect of the liver, lying between the inferior vena cava and the fossa for the ligamentum venosum, the remains of the ductus venosus, which in the fetus carried blood to the liver and inferior vena cava from the placenta.

The division into the four lobes just described is based on the gross anatomical appearance of the liver. This is not the functional division based upon the blood supply and biliary drainage. Upon a functional basis the liver may be divided into a right and left half by a plane rough-

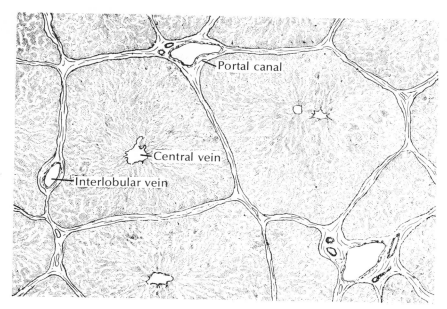

Fig. 12-15. Low magnification drawing of section of pig liver. (From Bevelander, G., and Ramaley, J. A.: Essentials of histology, ed. 7, St. Louis, 1974, The C. V. Mosby Co.)

ly passing from anterior to posterior through the fossa for the gallbladder and the caudate lobe. Generally speaking, the right half has a vascular supply and biliary drainage that are separate from the left half. In turn, each half may be further subdivided into a number of segments or areas, each having a fairly distinct vascular supply and biliary duct system.

Except for a small area on the posterior and superior surface of the right lobe the liver is entirely covered by peritoneum.

The liver has a connective tissue sheath from which fibrous bands pass deep into the substance of the gland. This is the hepatic capsule (capsule of Glisson). These bands, together with the branches of the blood vessels, divide the organ into many small hepatic lobules. In man the lobules are incompletely separated from each other. In the center of each lobule is a branch of the hepatic vein. Arranged about the periphery of each lobule are several portal canals. Each portal canal consists of connective tissue and branches of the portal vein, the hepatic artery, and the hepatic duct (Fig. 12-16). The secretory cells of the liver are arranged in curved plates radiating outward from the central vein. Bile is secreted into tiny bile capillaries between the secretory cells and is carried to the periphery of the lobules to a tributary of the

385

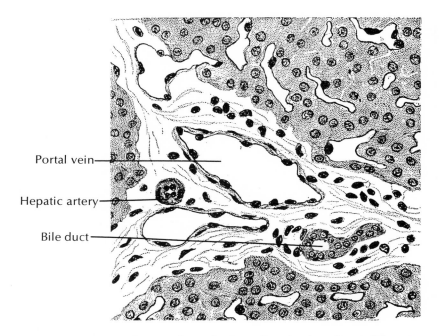

Portal vein

Hepatic artery

Bile duct

Fig. 12-16. Diagram of a portal canal. (From Bevelander, G., and Ramaley, J. A.: Essentials of histology, ed. 7, St. Louis, 1974, The C. V. Mosby Co.)

hepatic duct. Between the curved plates of liver cells are capillary blood sinuses that connect the terminal branches of the hepatic artery and portal vein with venules that drain into the hepatic veins. In the lining of these sinuses are macrophages, which in the liver are called Kupffer cells. Nerve fibers for the liver are derived from the vagus nerves and the celiac plexus. There is a nerve plexus along the hepatic artery.

The liver has many and varied functions and is essential to life. All liver cells look alike, and so far as is known, no special group of cells has any particular function. Each cell apparently is capable of performing any or all of the hepatic functions. Digested carbohydrates, mainly in the form of glucose, may be stored in the liver as glycogen, and when required, the glycogen is changed back to glucose. Therefore, the liver plays an important role in maintaining the proper level of blood sugar. Amino acids derived from digested protein are used by the liver to form various body proteins, or they may be consumed as fuel, and the resulting waste products are excreted by the liver. Digested fats may be added to the body stores or burned as fuel. The liver secretes bile and bile salts, which are necessary for digestive processes in the intestinal tract. The liver makes substances that are of primary importance in the mechanism of blood clotting, including fibrinogen and prothrombin. Various toxic substances that may be present in the blood stream are detoxified by the liver. Since some of the substances elaborated by the liver are secreted directly into the blood stream, the gland is regarded as an endocrine gland as well as an exocrine gland.

Because of its size the liver is a very important reservoir for storage of blood and body fluid. Also because of its size the liver contains a great deal of reticuloendothelial tissue. The Kupffer cells perform the various functions of macrophages.

Hepatic ducts and gallbladder

At the porta hepatis, bile ducts coming from the right and left portions of the liver unite to form a single hepatic duct. After the cystic duct coming from the gallbladder joins the hepatic duct, the tube is called the common bile duct (ductus choledochus), which empties into the second part of the duodenum.

The cystic duct passes to the right from its place of union with the hepatic duct. Its terminal dilated portion is the gallbladder. In performing a cholecystectomy, the surgeon removes the gallbladder and as much of the cystic duct as possible but must leave the common duct intact. If the common duct is destroyed or blocked, bile cannot be emptied into the duodenum and is then absorbed into the circulation; jaundice results and ultimately death if the obstruction is not relieved. If only the cystic duct is obstructed, as it may be by a gallstone, there is no jaundice, for bile flows freely from the liver through the common duct into the duodenum. The gallbladder concentrates and stores bile.

The gallbladder and the ducts have an inner mucous membrane coat, a middle coat of smooth muscle, and an outer layer of peritoneum. The outer layer of peritoneum may be partially missing in persons in whom the gallbladder is partly buried within the substance of the liver.

Circulation through the liver

Blood circulating through the liver is derived from two sources, the hepatic artery and the portal vein (see Fig. 9-28). The hepatic artery provides nourishment for the liver tissue.

The portal vein, draining the intestines, enters the liver at the porta hepatis and breaks up into branches that run through the connective tissue septa of the lobes as the interlobar vessels. The interlobar veins divide into interlobular veins that encircle and eventually penetrate the lobules, breaking up into fine capillaries the hepatic sinusoids. The hepatic sinusoids drain into the central vein. The central veins of other lobules unite, forming the hepatic veins, which eventually empty into the inferior vena cava. This circulatory pattern allows the liver cells ready access to nutrient-laden blood and also provides ready return to

387

the circulation when stored material, such as glycogen, needs to be released.

PANCREAS   The pancreas, which secretes pancreatic juice into the duodenum, is an important gland. It also has an endocrine secretion (insulin). It has a head within the curve of the duodenum and a long slender tail extending to the left, posterior to the stomach, as far as the spleen (Fig. 12-17). It is a retroperitoneal organ lying anterior to the inferior vena cava, aorta, and left kidney.

The pancreas usually has two ducts. The main one (Wirsung's) begins in the tail and passes through the length of the gland to join with the common bile duct in a dilated vestibule, Vater's ampulla, which opens into the duodenum at the main duodenal papilla (Vater's). The common bile duct and the main pancreatic duct may have two separate openings or a single common opening into the duodenum. There is also an accessory duct (Santorini's) that, when present, drains a portion of the head and empties into the duodenum by a separate opening, the minor duodenal papilla, about 2.5 cm above that of the main duct.

The pancreas is a compound tubuloalveolar gland having an immense number of small lobules. The lining is a simple columnar epithelium. The lobules are separated by a delicate connective tissue net-

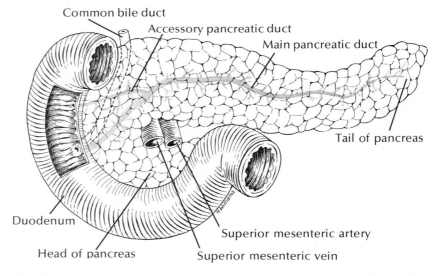

Fig. 12-17. Pancreas and duodenum. A window has been cut in the anterior wall of the duodenum to show the openings of the common bile duct and the pancreatic ducts into the lumen of the duodenum.

388

work. In among the tubules are small islands of granular cells arranged in irregular cords. Each island contains numerous capillaries. These collections of cells are the islands of Langerhans, which secrete insulin (Fig. 12-18).

The pancreas is richly supplied with blood that comes from branches of the celiac and superior mesenteric arteries. The superior pancreaticoduodenal artery is a branch of the hepatic; the inferior pancreaticoduodenal is a branch of the superior mesenteric; and there are some branches from the splenic artery. The venous drainage is into tributaries of the portal vein. Sympathetic nerves (thoracolumbar outflow) from outlying portions of the celiac ganglion supply the pancreas, and there are also fibers from the vagus nerves (cranial autonomic outflow). Sensory nerve fibers from the pancreas travel mainly with the sympathetic nerves back to the spinal cord. The nerves have a minor effect in regulating the activity of the pancreas. The principal control of pancreatic activity is from hormones.

For purposes of description the small intestine is divided into three arbitrary divisions: the duodenum, jejunum, and ileum. The duodenum is about 22 cm long (12 fingerbreadths), the jejunum 2 meters, and the ileum 3 meters. The whole length is perhaps 6 meters, but this varies greatly with the degree to which the muscle fibers are contracted.

SMALL INTESTINE

The wall in the small intestine has the following four layers:
1. The tunica mucosa, or mucous membrane, consists of a surface layer of simple columnar epithelium lying on a thin sheet of connective tissue, the lamina propria, and having superficial to

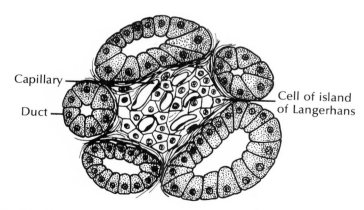

Fig. 12-18. Cellular structure of the pancreas showing several ducts in cross section and an island of Langerhans.

389

this a thin sheet of smooth muscle, the muscularis mucosae. There are many small tubular glands in the mucous membrane.

The mucous membrane has an immense number of small elevations, called villi, that give the surface a velvety appearance. Each villus is a long, slender, conelike projection having small blood vessels and a large lymphatic in the center. The body of each villus also contains some smooth muscle cells that upon contraction shorten the villus and upon relaxation allow it to elongate. The size and number of villi are greatest in the upper part of the jejunum and gradually decrease toward the ileocecal valve.

The mucous membrane also possesses numerous large, circular folds, called plicae circulares. These folds are best developed in the lower duodenum and upper jejunum. They are less

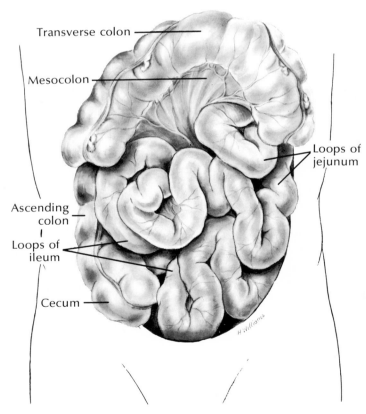

Fig. 12-19. Anterior view of intestines. The transverse colon has been turned superiorly to show the loops of jejunum. (Male, 53 years of age.)

numerous in the ileum and disappear near its distal end. The villi and plicae circulares together greatly increase the surface area of the mucous membrane of the small intestine.

Scattered along the mucosal surface of the small intestine are oval, flattened plaques of lymphatic tissue, called solitary lymph follicles, or nodules. In the lower ileum are groups of these minute lymph nodules forming aggregated lymph nodules, or Peyer's patches. A few of these may be found in higher areas of the small bowel.

2. The tela submucosa is composed of a strong layer of connective tissue.
3. The tunica muscularis has an outer longitudinal layer and an inner circular layer of smooth muscle. The longitudinal layer forms a continuous sheet around the entire small intestine.
4. The tunica serosa is composed of visceral peritoneum continuous with that of the mesentery. On the duodenum this coat is incomplete because much of this part of the intestine is retroperitoneal.

The duodenum receives several arterial branches from the celiac artery, but the remainder of the small intestine is supplied by the branches of the superior mesenteric artery. These branches lie within the mesentery and anastomose freely with each other, forming arterial arcades. Branches from these arcades anastomose, forming secondary arcades. The arteries to the jejunum form only one or two arches, but in the lower part of the mesentery the branches are much more complex, and the distal portion of the ileum may have as many as five sets of arches. The final arterial branches pass directly into the gut wall. The veins from the small intestine unite to form the superior mesenteric vein, one of the main tributaries of the portal vein.

The nerve supply to the small intestine comes from the celiac and superior mesenteric ganglia and from the vagus nerves. Within the wall of the gut the nerve fibers intermingle to form two extensive plexuses. Between the longitudinal and circular muscle layers of the tunica muscularis is the myenteric (Auerbach's) plexus, and in the tela submucosa is found the submucous plexus (Meissner's). There are sensory fibers, but the main conscious sensory impressions are those of pain when the wall is pulled, distended, or stretched.

The duodenum begins at the pylorus. It is a C-shaped tube, with the concavity toward the left, and the head of the pancreas lies within this concavity. It has three parts: a superior portion running to the right, a descending portion running inferiorly along the right side of the vertebral column, and an inferior portion running, at first, trans-

Duodenum

versely to the left in front of the inferior vena cava, aorta, and vertebral column and then turning superiorly and anteriorly to become the jejunum. The ducts of the liver and pancreas open into the descending portion of the duodenum. Only in the duodenum do the intestinal glands extend into the tela submucosa (Fig. 12-20).

Jejunum, ileum, and mesentery

The jejunum and ileum, or main portions of the small intestine, are suspended in the abdomen by the mesentery. This fan-shaped fold of peritoneum is attached to the posterior abdominal wall for about 15 cm and is obliquely directed from the left side of the second lumbar vertebra over the duodenum, aorta, inferior vena cava, and right ureter to the right lower border of the fifth lumbar vertebra. The free border of the mesentery is about 6 meters long to correspond with the length of

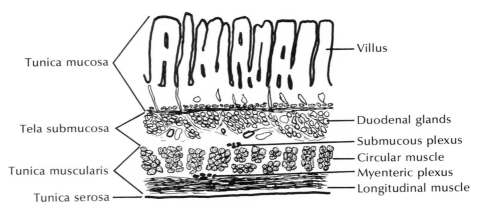

Fig. 12-20. Longitudinal section of duodenum.

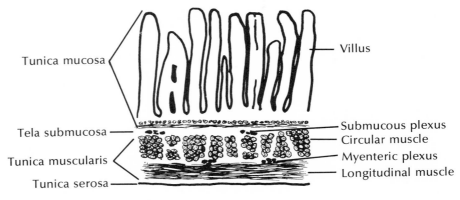

392   **Fig. 12-21.** Longitudinal section of jejunum.

the combined jejunum and ileum. Between the serous, or peritoneal layers of the mesentery are the superior mesenteric artery and vein with their branches, many lymphatic vessels and nodes, and nerve fibers.

The jejunum and ileum functionally are regarded as a single organ for it is here that the final processes of digestion occur and that most

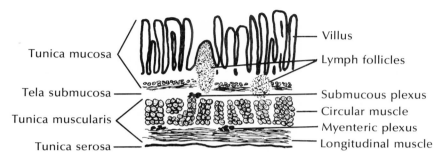

Fig. 12-22. Longitudinal section of ileum.

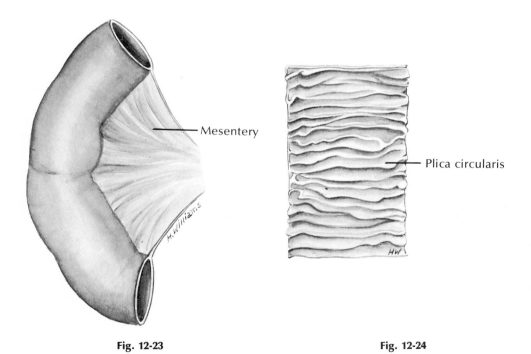

Fig. 12-23   Fig. 12-24

Fig. 12-23. Segment of jejunum. In this specimen the mesentery is well filled with fat, thus obscuring the vessels.
Fig. 12-24. Segment of jejunum, showing plicae.

393

of the products are absorbed from the digestive tract. There is no sharp line of demarcation between jejunum and ileum, but the various distinctions between typical portions of each may be summarized. Let us take a segment of proximal jejunum and of distal ileum and examine them closely. The mesentery of the jejunal segment is shorter and contains less fat. There is only one arterial arcade and the straight arteries running from the arcade to the intestinal wall are long and numerous. The mesentery of the ileal segment is longer, there is more fat, there are several arterial arcades, and the straight arteries are short and not so numerous. In general the jejunum has a richer blood supply than the ileum (Fig. 12-25). The jejunal mucosa is thicker, and the villi and the circular folds are more numerous and more complicated. The jejunum has a greater caliber than the ileum. There is a much greater surface area of the mucosa of the jejunum than there is

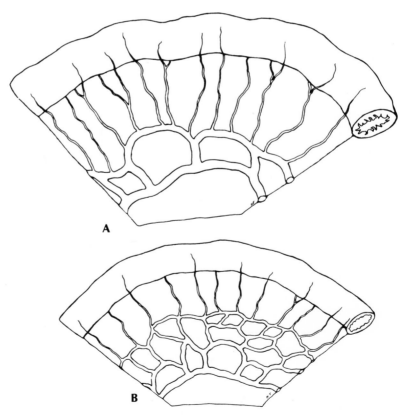

Fig. 12-25. Comparison of arterial supply of jejunum and ileum. **A,** Segment of jejunum. **B,** Segment of ileum.

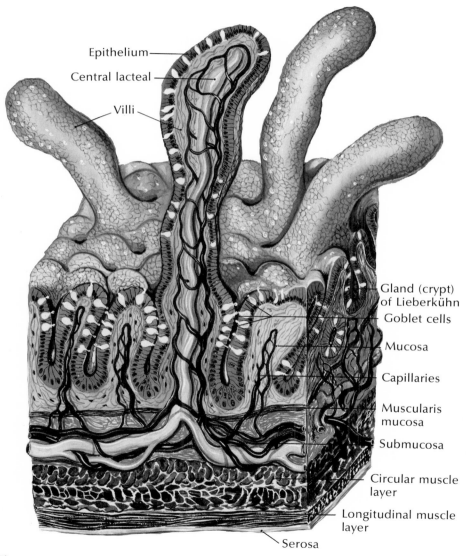

Epithelium

Central lacteal

Villi

Gland (crypt) of Lieberkühn

Goblet cells

Mucosa

Capillaries

Muscularis mucosa

Submucosa

Circular muscle layer

Longitudinal muscle layer

Serosa

Fig. 12-26. Section of the intestinal mucosa showing villi, central lacteal, and glands. (From Anthony, C. P., and Kolthoff, N. J.: Textbook of anatomy and physiology, ed. 8, St. Louis, 1971, The C. V. Mosby Co.)

395

in a section of ileum of the same length. The aggregate lymph follicles are larger and more numerous in the lower ileum.

The functions of the jejunum and ileum are essential to life. There is a margin of reserve, for a considerable segment of either may be removed surgically without endangering health, but if too much is resected the patient will die of deficient nutrition.

The position of the loops of small intestine varies with their distention and the progress of food matter through the bowel. The loops of jejunum occupy the superior left part of the abdominal cavity and the loops of the ileum the inferior right portion; some loops of the ileum usually extend inferiorly into the pelvic cavity.

LARGE INTESTINE   The large intestine begins in the inferior right portion of the abdominal cavity. It is continued on the right side of the abdomen as far as the undersurface of the liver. It then crosses to the left side by a festoonlike loop, turns inferiorly under the spleen, and continues down the left flank into the pelvic cavity where it ends at the anus. The beginning is called the cecum, on which the vermiform process (appendix) is a pocket. Following the cecum in order are the ascending colon, the hepatic flexure, the transverse colon, the splenic flexure, the descending colon, the iliac colon, the pelvic colon, the rectum, and the anal canal (see Fig. 12-10). With the exception of the appendix, rectum, and anal canal, the various portions have no delimiting characteristics and are merely names of location given for convenience of description.

The large intestine is distinquished from the small in the following ways:

1. The tunica mucosa is soft and velvety, but has no villi on the mucosal surface and no plicae circulares.
2. The longitudinal muscle layer of the tunica muscularis is not continuous, but is limited to three longitudinal bands that are visible on the surface as teniae coli.
3. The cecum, transverse colon, and pelvic colon regularly have mesenteries and therefore a complete tunica serosa. The ascending, descending, and iliac colons have a serosa only on the anterior surface unless they possess mesenteries, as sometimes happens.
4. There are many small tags of fat-filled peritoneum along the free border of the large gut called appendices epiploicae.
5. The walls of the transverse colon have definite rounded pouches, or sacculations, called haustra, which are separated from each other by semilunar folds. These are less well marked in the ascending and pelvic colons and poorly developed or ab-

sent in the descending and iliac colons. They do not exist in the cecum or rectum.

In summary, a loop of large bowel may be distinquished from a loop of small bowel by the presence of teniae coli, appendices epiploicae, and haustra.

The appendix, cecum, and proximal portion of the colon receive their arterial supply from the superior mesenteric artery; the remainder of the colon and the upper portion of the rectum receive arterial branches from the inferior mesenteric artery; and the distal end of the anal canal has arterial branches from the internal iliac artery. The superior rectal (hemorrhoidal) artery is a branch of the inferior mesenteric; the middle rectal (hemorrhoidal) is a branch of the anterior division of the internal iliac artery; and the inferior rectal (hemorrhoidal) is a branch of the internal pudendal artery (see Figs. 9-20 and 10-11).

The superior mesenteric vein has important tributaries from the veins of the proximal portion of the colon, and the inferior mesenteric vein drains blood into the portal system from the remainder of the colon and upper rectum. The two mesenteric veins anastomose with each other, and in the wall of the rectum the inferior mesenteric vein communicates with the veins of the distal end of the gut, which drain into the inferior vena cava. There is likewise an anastomosis between systemic and portal veins at the lower end of the esophagus, along the round ligament of the liver, and at the root of the mesentery (see Fig. 9-28).

The cecum, ascending colon, and proximal portion of the transverse colon receive nerve fibers from the superior mesenteric plexus and from the vagus nerves. The smooth muscle of the rest of the large gut receives fibers from the inferior mesenteric plexus and from pelvic ganglia. Sensory fibers from the intestine pass along the splanchnic nerves to the thoracic segments of the cord. Sensory fibers from the body wall go to the same segments. For this reason the pain of early appendicitis may seem to be in the pit of the stomach.

Cecum

The cecum is a multilocular pouch that lies inferior to the level of the ileocecal opening. It is about 5 cm long and during childhood is surrounded by peritoneum. In the adult the cecum often becomes adherent secondarily to the posterior wall of the abdominal cavity, and then it possesses a serous covering on its anterior wall only. On its anterior surface the tenia coli is well marked, terminates below on the appendix, and therefore serves as a guide in finding the appendix. The vermiform process, or appendix, is a slender tube attached to the base of the cecum. It varies greatly in length and position and usually has a

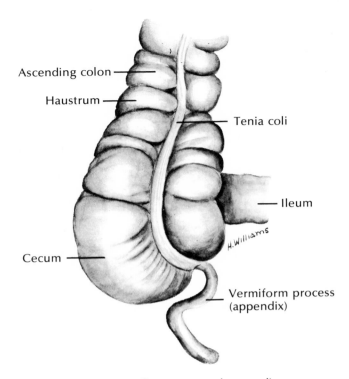

Ascending colon

Haustrum

Tenia coli

Ileum

Cecum

Vermiform process
(appendix)

H.Williams

Fig. 12-27. The cecum and appendix.

small mesentery of its own. The cavity of the appendix opens into that of the cecum (Fig. 12-27).

The opening of the ileum into the cecum is guarded by liplike folds. These folds are composed of mucous membrane and circular muscle bundles, forming a valvelike orifice that allows the contents to flow into the cecum but not back into the ileum.

Ascending colon

The ascending colon extends from the level of the ileocecal valve superiorly to the hepatic flexure. It is variable in length but is usually about 15 cm long and as a rule has a larger caliber than the descending colon. It usually has no peritoneum on its posterior surface and therefore no mesentery. The lower portion is close to the anterior abdominal wall, but the upper portion lies deeper behind the right lobe of the liver and in front of the anterior surface of the right kidney.

Transverse colon

The transverse colon passes in a long loop inferior to the stomach and is about 50 cm long. It begins at the hepatic flexure, passes transversely across the abdominal cavity, and ends at the splenic flexure

398

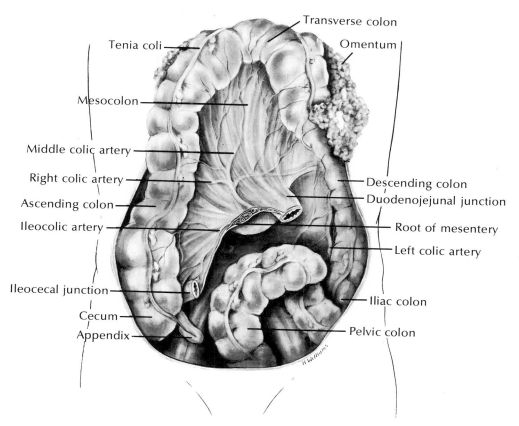

Tenia coli

Transverse colon

Omentum

Mesocolon

Middle colic artery

Right colic artery

Ascending colon

Ileocolic artery

Descending colon

Duodenojejunal junction

Root of mesentery

Left colic artery

Ileocecal junction

Cecum

Appendix

Iliac colon

Pelvic colon

Fig. 12-28. Colon and root of mesentery. The transverse colon has been turned superiorly to show the duodenojejunal junction. The iliac and pelvic colon, named portions of the sigmoid colon, are also shown. (Male, 53 years of age.)

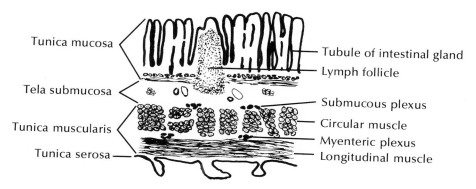

Tunica mucosa

Tela submucosa

Tunica muscularis

Tunica serosa

Tubule of intestinal gland

Lymph follicle

Submucous plexus

Circular muscle

Myenteric plexus

Longitudinal muscle

Fig. 12-29. Longitudinal section of transverse colon.

399

near the spleen. This portion has a mesentery, the transverse meso-colon. In the adult the mesocolon is usually blended with the greater omentum. The peritoneum forming the mesocolon is reflected from that which covers the pancreas. The midportion of the transverse co-lon is freely movable and varies greatly in its position and in the length of its mesentery. At either end the mesocolon becomes much shorter and disappears at either flexure. Both the hepatic and splenic flexures are well anchored to the posterior abdominal wall and vary little in position. The splenic flexure usually lies at a somewhat higher level than the hepatic.

Descending colon

The descending colon is about 15 cm long, ordinarily has no mesentery, but is firmly attached to the left posterior wall of the abdominal cavity. In diameter it is usually much smaller than the as-cending colon.

Iliac colon

The iliac colon is that portion lying on the medial surface of the left iliacus muscle; it is about 15 cm long and usually has no mesentery. It is quite often considered as a portion of the descending colon and is not described separately.

Pelvic colon

The pelvic colon begins where the bowel passes over the pelvic brim into the pelvic cavity. This portion is about 40 cm long and has a well-developed mesentery, the pelvic mesocolon. This loop of bowel varies greatly in length and therefore in position, but usually remains within the pelvic cavity. It makes a curve within the pel-vis that is somewhat S-shaped and is therefore often called the sigmoid colon, and its mesentery is called the mesosigmoid. The longitudinal muscle bundles of the tunica muscularis spread out so that in the dis-tal portion of the pelvic colon the longitudinal muscle layer becomes continuous, and teniae coli and haustra disappear. The area of transi-tion from sigmoid colon to rectum is frequently called the recto-sigmoid.

Rectum

The rectum has no mesentery, no appendices epiploicae, and no haustra. At its beginning it is covered by peritoneum on the anterior surface, but inferiorly has no peritoneal covering at all. It lies on the anterior surface of the sacrum and coccyx, surrounded by pelvic fas-cia. It is curved somewhat from side to side and from anterior to poste-rior, but none of the curves is acute (Fig. 12-30). In men it lies pos-terior to prostate gland and bladder and in women posterior to the uterus and vagina. There are several crescentic folds in the lateral walls of the rectum that project into its cavity. The terminal portion

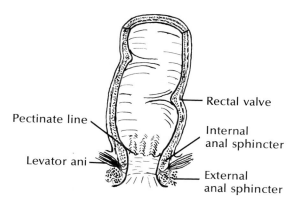

Pectinate line

Levator ani

Rectal valve

Internal
anal sphincter

External
anal sphincter

Fig. 12-30. Diagram of vertical section of rectum and anal canal.

narrows rapidly, and the mucous membrane has a number of vertical folds, called rectal columns, with spaces between, called rectal sinuses. The veins present in the mucosa covering the rectal columns frequently become dilated, thus forming internal hemorrhoids. A line drawn around the rectum at the base of the rectal columns is undulating or wavy and is called the pectinate, or dentate, line. This line is frequently used by anatomists and surgeons to mark the junction of the rectum and anal canal. The name rectum would imply that this portion of the bowel is straight. In many animals this is true, but in man it is not. For convenience the name is used in human anatomy.

The anal canal, a narrow passage between two levator ani muscles, is about 2.5 cm long. These two muscles form a muscular diaphragm in the floor of the pelvic cavity. They are attached to the lateral walls of the pelvic girdle and meet in the midline in a raphe extending from the coccyx posteriorly to the midpoint of the perineum anterior to the anus. The anal canal is directed posteriorly and inferiorly, and in the recumbent position often forms an angle with the horizontal of as much as 45°. The lining of the anal canal is stratified squamous epithelium.

Some descriptions of this area include the terminal part of the rectum containing the rectal columns and sinuses as the first part of the anal canal and therefore refer to these structures as anal columns and anal sinuses.

The levator ani muscles act as a sphincter of the gut, but there are in addition two other sphincters: (1) an internal sphincter, which is a thickened portion of the circular muscle layer of the tunica muscularis and therefore smooth or involuntary muscle, and (2) an external sphincter composed of small bundles of striate or voluntary muscle lying beneath the skin about the anus.

Anal canal

401

REVIEW QUESTIONS

1. What structures bound the mouth?
2. Describe the soft palate.
3. Describe the hard palate.
4. Describe the tongue.
5. Name the extrinsic muscles of the tongue. Give one function of each.
6. Name the salivary glands. Where is each located? What is the source of the secretory nerve fibers to each?
7. How many teeth are in the deciduous dentition? How many in the permanent dentition?
8. Name the muscles of mastication. Give one function of each.
9. Describe the pharynx.
10. Name the muscles of the pharynx. How do they function in the act of swallowing?
11. Give the location of the various tonsils.
12. What structures form the wall of the abdominal cavity?
13. What is meant by a retroperitoneal organ?
14. Describe the wall of the stomach.
15. What are the three subdivisions of the small intestine?
16. Give two functions of the pancreas.
17. Describe the liver.
18. Describe the gallbladder.
19. How may the large intestine be distinguished from the small intestine?
20. What are the subdivisions of the large intestine?
21. Describe the cecum.
22. Describe the rectum.
23. What is the function of the gallbladder?
24. How may a segment of proximal jejunum be distinguished from a segment of distal ileum?
25. List the ligaments of the liver.
26. Discuss circulation through the liver.

CHAPTER 13

THE URINARY SYSTEM

The urinary system consists of a pair of kidneys, which secrete urine; a pair of ureters, which convey the urine from the kidneys to the bladder; a bladder, which holds the urine; and a urethra, which carries the urine to the exterior. The urethra is much longer in men than in women, but otherwise there are no sexual differences in the urinary system (Fig. 13-1).

In life the kidney is a dark reddish-brown color that shows through the glistening, translucent capsule. The shape of the kidney is so characteristic that it needs little description. The convex border of the kidney is on the lateral side, and the concave border is turned toward the vertebral column. On the concave border is a deep excavation in the substance of the organ, called the renal sinus, the opening of which is the hilus of the kidney. The renal vessels enter and leave the kidney through the hilus, whereas the renal pelvis, the dilated superior end of the ureter, is located partially within the renal sinus. The suprarenal gland fits like a cap on the superior end of the kidney (Fig. 13-2). The right kidney may be a little lower than the left. The inferior border of the kidney is about 3.5 cm above the level of the iliac crest when the body is erect; the organ ascends somewhat in the horizontal position.

The thin, smooth capsule closely enveloping the kidney is called the tunica fibrosa, or renal capsule proper. External to this is a considerable mass of mixed connective and fatty tissue, within which the kidney is embedded. The fatty tissue is sometimes called the adipose capsule, or perirenal fat, and the fibrous tissue is called the renal fascia, or capsule. This fibrous and fatty tissue helps to keep the kidneys

KIDNEY

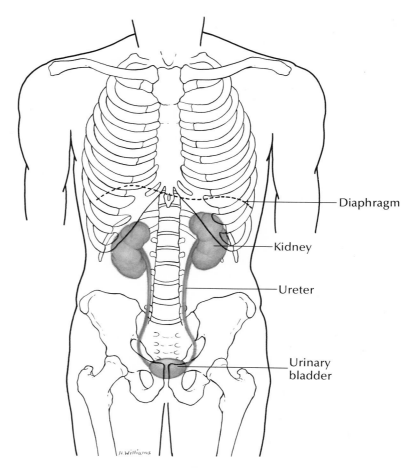

Fig. 13-1. The position of the urinary system.

in their normal position. Anterior to the kidneys is the parietal peritoneum, and posterior to the kidneys are the deep muscles of the back. Hence, the kidneys are retroperitoneal.

Deep to the tunica fibrosa, the cortex of the kidney forms a complete peripheral layer and extends, in places, medially to reach the renal sinus. These extensions of cortex, the renal columns, are separated from one another by the renal pyramids, which constitute the medulla. Each pyramid has its base placed against the cortical layer and its apex projecting into the sinus as a renal papilla (Fig. 13-4).

Each kidney has an average of ten renal pyramids, one or more of which empties into one of nine minor calyces. The minor calyces unite to form two or occasionally three major calyces, the confluence of

404

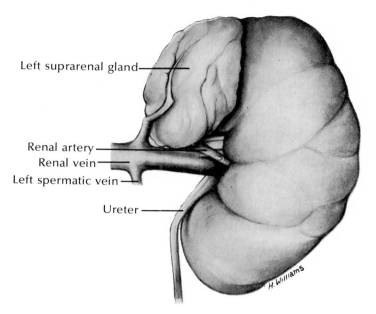

Fig. 13-2. Left kidney and suprarenal gland, anterior view.

Left suprarenal gland

Renal artery
Renal vein
Left spermatic vein

Ureter

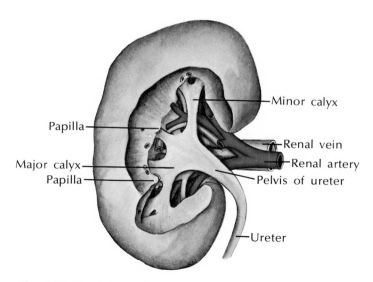

Papilla

Major calyx
Papilla

Minor calyx

Renal vein
Renal artery
Pelvis of ureter

Ureter

Fig. 13-3. The left renal pelvis and calyces, posterior view.

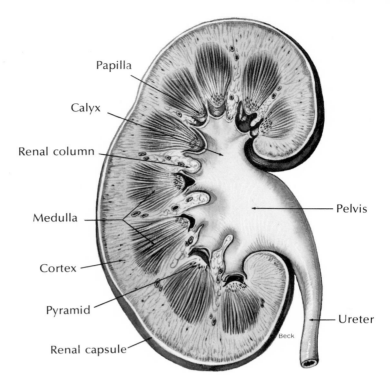

Papilla

Calyx

Renal column

Medulla

Cortex

Pyramid

Renal capsule

Pelvis

Ureter

Beck

Fig. 13-4. Coronal section through the right kidney. (From Anthony, C. P., and Kolthoff, N. J.: Textbook of anatomy and physiology, ed. 8, St. Louis, 1971, The C. V. Mosby Co.)

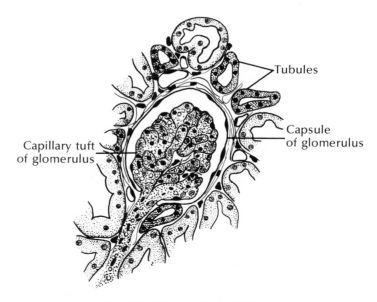

Tubules

Capsule
of glomerulus

Capillary tuft
of glomerulus

406

Fig. 13-5. Glomerulus of kidney.

which forms the renal pelvis, or the superior dilated portion of the ureter. The medulla has a more striated appearance than the cortex and is
deeper red in color. The cortex is granular and has a pale red color.
This granular appearance is due to an immense number of kidney corpuscles. Each corpuscle is composed of a glomerulus, or loop of capillaries, surrounded by a thin-walled sac, or capsule, of epithelial tissue (Bowman's capsule) (Fig. 13-5). The capsule opens into a tubule
that, after a tortuous course through cortex and medulla, opens into
the renal sinus. Blood laden with waste material enters the hilus
through the renal artery, which breaks up into many small radiating
branches terminating in the capillaries of the renal corpuscles. From
the renal corpuscles, waste material is passed into the capsule of the
glomerulus. The blood passes into veins that radiate toward the hilus
to form the tributaries of the renal veins. The substance of the kidney

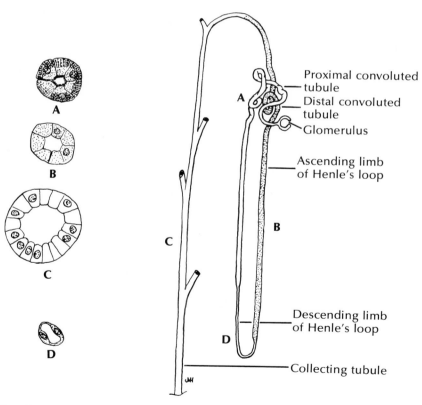

Fig. 13-6. A single glomerulus and tubule. On the left are diagrams of the
cross section of the tubule at four levels, indicated by the letters, *A, B, C,*
and *D.*

407

is therefore formed of blood vessels and tubules within a small amount of framework composed of connective tissue.

A renal, or uriniferous, tubule has a very characteristic design. Soon after its beginning at the capsule of the glomerulus it becomes coiled, forming the proximal convoluted tubule, which in turn connects with Henle's loop. The ascending and descending limbs of the loop pass in a straight line through the medulla of a pyramid toward the hilus and are connected by a short curved piece. The ascending limb is followed by a distal convoluted portion that in turn empties into the collecting tubule that passes through the pyramid and carries the urine into the pelvis of the ureter (Fig. 13-6).

In the renal tubules certain substances such as water and minerals are resorbed into the blood stream, thus maintaining a constant balance within the body. The urine in the renal pelvis contains waste material and any excess of water and other substances.

Within the substance of the kidney the renal artery gives off interlobar arteries, which lie between the pyramids, and these in turn form a series of incomplete arches, the arciform, or arcuate, arteries, cross-

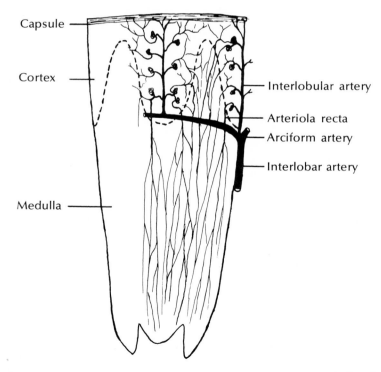

Capsule

Cortex

Interlobular artery

Arteriola recta

Arciform artery

Interlobar artery

Medulla

Fig. 13-7. The arterial supply of glomeruli and tubules. The kidney section has been drawn wider and shorter than it actually is.

408

ing the base of the pyramids. Radiating laterally toward the surface of the kidney from the arciform arteries are the interlobular arteries. These give off the afferent vessels to the glomeruli (Fig. 13-7). The efferent vessels from the glomeruli break up into a second set of capillaries about the convoluted tubules. From these, blood passes into the venous system of the kidney. Other vessels, the arteriolae rectae or straight arterioles, radiate inward from the efferent glomerular arteries.

The renal arteries are branches of the abdominal aorta, and the renal veins drain into the inferior vena cava. Frequently there are accessory renal blood vessels. The nerves to the kidney are small branches that come from a plexus of fibers about the renal artery and accompany arterial branches into the renal substance. Sensory fibers from the kidney are probably carried by the tenth, eleventh, and twelfth thoracic nerves; autonomic fibers, from splanchnic and possibly vagus nerves, control the vascular supply of the kidney.

In the fetus each renal pyramid forms a distinct lobe. Occasionally these lobes persist more or less distinctly into adult life.

URETER

The ureter is about 25 cm long. It begins as a funnel-shaped tube, the renal pelvis, located partially in the renal sinus. In the renal sinus, the ureter is represented by a number of thin-walled tubes, called major and minor renal calyces (Figs. 13-3 and 13-4). The mucosa of these structures has an epithelium continuous with the epithelium lining the renal tubules. At the level of the inferior border of the kidney the pelvis of the ureter narrows and is converted into a thick-walled tube intimately attached but posterior to the parietal peritoneum. It passes inferiorly parallel to the vertebral column on the muscles of the posterior abdominal wall and usually just over the tips of the transverse processes of the lumbar vertebrae. Within the pelvic cavity the ureter turns anteriorly and medially to enter the bladder from below. Where they open into the bladder, the ureters are about 5 cm apart (Fig. 13-8). In women the uterine artery crosses over the ureter, just before its termination, and in ligating the artery during removal of the uterus, a surgeon must take care to avoid injury to the ureter. In men the ductus deferens crosses over the inferior end of the ureter at the same site as the uterine artery in women.

The lumen of the ureter, although variable in size, is physiologically narrowed at two sites: (1) the uteropelvic junction and (2) the entrance of the ureter into the bladder. Small kidney stones, or renal calculi, may lodge at either of the constrictions giving rise to dilation of the ureter or renal pelvis (hydronephrosis) and to extreme pain, or renal colic.

The superior end of the ureter receives its arterial blood from branches of the renal artery; the inferior end receives blood from the arteries that supply the urinary bladder, and the midportion receives small arterial branches from the spermatic artery, aorta, or common iliac artery. There is a free anastomosis of these various small arteries within the wall of the ureter itself. The nerve fibers supplying the ureter follow along the arteries and come from the thoracolumbar and sacral autonomic outflows.

The wall of the ureter has three coats:

1. The tunica mucosa has a number of layers of epithelial cells, continuous inferiorly with the mucous membrane of the bladder and superiorly with the lining of the renal pelvis into which open the renal tubules.

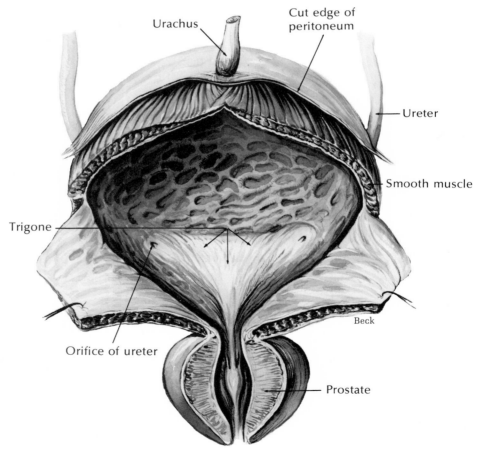

Fig. 13-8. The male urinary bladder, cut to show the interior. (From Anthony, C. P., and Kolthoff, N. J.: Textbook of anatomy and physiology, ed. 8, St. Louis, 1971, The C. V. Mosby Co.)

2. The tunica muscularis is composed of smooth muscle bundles, some arranged in circular fashion and some longitudinal, with bands of connective tissue between them.
3. The tunica adventitia is an outer layer of connective tissue.

The urinary bladder is a hollow, muscular viscus lying in the midline external to the parietal peritoneum and posterior to the symphysis pubis. In men it lies anterior to the rectum and superior to the prostate gland, and in women it lies anterior to the uterus and vagina (see Figs. 15-2 and 16-3). A fibrous cord passes superiorly beneath the peritoneum from the apex of the bladder to the umbilicus. This is the median umbilical ligament and is the remains of an embryonic passage, the urachus. The floor (base or trigone) of the bladder is triangular in outline, with a ureter opening at each corner of the base posteriorly and the urethra opening at the apex inferiorly. The base of the bladder has a relatively smooth surface that changes but little in size no matter whether the viscus is full or empty, but the remainder of the wall is thrown into folds when the bladder is empty. When the viscus is distended with urine, its wall is smooth. The bladder is capable of considerable distention, but is usually emptied when it contains some 350 ml of urine, though it can contain 600 ml without too great discomfort. As the bladder distends, it pushes its way superiorly between the abdominal wall and the parietal coat of peritoneum. In great distention the fundus may almost reach the level of the umbilicus.

Since the anterior surface of the bladder is not covered with peritoneum, it is possible, if the organ is distended, for the surgeon to cut through the anterior abdominal wall just superior to the symphysis and enter the cavity of the bladder without opening the peritoneal cavity.

The wall of the bladder has four coats:

1. The tunica mucosa has transitional epithelium.
2. The tela submucosa is composed of fibrous connective tissue with a considerable number of elastic fibers.
3. The thick tunica muscularis is composed of smooth muscle. There are many interlacing bundles of muscles, but these are not arranged into definite layers. At the outlet of the bladder the smooth muscle bundles are not arranged to form a definite sphincter muscle. The tunica muscularis of the bladder is continuous with the smooth muscle layer of the urethra.
4. The outer coat is tunica serosa where the bladder is covered with peritoneum and elsewhere is tunica adventitia or fibrous connective tissue.

Branches derived from the internal iliac artery pass into the bladder from either side and are accompanied by nerve fibers from the upper lumbar nerves (thoracolumbar autonomic outflow) and from the third and fourth sacral nerves (sacral autonomic outflow). Sensory fibers from the bladder accompany these motor nerve fibers.

URETHRA

In women the urethra is a simple tube about 4 cm long passing inferiorly behind the symphysis, through the urogenital diaphragm, and emptying between the labia minora, anterior to the vagina, and posterior to the clitoris. As it passes through the urogenital diaphragm, it is surrounded by a sphincter of striate muscle, the sphincter of the membranous urethra, or a voluntary sphincter.

The wall of the urethra has an inner mucous membrane layer, a thin submucous coat, and a thick muscular layer.

In men the urethra is much longer. It has three portions: a prostatic portion about 2.5 cm long, a membranous portion about .5 cm long passing through the urogenital diaphragm, and a cavernous portion within the corpus spongiosum. The membranous portion in men has a voluntary sphincter, as in women.

The coats of the urethra in men are the same as those in women, but there are certain male sex glands that empty their secretions into the urethra (see discussion in Chapter 16).

Because of illness or injury it is occasionally impossible to relax the sphincter and thus to empty the bladder. Catheterization is then necessary. This is easy in women because the urethra is short and straight. It is more difficult in men because the urethra has an S-shaped course. The first curve is the downward passage through the prostate; the second curve is produced by the pendulous penis. There is no second curve in the erect organ.

It is possible for a surgeon to pass a hollow tube (a cystoscope) through the urethra into the bladder and by means of a complicated system of mirrors and lights to examine the mucosa of the bladder, to perform operations within the organ, and to catheterize each ureter separately.

REVIEW QUESTIONS

1. What structures form the urinary system?
2. Describe the structure of a ureter.
3. Describe the urinary bladder.
4. What are the various portions of a renal tubule?
5. The renal arteries are branches of what artery? To what vein do the renal veins drain?
6. What are the three portions of the male urethra?
7. What is catheterization of the urinary bladder?
8. Describe the arterial supply to the ureter.
9. Where is the striate sphincter of the urethra located?
10. Describe a glomerulus of the kidney.

CHAPTER 14

THE SKIN AND SUBCUTANEOUS TISSUES

The skin is the outer covering of the body. At the margins of the eyelids it is continuous with the conjunctiva. At other openings on the body surface, such as the mouth, nose, and anus, it is continuous, with mucous membrane linings. The skin contains blood vessels, sebaceous (oil) and sudoriferous (sweat) glands, and the endings of sensory nerves. In certain areas of the body modified skin cells form nails and hair.

Skin is composed of two main layers, or strata: (1) a superficial sheet of stratified squamous epithelium, called the epidermis or cuticle, and (2) a deeper layer of connective tissue, called the dermis, corium, or true skin. The epidermis is subdivided by histologists into five layers (Fig. 14-1). The deepest stratum is called the germinative stratum, or malpighian layer. The next is the prickle cell layer, or stratum spinosum. The third is the stratum granulosum, the cells of which contain many pigment granules. A thin stratum lucidum is the fourth layer and is composed of clear amorphous material. The fifth and outermost layer, the stratum corneum or cornified layer, is composed of many layers of closely packed squamous cells that have lost their nuclei. The surface layers of squamous cells are being shed constantly and replaced by deeper cells.

The epidermis contains no blood vessels (Fig. 14-2). The dermis is composed of interlacing bundles of fibrous and elastic tissue that gradually blend with the areolar subcutaneous tissue. Over most of the body the outer surface of the dermis is folded into irregular ridges forming papillae, with the deeper cell layers of the epidermis filling

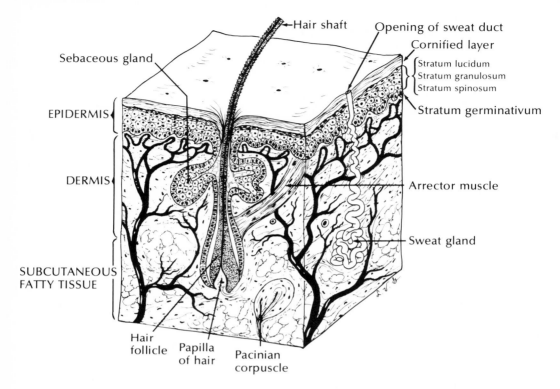

Fig. 14-1. Illustration of a section of human skin showing the several layers and many of the other structures appearing in skin. (Modified from Schottelius, B. A., and Schottelius, D. D.: Textbook of physiology, ed. 17, St. Louis, 1973, The C. V. Mosby Co.)

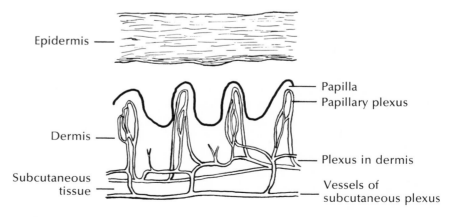

Fig. 14-2. Arterioles of skin. The deeper layers of the cuticle have been left blank.

414

in the spaces between the papillae. Embedded within the dermis are sweat glands, sebaceous glands, and hair shafts. Very small blood vessels, lymphatics, and nerve fibers have their endings in the dermis. In the subcutaneous tissue small arteries form an arterial plexus from which small vessels pass into the dermis and form another plexus under the papillae.

The color of the skin varies with the amount of pigment in the cells of the epidermis and with the blood supply. According to the amount of pigmentation of the skin, mankind is divided into various groups: white, yellow, brown, and black. The skin is more deeply pigmented in certain parts of the body, such as the perineum, armpits, areolae of the nipples, and the exposed surfaces of the body. It may also become more deeply pigmented in any part of the body subjected to direct rays of the sun. In old age the skin becomes more deeply pigmented with yellow and frequently contains irregular brown areas. In obstruction of the common bile duct the skin may become a dark brown.

The deeper layers of the skin contain many small blood vessels that, in health, give a pink tint to the skin. If the blood is poorly oxygenated, the resulting blue tint is known as cyanosis. After death, the body surface becomes whitened in areas where the blood has drained away and a bluish purple in areas that contain stagnant blood.

The skin varies in thickness, that covering the exposed areas of face and hands being thicker than that on the areas protected by clothing. The soles of the feet are calloused, and the hands of a laborer are really horny in character. The protected skin surface of the inner side of the arms and legs is more delicate than that on the outer surface. The skin of a person in poor health is usually dryer and more sensitive than that of a person in robust health. An invalid or an unconscious person may suffer a severe burn from a hot-water bottle at a temperature that would not harm a well person. The skin of a person with a hypothyroid disorder (one having an underactive thyroid gland) is thick, dry, and leathery. The skin of a person with a hyperthyroid disorder (one having an overactive thyroid gland) is warm, moist, and flushed. The skin is a delicate indicator of health and of encroachments on functional efficiency.

The skin is quite elastic and in most areas, particularly over the extensor side of joints, is freely movable. In certain areas, such as palms and soles and on the flexor side of joints, the skin is bound to the underlying structures, thus producing the flexor folds. On the palms and soles the epidermis forms ridges that produce the characteristic and distinctive patterns seen in the skin over the terminal phalanges. These patterns remain constant throughout life and form the basis for identification by fingerprints.

HAIR
Hair grows from certain specialized cells of the skin. The color of the hair changes with age, the white hair of the aged being due to loss of pigment.

In both sexes there are well-marked areas of hair on the scalp, the eyebrows, the eyelids, and at the anterior openings of the nose. At puberty, hair appears in the armpits, around the genitalia of both sexes, and on the face of men. In women the genital hair is confined to the labia majora and to a small triangular area over the symphysis. In men the area covered by hair extends upward to the umbilicus, and there is usually a hairy area on the chest as well. The palms and soles have no hair, but the parts of the body not already mentioned are sparsely provided with scattered hairs, larger and more numerous in the male.

A small bundle of smooth muscle, the arrector pili, is attached to certain hair shafts (Fig. 14-1). When their muscles contract, the hairs stand more nearly erect, and the consequent small wrinkles of skin give the appearance known as "goose flesh." The arrector pili muscles are innervated by sympathetic nerve fibers.

SEBACEOUS GLANDS
Wherever there are hairs, there are small glands that secrete sebum, an oily substance. In certain areas, particularly on the nose, where the hairs are quite small, the sebaceous glands are large. If the outlet of a gland becomes blocked, a sebaceous cyst results.

The tarsal glands, lying within the tarsus of each eyelid, are modified sebaceous glands. These are also known as meibomian glands, and occasionally a meibomian cyst occurs when the outlet of a gland is blocked. An infection of one of these glands produces a stye (Fig. 14-3).

SUDORIFEROUS GLANDS
There are sweat, or sudoriferous, glands distributed over the entire body; they are more abundant in the palm of the hand, the sole of the foot, and in the armpit than on the rest of the body surface. The sweat glands are an important part of the heat-regulating mechanism of the body and also act as excretory organs.

The ceruminous glands of the external ear canal, which secrete wax, are modified sudoriferous glands. The ciliary glands, located in the eyelids behind the eyelashes, are also modified sweat glands.

NAILS
Nails are produced by specialized skin cells on the dorsal aspect of the terminal phalanges of fingers and toes. The hoofs and claws of other animals are similar structures. Nails protect the ends of the fingers and form a stiff backing to the soft sensitive pulp of the fingertips. The stubby finger ends seen in persons who continually bite their nails result from the loss of this stiffening.

The appearance of the nails changes with age and with fluctuations in health. In healthy young adults they should be smooth and free from ridges or grooves and should be neither too brittle nor too soft. In illness the nails become rigid and grooved and are easily broken and torn. In old age, they are likely to be brittle, rather opaque, thickened, and roughened.

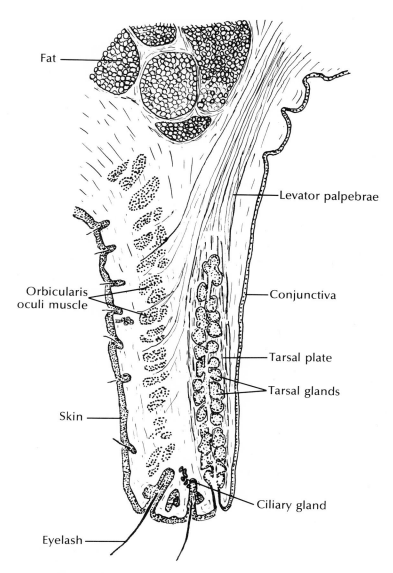

Fig. 14-3. Diagrammatic section through upper eyelid to show relationships of major structures. (From DiDio, L. J. A.: Synopsis of anatomy, St. Louis, 1970, The C. V. Mosby Co.)

**SUPERFICIAL
FASCIA**

Beneath the skin is a layer of loose connective tissue filled with fat. The thickness of this layer varies in different parts of the body and also varies with age, health, and sex. This tissue is also called the sub-cutaneous tissue, or the panniculus adiposus (Figs. 14-4 to 14-9).

Healthy infants of both sexes have a thick subcutaneous tissue well filled with fat that is rather evenly distributed over the entire body, thus giving the baby its round, chubby appearance. When the fat is particularly abundant, the skin lies in folds. After the child begins to walk, there are changes in the distribution of fat, which is nowhere very abundant, both boys and girls tending to lose the chubby appearance of infancy.

In adolescence a sex difference is apparent in the distribution of

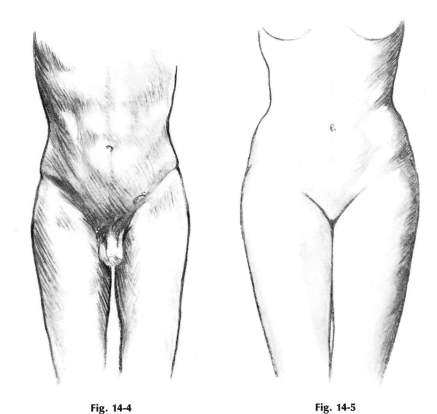

Fig. 14-4   **Fig. 14-5**

Fig. 14-4. Male figure, anterior view. Note absence of fat pads. (After John Millard.)

Fig. 14-5. Female figure, anterior view, showing contours produced by fat pads. (After John Millard.)

418

fat; women develop fat pads over the shoulders, buttocks, lateral side of the thighs, the symphysis pubis, and the breasts. The fat pads in men are thinner and more evenly distributed over the body.

In middle life both sexes tend to accumulate reserves of fat in their subcutaneous tissues. In old age the fat is lost and, because of loss of elastic tissue from its deeper layers, the skin becomes wrinkled, folded, and flabby.

Subcutaneous tissue of the eyelids, the areolae of the breasts, the penis, the scrotum, and the clitoris contains no fat.

The subcutaneous tissue acts as a storehouse for reserves of fat, as

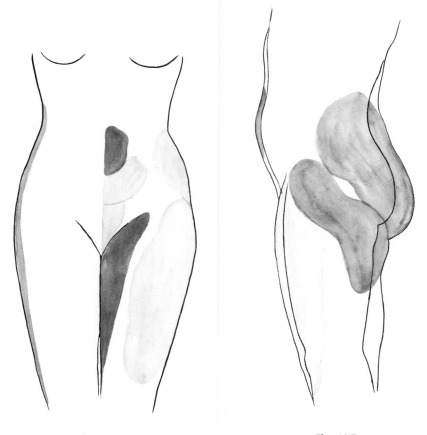

Fig. 14-6   **Fig. 14-7**

Fig. 14-6. Fat pads of female. On the left side of the figure, pads are shown in anterior view and on the right side the thickness in cross section. (After John Millard.)

Fig. 14-7. Fat pads of female, lateral view. The outline of the male is superposed. (After John Millard.)

419

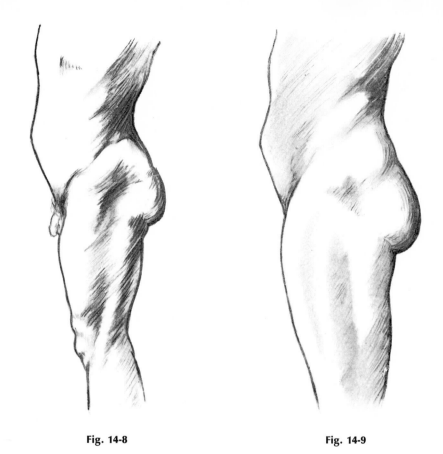

Fig. 14-8   **Fig. 14-9**

Fig. 14-8. Male figure, lateral view. Note absence of fat pads. (After John Millard.)

Fig. 14-9. Female figure, lateral view, showing contours produced by fat pads. (After John Millard.)

a protective layer for the deeper structures, as a loose tissue in which blood vessels and nerves may freely ramify, and as a temporary reservoir for excess body fluid (Figs. 14-10 to 14-13).

DEEP FASCIA   Beneath the superficial fascia is a thin layer of rather dense white connective tissue that contains little or no fat and is called the deep fascia. It forms an investment for muscles, and from its deep surface sheets of fascia pass inward to form intermuscular septa. This layer has certain thickenings that have been described elsewhere as ligaments and retinacula. It should be clearly kept in mind that no fascia is a discrete structure, but that fasciae are everywhere continuous and that certain areas or thickenings are given names for convenience in

420

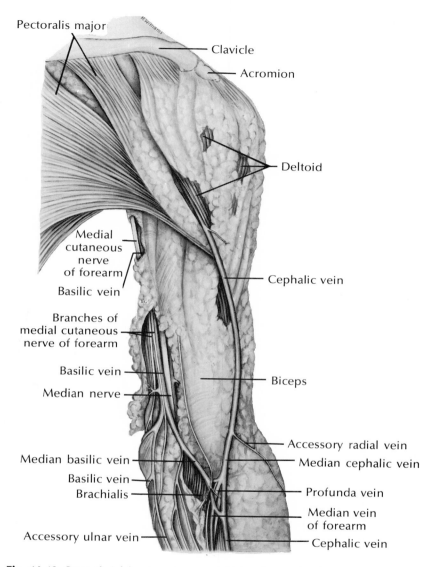

Pectoralis major

Clavicle

Acromion

Deltoid

Medial
cutaneous
nerve
of forearm

Cephalic vein

Basilic vein

Branches of
medial cutaneous
nerve of forearm

Basilic vein

Biceps

Median nerve

Accessory radial vein

Median basilic vein

Median cephalic vein

Basilic vein

Brachialis

Profunda vein

Median vein
of forearm

Accessory ulnar vein

Cephalic vein

Fig. 14-10. Superficial fascia, nerves, and blood vessels of anterior aspect of the left arm. (Male, 87 years of age.)

anatomical descriptions. Some of these bands of deep fascia, such as the iliotibial tract, thoracolumbar fascia, and plantar aponeurosis, are among the most important supporting structures of the body.

In various places in the subcutaneous tissue there develop small closed sacs, called bursae, filled with a clear fluid and lined with syno-   **BURSAE**

vial membrane. These bursae are usually found over bony prominences and beneath tendons. There is always one such bursa over the
olecranon of the ulna, one over the ischial tuberosity, and several about
the knee joint. If the skin over a bursa is chronically irritated, the
amount of fluid in the sac is increased, rendering the bursa large and

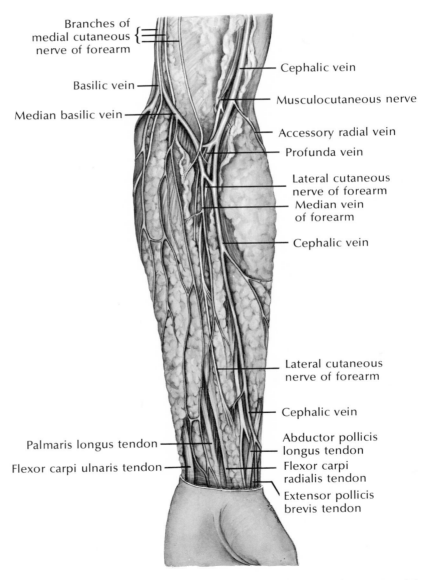

Fig. 14-11. Superficial fascia, nerves, and blood vessels of volar aspect of the
left forearm. (Male, 87 years of age.)

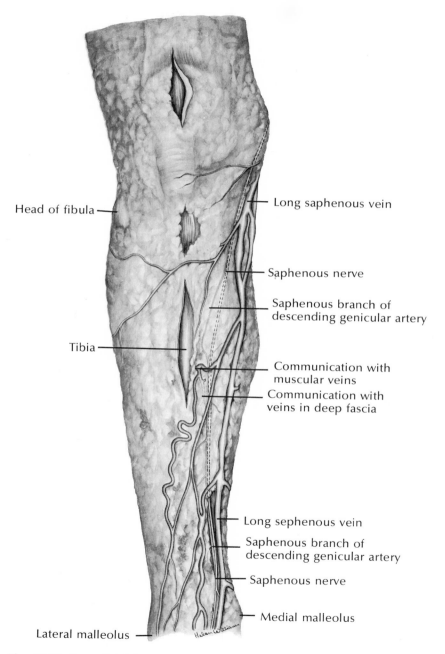

Head of fibula—

Long saphenous vein

Saphenous nerve

Saphenous branch of
descending genicular artery

Tibia—

Communication with
muscular veins

Communication with
veins in deep fascia

Long sephenous vein

Saphenous branch of
descending genicular artery

Saphenous nerve

Medial malleolus

Lateral malleolus—

Fig. 14-12. Superficial fascia, nerves, and blood vessels on anterior aspect
of left leg. (Male, 62 years of age.)

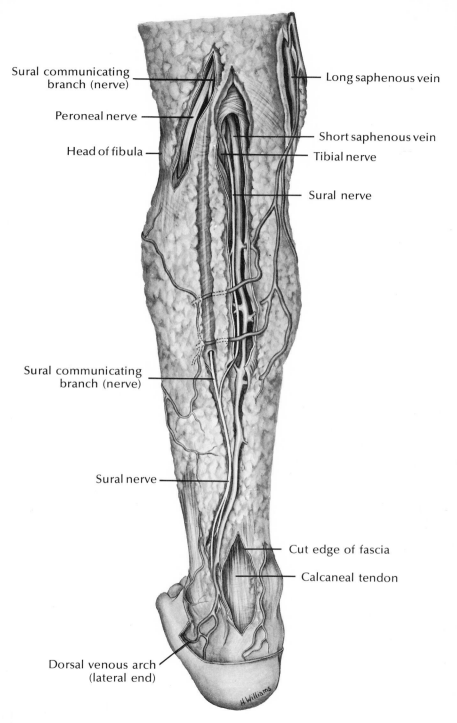

Sural communicating
branch (nerve)

Peroneal nerve

Head of fibula

Long saphenous vein

Short saphenous vein

Tibial nerve

Sural nerve

Sural communicating
branch (nerve)

Sural nerve

Cut edge of fascia

Calcaneal tendon

Dorsal venous arch
(lateral end)

Fig. 14-13. Superficial fascia, nerves, and blood vessels on posterior aspect
of left leg. (Male, 62 years of age.)

tense, a condition known as bursitis. The fluid may even become infected, transforming the bursa into an abscess.

In areas where muscle tendons pass beneath specialized thickenings of the deep fascia, such as the retinacula at the wrist and ankle,
sheaths are found surrounding the tendons. These sheaths are closed
tubular sacs, similar to bursae, having an inner layer closely applied to

**TENDON
SHEATHS**

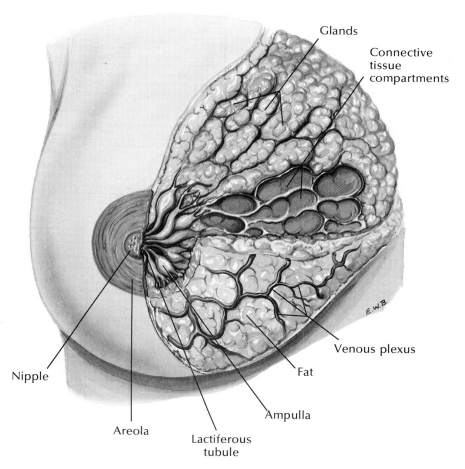

Fig. 14-14. Anterior view of the breast. The skin has been removed in the
lower right quadrant to reveal the plexus overlying the adipose (fatty) tissue.
In the upper right quadrant the adipose tissue has been removed to show
the alveoli of the glands. The glands have been removed in a small area to
reveal the connective tissue compartments that separate the lobules. (From
Anthony, C. P., and Kolthoff, N. J.: Textbook of anatomy and physiology,
ed. 8, St. Louis, 1971, The C. V. Mosby Co.)

425

the tendon and an outer layer attached to the walls of the channel through which the tendon runs. These sheaths enable the tendons to glide back and forth more easily.

MAMMARY GLAND

Each breast is a glandular organ located in the subcutaneous tissue of the anterior chest wall, overlying the pectoralis muscles, and extending from the second to the sixth ribs. The nipple is situated near the summit of the breast and, although variable, tends to lie at the level of the fourth intercostal space.

Each mammary gland is composed of 15 to 20 separate compound tubular alveolar glands (lobes). Dense connective tissue with large accumulation of fat surrounds the lobes and subdivides them into lobules. Thickened bands of connective tissue (suspensory ligaments of Cooper) attach the skin of the breast to the underlying deep fascia. It is the presence of these connective tissue attachments that leads to dimpling of the skin over an area of carcinoma of the breast. As the tumor enlarges, the connective tissue bands become taut, and the skin is retracted. The breasts are hemispherical in shape, but on the upper lateral quadrant there is projecting portion (axillary tail) extending toward the armpit (see Fig. 10-7).

The nipple contains minute openings for the milk ducts, one from each lobe. The distal portion of each duct, dilated, is named the ampulla. Surrounding the nipple is a circular band of pigmented skin, called the areola. In women who have had no children it is brownish-pink in color. The color changes to a deep brown during the early months of pregnancy, and this pigmentation is retained thereafter. Also concentrated in the areola are sensory nerve endings, stimulation of which causes contraction of smooth muscle in the areola and nipple, resulting in hardening and protrusion of the nipple. Such a reaction can be elicited by either temperature (cold), tactile, or sexual stimulation.

The breast receives its arterial supply from branches of the internal thoracic, lateral thoracic, or intercostal arteries. The nerve supply is furnished by branches of the fourth through sixth intercostal nerves. Although the lymphatics of the breast are numerous, the chief drainage pattern is into the axillary group of lymph nodes (see Fig. 10-7).

During childhood the breasts are small and show little sex differentiation. In men the nipple is distinct though small, but the glandular portion of the breast is rudimentary. Growth of the milk-producing system in women is dependent on numerous hormonal factors that interact during two chronologic events, puberty and pregnancy. Overall, the major influences on the breast growth at puberty or pregnancy are estrogen and progesterone. During gestation only nonmilk (colostrum) is produced. At birth, milk is produced by the milk-secretory cells, acting much like sweat glands. Once the flow of milk is initiated, milk is secreted into the lumen of the alveolus while contraction of myoepithelial cells surrounding the alveoli empty the alveolar lumen, thereby enhancing further milk secretion.

Galactorrhea. Galactorrhea refers to the nonphysiologic and inappropriate secretion of milky fluid that is either not related to pregnancy or is persistent and excessive to the needs of the neonate. Although physiology is not the domain of this book, it is important to realize that the quantity of secretion is not an important criterion, any galactorrhea demands evaluation. The final common pathway leading to the condition is thought to be an inappropriate augmentation of an anterior pituitary hormone, prolactin. This condition can be caused by a multitude of factors; however, one factor that must be ruled out is a pituitary tumor.

REVIEW QUESTIONS

1. What are the two main layers of the skin?
2. Give four factors that influence the color of the skin.
3. Name two types of glands associated with the skin, and name the substance secreted by each.
4. What are four functions of subcutaneous tissue?
5. How does deep fascia differ from superficial fascia?
6. Describe the mammary gland.
7. Describe a fingernail.
8. What is the function of a tendon sheath?
9. What is a subcutaneous bursa? Give three locations where such bursae may be found.
10. Describe the difference in the distribution of hair in adult men and in adult women.
11. Discuss galactorrhea.

CHAPTER 15

THE FEMALE
REPRODUCTIVE SYSTEM

The female reproductive organs include a pair of ovaries, two uterine tubes, a uterus, a vagina, and the external genitalia, composed of the labia majora, labia minora, clitoris, bulb of the vestibule, and the vestibular glands. The orifice is called the vulva. The vestibule is a capacious pocket about 5 cm deep connecting the vulva with the vagina and delimited from the vagina by an incomplete septum, called the hymen.

OVARY   The ovary is a solid gland about 3.5 cm long lying on the lateral wall of the pelvic cavity and attached by a fold of peritoneum, the mesovarium, to the broad ligament of the uterus. A round cord, called the ligament of the ovary, passes from the ovary to the uterus near the attachment of the uterine tube. The margin of the broad ligament between the ovary and the fimbriated end of the uterine tube on the one hand and the lateral pelvic wall on the other is called the infundibulo-pelvic ligament.

The free surface of the ovary has an outer layer of low columnar or cuboidal epithelium continuous with the mesothelium of the peritoneum. The substance of the gland, subdivided by strands of connective tissue through which run blood vessels and nerves, is composed of columns and nests of germinal epithelial cells. The ova are formed from the germinal epithelium. A nest of cells increases in size and number, and the cells assume a definite arrangement. The outer cells form a stratified columnar wall about a clear central cavity filled with fluid.

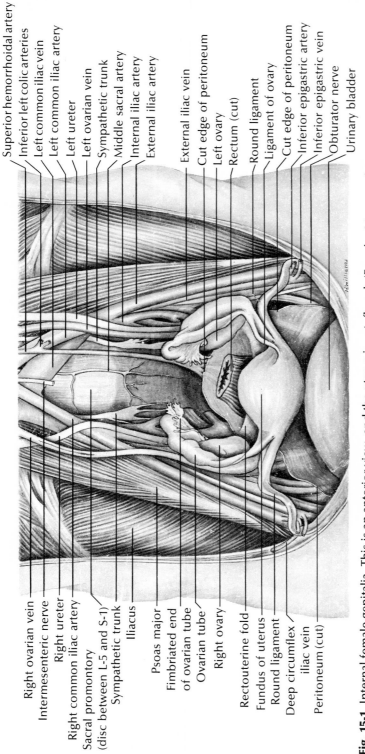

Superior hemorrhoidal artery
Inferior left colic arteries
Left common iliac vein
Left common iliac artery
Left ureter
Left ovarian vein
Sympathetic trunk
Middle sacral artery
Internal iliac artery
External iliac artery

External iliac vein
Cut edge of peritoneum
Left ovary
Rectum (cut)
Round ligament
Ligament of ovary
Cut edge of peritoneum
Inferior epigastric artery
Inferior epigastric vein
Obturator nerve
Urinary bladder

Right ovarian vein
Intermesenteric nerve
Right ureter
Right common iliac artery
Sacral promontory
(disc between L-5 and S-1)
Sympathetic trunk
Iliacus

Psoas major
Fimbriated end
of ovarian tube
Ovarian tube
Right ovary

Rectouterine fold
Fundus of uterus
Round ligament
Deep circumflex
iliac vein
Peritoneum (cut)

Fig. 15-1. Internal female genitalia. This is an anterior view, and the uterus is anteflexed. (Female, 31 years of age.)

429

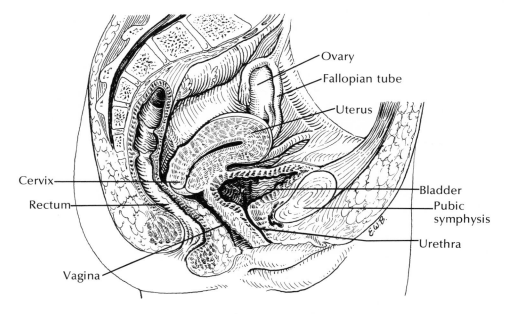

Fig. 15-2. Diagram of female genital organs. (Adapted from Schottelius, B. A., and Schottelius, D. D.: Textbook of physiology, ed. 17, St. Louis, 1973, The C. V. Mosby Co.)

The remaining cells collect into a mass, forming a thickening of one area of the wall. Such a structure is known as an ovarian (graafian) follicle. One of the cells of the inner mass is destined to become the ovum. When the ovum is ripe, the follicle ruptures and the ovum escapes from the ovary into the peritoneal cavity, from which it is picked up by the trumpet-shaped termination of the uterine tube.

The ruptured follicle collapses, and the cavity becomes filled with a yellow-colored material and is known as a corpus luteum (yellow body). If a pregnancy occurs, the corpus luteum becomes larger during the pregnancy. Ultimately a corpus luteum becomes smaller, loses its color and becomes a corpus albicans (white body), and finally disappears. In a young woman the ovary is smooth, but in old age it becomes shrunken and wrinkled.

The ovarian arteries are a pair of long, slender vessels arising from the anterior aspect of the aorta just inferior to the level of origin of the renal arteries. They pass inferiorly, posterior to the peritoneum, through the infundibulopelvic ligament, and into the ovary between the folds of the mesovarium, where they anastomose with branches of the uterine artery. Each ovarian artery is accompanied by a plexus of veins, which on the left side empties into the left renal vein and on the

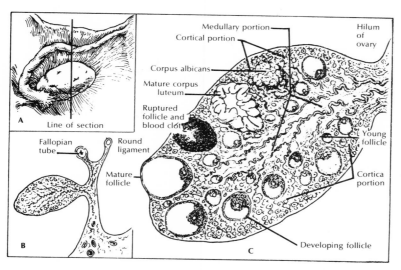

Fig. 15-3. Ovarian structures and relations. **A,** Surface relations of ovary, tube, and round ligament and the line of section for **B. B,** Attachment of the ovary to the broad ligament at the hilus and, incidentally, the relative locations of the tube and round ligament. **C,** Diagrammatic representation of the details of ovarian structure. The blood vessels, lymphatics, and nerves enter at the hilus and, with their connective tissue supports, extend through the center of the ovary, forming the medullary portion. From this central location, nutrition, drainage, and nerve control are supplied to the cortical portion, which is the special functioning part of the ovary. (From Crossen, R. J.: Diseases of women, St. Louis, The C. V. Mosby Co.)

right into the inferior vena cava. The ovarian nerves contain sensory fibers and filaments of the thoracolumbar outflow that accompany the arteries and pass through the aortic and renal plexuses. These vasomotor nerve fibers go to the blood vessels of the ovary. There is no known parasympathetic supply to the ovary.

The ovary is also classified as an endocrine gland (see discussion in Chapter 8).

The uterine tube, fallopian tube, or oviduct is the passage by which the ovum travels from the ovary to the cavity of the uterus. It is about 10 cm long and is attached to the broad ligament of the uterus by a fold of peritoneum, the mesosalpinx. The end of the tube near the ovary has a trumpet-shaped opening with a fringelike border. This opening with its fringe of fingerlike processes, or fimbriae, overhangs the ovary but is not usually directly connected with it.

The uterine tube has the following coats:

1. A tunica mucosa continuous with the inner coat of the uterus,

UTERINE TUBE

431

but having many complex longitudinal folds, or plicae, the epithelium being columnar and in some areas ciliated

2. A tela submucosa of connective tissue
3. A tunica muscularis of two strata of smooth muscle (poorly separated from each other), one longitudinal and one circular in arrangement, the longitudinal fibers being outside the circular
4. An outer tunica serosa covered with peritoneum

The uterine tube is supplied by arterial branches from the uterine and ovarian arteries, and nerve fibers come from the branches that supply the ovary. The venous drainage is into uterine and ovarian veins.

The uterine tube becomes narrower as it nears the uterus; it is about 1 mm in diameter where it passes through the uterine wall. The ovum is fertilized in the uterine tube and passes into the uterus, where it is implanted in the uterine wall. If the fertilized ovum is unusually large or if the medial end of the tube is constricted, the ovum may become implanted in the tube and a tubal pregnancy results.

UTERUS   The uterus is a thick-walled, muscular organ in the anterior part of the pelvic cavity, lying between the bladder anteriorly and the rectum posteriorly. It is a pear-shaped organ about 7.5 cm long, 5 cm wide, and 2.5 cm thick in a nonpregnant adult woman. For descriptive purposes it is divided into four parts. The inferior one third consists of the cervix, or neck, and the isthmus. The cervix is the portion passing through the pelvic floor and extending into the vagina. The isthmus is a constricted portion superior to the cervix and is called the lower uterine segment by obstetricians. The superior two thirds of the uterus consists of the corpus, or body, and the fundus. The fundus is the dome-shaped portion extending above the place of attachment of the uterine tubes. The cavity of the uterus is quite small; its outline is triangular with the base superior. The uterine tubes open into each angle of the base. The inferior end, or apex, of the uterine cavity opens through the cervix into the vagina. This opening is called the os, or mouth, of the uterus (Fig. 15-4).

Usually the long axis of the uterus points anteriorly and superiorly in the anteverted position, and the body of the uterus is slightly bent on the cervix, producing anteflexion. Often the fundus lies a little to one side of the midline, usually toward the right.

The uterus, however, is not fixed in one position but can be moved easily in all directions. It is pressed posteriorly in the pelvis by an enlarging bladder and anteriorly when the upper part of the rectum is distended. The uterus, therefore, possesses normally a considerable range

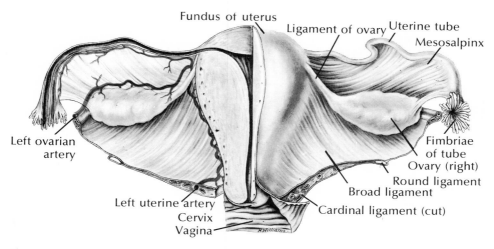

Fundus of uterus
Ligament of ovary
Uterine tube
Mesosalpinx
Left ovarian artery
Fimbriae of tube
Ovary (right)
Round ligament
Broad ligament
Left uterine artery
Cervix
Vagina
Cardinal ligament (cut)

Fig. 15-4. Posterior view of uterus and associated structures. On the left side of the drawing the posterior portion of the uterus has been removed to show the cavity, and the left uterine tube has been opened longitudinally.

of mobility, and only when found beyond the normal range can the uterus be said to be misplaced. Posterior placement of the uterus occurs in two forms, retroversion and retroflexion. In retroversion the body of the uterus is tilted posteriorly and the cervix points anteriorly. In retroflexion the body of the uterus is bent posteriorly with little or no change in the position of the cervix. Seldom does such malposition cause symptoms or interfere with conception.

Prolapse of the uterus is a condition in which the uterus sinks decidedly below its normal level in the pelvis, a condition referred to as "falling of the womb."

The cervix of the uterus is surrounded by the visceral fascia of the pelvis, but the corpus and fundus are clothed anteriorly and posteriorly by visceral peritoneum, continuous on each side with the broad ligament, which attaches the uterus to the sides of the pelvic cavity. The uterine artery, a branch of the internal iliac artery, passes through the base of the broad ligament to be distributed throughout the uterine wall. Within a fold of the broad ligament is a flattened band of fibromuscular tissue, the round ligament of the uterus, which passes from the uterus through the anterior abdominal wall by way of the inguinal canal to terminate in the labium majus. Occasionally an outpouching of the parietal peritoneum accompanies the round ligament through the inguinal canal as the canal of Nuck and may be the site of an inguinal hernia (Fig. 15-1).

The superior portion of the broad ligament has a covering of vis-

433

ceral peritoneum on either side, with some areolar connective tissue between. In the inferior portion of the ligament surrounding the uterine artery and veins, the connective tissue gradually increases in amount. At the base of the broad ligament is a strong, dense mass of connective tissue, called the cardinal, or lateral uterosacral, ligament, which runs on either side from the cervix of the uterus to the wall of pelvic cavity. There is also a heavy band of connective tissue running posteriorly on either side of the midline, from the cervix to the sacrum, called the (posterior) uterosacral ligament. The cardinal and uterosacral ligaments have some smooth-muscle fibers in addition to the connective tissue and are very important supports for the uterus and adjacent structures.

The uterine wall has three layers (Fig. 15-5):

1. An inner tunica mucosa (frequently called the endometrium) having columnar epithelium (some ciliated) and tubular glands and becoming, at the cervix, continuous with the stratified squamous epithelium of the vagina

2. A tunica muscularis (frequently called the myometrium) a thick

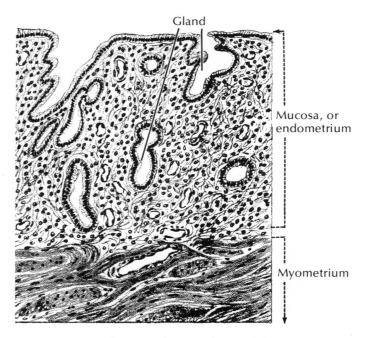

Gland

Mucosa, or endometrium

Myometrium

Fig. 15-5. Mucosa and part of muscularis of human uterus. (From Bevelander, G., and Ramaley, J. A.: Essentials of histology, ed. 7, St. Louis, 1974, The C. V. Mosby Co.)

layer of interlacing bands of smooth muscle with fibers running longitudinally, circularly, and diagonally

3. A tunica serosa covered with visceral peritoneum

During pregnancy the uterus greatly increases in size. Not only does the cavity enlarge, but the muscular walls also become much thicker. After delivery the uterus shrinks rapidly and under normal conditions should reach its nonpregnant size in six weeks. The mucous membrane of the uterus becomes thicker and more vascular during pregnancy, and it is into this layer that the placenta is implanted.

The mucous membrane also thickens and becomes more vascular before menstruation. During menstruation the surface layers are shed, but these are quickly regenerated at the end of menstruation.

The uterus receives fibers from the hypogastric plexus (thoracolumbar autonomic outflow) and from the sacral nerves (sacral autonomic outflow). Sensory fibers go mainly to the ninth through the twelfth thoracic segments of the spinal cord; however, fibers concerned with pain from the cervix apparently run into the sacral portion of the cord.

Pregnancy, which normally occurs in the uterus, may occur at other sites, a condition known as ectopic gestation. It is usually extrauterine and most commonly tubal. Other ectopic sites include (1) the ovary, (2) the abdominal cavity, (3) the cervix uteri.

VAGINA

The vagina is a passage connecting the cervix of the uterus with the vestibule of the vagina. It lies anterior to the rectum and posterior to the urethra and bladder and is about 7.5 cm long. Because the anterior and posterior walls lie in contact with each other, the cavity is reduced to a narrow cleft capable of great distention in childbirth (Fig. 15-2).

Since the cervix projects into the vagina from above, the posterior wall of the vagina is longer than the anterior, and on either side of the cervix is a recess, called the lateral fornix. The upper part of the posterior wall of the vagina is in contact with the peritoneum, which forms a pouch posterior to the uterus and anterior to the rectum, the rectouterine pouch (pouch of Douglas). Infections of this region may be drained by the surgeon, making an incision upward from the vagina. An abdominal ectopic pregnancy usually occurs in the rectouterine pouch.

In the perineum, between the vestibule and rectum, is a fibromuscular mass, called the perineal body, or gynecologic perineum (see Fig. 5-48). Numerous perineal muscles find attachment at this point; these form a sphincter for the vestibule. In childbirth this mass may be weakened or even extensively torn. Episiotomy is an incision designed

435

to substitute a clean cut for a ragged tear. A median episiotomy, the one most commonly used, is made along the perineal raphe to within 1.5 cm of the anus, an area that is easily and accurately repaired. The scar tissue resulting from the healing of this wound is not elastic, and thus the circumference of the vulva may be increased. Using the operation called perineorrhaphy, a surgeon seeks to reconstruct the perineal body.

The wall of the vagina has an inner lining of stratified squamous epithelium, a muscular layer of interlacing longitudinal and circular smooth-muscle bundles, and an outer connective tissue layer that blends with that of surrounding structures. The wall of the vagina usually possesses many folds. Near the outlet there is a striate sphincter (the bulbospongiosus muscle).

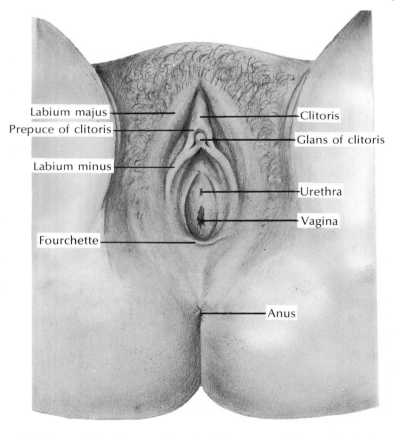

Fig. 15-6. External female genitalia. The labia majora have been parted to show deeper structures.

The labia majora are a pair of rounded folds of skin lying on each side of the vestibule and continuous with each other anteriorly through the mons pubis (Fig. 15-6). The mons is an elevation of the lower portion of the abdomen over the symphysis pubis caused by an accumulation of adipose tissue in the subcutaneous fascia. This fatty tissue is prolonged as a fingerlike projection into each labium majus. The skin of the labia majora and mons is covered by hair after adolescence.

The labia minora are a pair of smaller folds of skin lying on each side within the labia majora. Anteriorly, the lesser labia are continuous with the prepuce, or fold of skin covering the glans of the clitoris. The skin of the labia minora is smooth and hairless; it is continuous with the mucous membrane lining of the vagina. The labia minora have a central core of connective tissue but contain no fat.

The vestibule of the vagina is the space between the labia minora and inferior to the clitoris. It contains the openings of the urethra, vagina, and ducts of the vestibular glands. The labia minora are connected behind by a thin shelf of tissue, called the fourchette, a structure that is destroyed by the first parturition.

The clitoris is a C-shaped cylindrical mass composed of two small cylinders of erectile tissue placed side by side, the corpora cavernosa clitoridis. Posteriorly the two corpora diverge, forming the crura of the clitoris, and each is attached to the pubic arch. The clitoris is attached by means of a suspensory ligament to the anterior aspect of the symphysis pubis. The glans is a small mass of erectile tissue capping the free ends of the corpora cavernosa. The erectile tissue of the glans is continuous on the inferior aspect of the corpora cavernosa with a bilateral mass of erectile tissue, the bulb, in the walls of the vestibule. The clitoris, unlike the penis of the male, is not traversed by the urethra.

The greater vestibular glands, or glands of Bartholin, lie one on each side of the vestibule posterior to the bulb. They open into the vestibule between the fold of the labium minus and the hymen. The lesser vestibular glands are microscopic mucous glands emptying into the anterior part of the vestibule.

Contraception, the prevention of conception, or impregnation, short of abstinence during the expected time of ovulation (rhythm), is most effective with the following methods: (1) vaginal diaphragm, (2) oral medication to inhibit ovulation, and (3) intrauterine devices (IUD) to prevent implantation of the conceptus.

A diaphragm prevents the deposition of the ejaculate into the cervical canal, thus prohibiting sperm and seminal fluid from entering the uterus. Oral contraception utilizes the low-cost availability of progesterone and estrogen, since the appropriate combination of these two hormones inhibits ovulation, thereby preventing both tubal or intrauterine pregnancies. Intrauterine devices, placed in the uterus, apparently mobilize a leukocyte reaction with the macrophages destroying sperm and possibly acting on the blastocyst. With IUDs in place, only a very few intrauterine pregnancies (approximately 2%) have occurred; however, tubal pregnancies, although uncommon, can still occur. As an emergency type of treatment, postcoital contraception with diethylstilbestrol within 72 hours of sexual intercourse has proven to be effective in preventing pregnancy.

REVIEW QUESTIONS

1. What structures are included in the female reproductive system?
2. Where do the ovarian arteries arise?
3. Where do the ovarian veins drain?
4. Describe the uterine tube.
5. Describe the layers of the wall of the uterus.
6. In the base of the broad ligament what is the relation of the ureter to the uterine artery?
7. Where does fertilization of the ovum occur normally?
8. Where are the cardinal ligaments located?
9. Describe the clitoris.
10. How do the labia majora and labia minora differ?
11. What is the function of the cardinal ligament?
12. Describe the nerve supply to the ovary.
13. Where is the ovary located?
14. What is the mesovarium?
15. What is the mesosalpinx?
16. Discuss malposition of the uterus.
17. Describe three methods of contraception.
18. Discuss ectopic pregnancy.

CHAPTER 16

THE MALE
REPRODUCTIVE SYSTEM

The male reproductive system includes the testes with their ducts, the epididymis and ductus deferens, the scrotum, the penis, the prostate gland, the bulbourethral glands, and the urethra (Fig. 16-1).

The testis, or testicle, the male reproductive gland, is an oval organ about 5 cm long. The epididymis, which is the first part of the duct to the testis, is a convoluted tube massed into a comma-shaped structure attached to the posterior aspect of the testis. The duct emerges from the epididymis as the ductus deferens.

TESTIS

The testis has an outer coat, the tunica albuginea, composed of dense, white fibrous tissue, from the inner surface of which fibrous septa pass deep into the substance of the gland, separating it into wedge-shaped lobules. The septa end posteriorly in a mass of fibrous tissue, called the mediastinum testis. The arteries, veins, nerves, and lymph vessels pass through this mass to supply the testis.

The fibrous structures just described form the framework of the testis; interspersed among them is the parenchyma of the testis. The parenchyma is composed of very numerous, small coiled seminiferous tubules that look like fine threads. The germinal epithelium lining these seminiferous tubules produces the spermatozoa, or male reproductive cells.

The seminiferous tubules empty their reproductive cells into other tubules in the mediastinum testis, which form the rete testis. The epididymis is composed of closely coiled tubules that receive the repro-

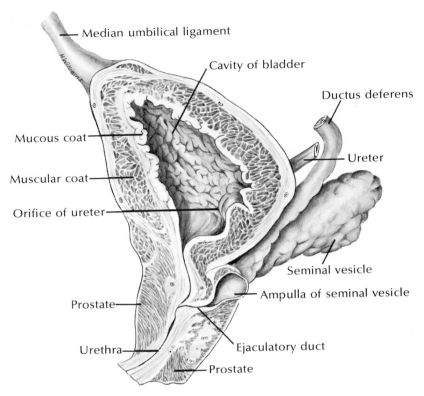

Fig. 16-1. Sagittal section through male bladder and prostatic urethra. The left half has been removed.

ductive cells from the rete testis and after a very tortuous passage empty them into the ductus deferens of the spermatic cord.

The arteries supplying the testes arise from the abdominal aorta. The vein of the right testis drains into the inferior vena cava, and that of the left testis drains into the left renal vein. The lymphatics of the testes drain into lymph nodes around the aorta. These vessels accompany the ductus deferens in the spermatic cord. The vascular and nerve supplies of the testes are entirely independent of that of the scrotum. The blood vessels of the testes receive vasomotor fibers from the thoracolumbar outflow. There is no known parasympathetic nerve supply to the testes. Visceral sensory fibers accompany the thoracolumbar fibers.

Early in fetal life there is an evagination of a tube of peritoneum through each inguinal canal into the scrotum, called the vaginal process of the peritoneum. Each testis and associated epididymis originally lie posterior to the parietal peritoneal coat of the abdominal

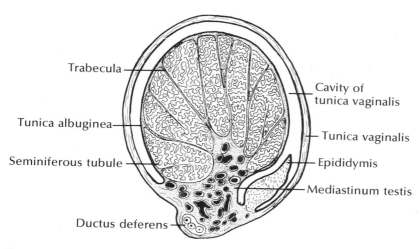

Fig. 16-2. Transverse section of testis and epididymis.

cavity. Late in fetal life the testes descend posterior to the peritoneum and pass into the scrotum. Then the vaginal process disappears except for the portion adjacent to the testis. This portion is called the tunica vaginalis of the testis; it is lined with serous membrane and has a parietal and a visceral layer. If this closed sac is distended with fluid, it is called a hydrocele. Occasionally the vaginal process persists, and it may be the site of an inguinal hernia. The vaginal process is also present in women, but it usually disappears entirely.

The three coverings received by the testis as it passes into the scrotum from the inguinal canal are discussed under inguinal canal in Chapter 5 (see Fig. 5-46).

The ductus deferens (vas deferens) is about 45 cm long. It passes from the inferior end of the epididymis superiorly within the spermatic cord through the inguinal canal into the abdominal cavity. It lies just outside the parietal peritoneum, passes over the pelvic brim into the pelvic cavity, and continues its course posterior to the bladder. Here the end of the duct dilates to form the ampulla and joins the duct of the seminal vesicle to form the ejaculatory duct. The ductus deferens has an inner mucous coat, a middle muscular coat, and an outer fibrous coat. It can be palpated within the spermatic cord as a firm, slender cord about as thick as the lead of a pencil.

The seminal vesicles are a pair of convoluted tubes partly covered by peritoneum and lying posterior to the bladder. One end empties into the ejaculatory duct and the other terminates as a blind pouch. The

**DUCTUS
DEFERENS AND
SEMINAL VESICLE**

441

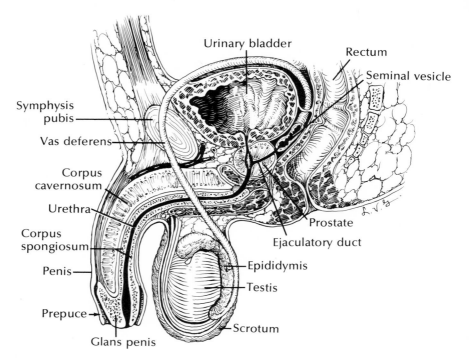

Fig. 16-3. Illustration of male genital organs. (From Schottelius, B. A., and Schottelius, D. D.: Textbook of physiology, ed. 17, St. Louis, 1973, The C. V. Mosby Co.)

seminal vesicles secrete a fluid that bathes the spermatozoa passing through the ductus deferens. To this is added the secretion of the prostate, and thus the seminal fluid is formed.

The ejaculatory duct is a slender tube about 2.5 cm long passing through the substance of the prostate to open into the urethra close to the orifices of the prostatic ducts.

The spermatic cord is composed of the ductus deferens and the testicular vessels and nerves surrounded by connective tissue. The veins from the testes are numerous and form the pampiniform plexus. If these veins become dilated, a condition known as varicocele results. The veins of each plexus ultimately unite to form a single testicular vein.

SCROTUM   The scrotum is a sac composed of skin and subcutaneous tissue. The skin is more heavily pigmented than that covering the general body surface and after adolescence is covered with hair. The subcutaneous tissue contains no fat but does contain scattered fibers of smooth muscle, the dartos muscle innervated by the genitofemoral nerve.

442

When its fibers are contracted, the walls of the scrotum are wrinkled, and the testes are held close up to the perineum. When the fibers are relaxed, the scrotum is pendulous and the wrinkles disappear. The left testis usually hangs lower than the right.

There is a ridge on the surface of the midline of the scrotum, called the raphe, which is continued anteriorly on the inferior surface of the penis and posteriorly toward the anus. The scrotum is incompletely divided by a median septum into two cavities, one for each testis.

The scrotal arteries are branches of the pudendal vessels, which supply the perineum, and the sensory nerves come from the pudendal nerves. The lymphatics drain into the inguinal nodes, and the veins drain into vessels accompanying the pudendal arteries. The scrotum may be injured or infected without involvement of the testis.

PENIS

The penis is composed of three columns of erectile tissue surrounded by skin and a thin layer of subcutaneous tissue. The skin of the penis, like that of the scrotum, is more pigmented than the skin of the body but is free of hair except near the root. The subcutaneous tissue contains no fat and attaches the skin loosely to the underlying structures. At the distal end the skin forms a free fold, the preputium, prepuce, or foreskin, that contains a sphincter similar to the dartos muscle of the scrotum. The lining of the prepuce is continued over the glans in intimate union with the substance of the glans.

The corpora cavernosa penis are two fused cylinders of erectile tissue forming the bulk of the shaft of the penis. The line of fusion is marked by a median septum and on the dorsal surface by a groove. The suspensory ligament of the penis extends from the loose fibrous tissue of the penis to the symphysis of the pubis. Posteriorly, the corpora cavernosa penis diverge as the crura of the penis, and each crus is attached to the pubic arch.

The corpus spongiosum penis (corpus cavernosum urethrae) is a cylinder of erectile tissue softer in consistency than the corpus cavernosum penis. At the distal end it is enlarged to form the glans, which caps the ends of the corpora cavernosa penis. Posteriorly, it is also enlarged to form the bulb of the urethra, which lies in the midline between the two diverging corpora cavernosa penis. The urethra enters the bulb and traverses the entire length of the corpus spongiosum penis, ending in the glans.

Each corpus cavernosum penis has an outer covering, the tunica albuginea, formed of dense fibrous connective tissue. The erectile tissue is a spongelike mass of blood sinuses lined with endothelium. The corpus spongiosum penis has a less strong outer coat (Fig. 16-4).

The arteries of the penis, which are branches of the internal pu-

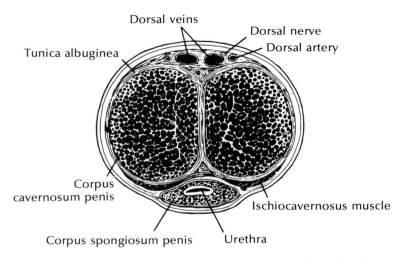

Dorsal veins

Dorsal nerve

Dorsal artery

Tunica albuginea

Corpus
cavernosum penis

Ischiocavernosus muscle

Corpus spongiosum penis   Urethra

Fig. 16-4. Cross section of shaft of penis. This specimen has a double dorsal vein. A single vein is more common.

dendal artery, are (1) the deep artery of the penis to the corpora cavernosa penis, (2) the artery of the bulb to the corpus spongiosum penis, and (3) the dorsal artery of the penis to the tunica albuginea and to the glans. The veins drain into the venous plexus on either side of the prostate gland, and the lymphatics drain into the superficial inguinal nodes.

The nerves come from the second, third, and fourth sacral nerves (sacral autonomic outflow) and from the lower part of the hypogastric plexus (thoracolumbar autonomic outflow). Sensory impulses go to the sacral segments of the cord.

PROSTATE GLAND

The prostate gland lies between the bladder and the rectum, surrounding the first part of the urethra. Superiorly, it is covered by the wall of the bladder; on each side is a rich plexus of veins coming from the penis, and inferiorly, it is supported by the pelvic fascia. The capsule of the prostate is poorly defined, but there is an interlacing structure of connective tissue and smooth muscle on the surface of the gland, which sends septa deep into the substance. Glandular epithelium is found in the lobules between the septa. The secretion of the prostate is emptied by a number of small ducts into the prostatic urethra.

Frequently in older men the prostate enlarges. The portion that lies between the ejaculatory ducts may form a projecting tongue more or less completely blocking the urethra like a ball valve.

444

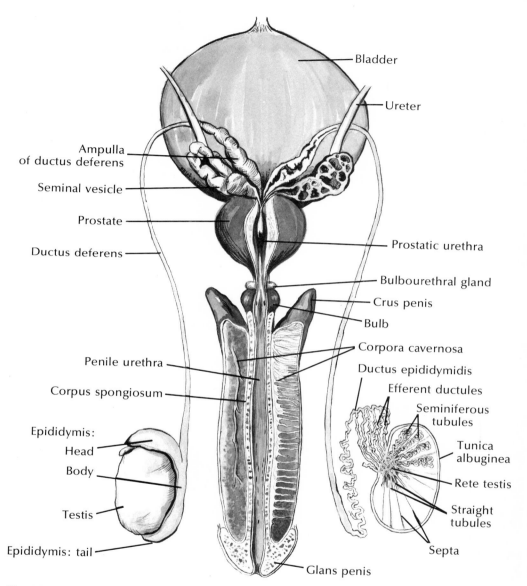

Fig. 16-5. Diagrammatic representation of the major parts of the male reproductive organs, as seen posteriorly. The structures covering the urethra
posteriorly have been removed. The seminal colliculus, representing the
termination of the ejaculatory ducts, has been detached from the posterior
wall and is left hanging in the prostatic urethra. Each of the corpora cavernosa has been sectioned longitudinally, as has the corpus spongiosum. The
openings of the bulbourethral glands are shown lateral to their actual position in the floor of the bulbar urethra. (From DiDio, L. J. A.: Synopsis of
anatomy, St. Louis, 1970, The C. V. Mosby Co.)

A sheath of fibrous tissue formed from the visceral pelvic fascia surrounds the prostate. From this sheath the prostate can be shelled out in the operation of prostatectomy.

BULBOURETHRAL GLANDS

The bulbourethral, or Cowper's, glands are a pair of small glands about the size of a pea, placed one on each of the membranous portion of the urethra, just posterior to the bulb. Each empties by a single duct into the third part of the urethra just beyond the bulb.

URETHRA

The urethra is a tube that extends from the bladder to the exterior.

The male urethra extends from the neck of the bladder to the external urethral orifice and serves as a passageway for urine and semen. It can be divided into three parts: prostatic, membranous, and penile (Fig. 16-5). The prostatic portion, running through the prostate gland, receives the openings of the ejaculatory ducts. The membranous portion passes through the urogenital diaphragm, and the penile portion traverses the length of the corpus spongiosum.

The female urethra extends from the neck of the bladder to the external urethral orifice and corresponds to the prostatic and membranous portions of the male urethra.

ERECTION AND EJACULATION

In response to psychic or physical stimuli or both, efferent impulses from the sacral outflow (parasympathetic) cause relaxation and subsequent enlargement of the arteries supplying the penis. The increased blood supply engorges the cavernous tissue, which in turn squeezes the deep dorsal vein(s) against the deep fascia of the penis. Venous return from the erectile tissue is therefore reduced and erection occurs.

Ejaculation, which is the release of semen containing the male reproductive cells, is under the control of the thoracolumbar outflow (sympathetic) division of the autonomic nervous system. Approximately 3.5 ml of semen, or seminal fluid, is expelled per orgasm. Semen consists of the following: (1) sperm (350 million per ejaculate) and fluid secreted by the testes and epididymides, which constitute 5% of the total fluid volume, (2) fluid secreted by the seminal vesicles, 30% of the total fluid volume, (3) fluid secreted by the prostate gland, 60% of the total fluid volume, and (4) fluid secreted by the bulbourethral glands, 5% of the total fluid volume. The seminal fluid not only acts as a carrying medium but also activates the sperm, which until release are nonmotile. Sperm are stored only in the epididymides and once released are passed via rhythmic muscular contractions of the ductus deferens to the prostatic urethra.

VASECTOMY

Vasectomy, the excision of a segment of the vas deferens, is a relatively recent addition to the methods of achieving birth control. With this method, sperm produced in the testes, cannot be conveyed to the outside.

REVIEW QUESTIONS

1. What structures are included in the male reproductive system?
2. Where do the testicular arteries arise?
3. Where do the testicular veins drain?
4. What is the function of the seminiferous tubules?
5. What is the function of the seminal vesicles?
6. Describe the penis.
7. What is the function of the prostate gland?
8. What is the dartos muscle?
9. What is the vaginal process of the peritoneum? In the male adult, what portion persists?
10. Trace the path of a spermatozoon from the seminiferous tubule to the urethra.
11. Discuss the mechanism of erection and ejaculation.

CHAPTER 17

SURFACE ANATOMY

I t is the purpose of this chapter to discuss the more prominent surface features of the regions of the body and to emphasize the large
number of structures that may be identified by palpation through the
skin.

HEAD   Just anterior to the auricle, the pulsation of the superficial temporal artery is felt. The anesthetist frequently uses this vessel in taking
the pulse. The frontal branch of the temporal artery often stands out
as a tortuous ridge that, in elderly people, runs over the temple. Along
the inferior border of the mandible, about one third of the way forward
from the angle, the facial artery may be felt passing over the bone to
reach the cheek.

If the teeth are firmly clenched, the temporal muscle may be ob-
served as a bulging in the temple, and the masseter, as a bulging
near the angle of the lower jaw. The mandibular contour is easily
felt through the skin. The zygomatic arch, a bridge of bone forming
the framework of the cheek, may be palpated along its entire length
from a point just anterior to the ear to a point on the side of the face
inferior to the eye. About one fingerbreadth below this arch and parallel
to it, the duct of the parotid gland passes anteriorly on the surface of
the masseter muscle and may be rolled under the finger.

If one places a finger just anterior to the opening of the external
ear, the condyle of the mandible can be felt sliding posteriorly and
anteriorly in movements of the lower jaw.

Posterior to the ear a lymph node of the retroauricular group may
be identified as it lies on the mastoid process. In infections of the scalp

448

this node becomes enlarged and tender. The submandibular (sub-maxillary) lymph nodes can be felt along the inferior border of the mandible and are usually enlarged and tender in upper respiratory infections.

On each side of the larynx the pulsations of the common carotid artery can be both felt and seen. If the collar is too tight or muscular effort is considerable, the veins of the neck, paritcularly the external jugular, become large and obvious.

Muscular resistance to the pressure of a hand under the chin brings into prominence the entire length of the sternocleidomastoid muscles, which can then be palpated from origin to insertion. The suprasternal or jugular notch is the small hollow in the midline just superior to the sternum and between the medial ends of the clavicles (see Fig. 5-3).

The most prominent structure in the midline of the neck is the anterior margin of the thyroid cartilage, or the Adam's apple, which is larger in men than in women. Superiorly the hyoid bone can be traced posteriorly to each end, or greater cornu. Inferior to the thyroid cartilage the anterior band of the cricoid cartilage can be felt and inferior to that the upper rings of the trachea, or windpipe. Frequently the isthmus of the thyroid gland can be felt crossing the trachea. If the gland is enlarged, it bulges anteriorly in the inferior part of the neck.

Between the muscular columns at the back of the neck the external occipital protuberance of the skull is easily located. In the midline inferiorly, and sunk between the columns, is the ligamentum nuchae, passing inferiorly to the spine of the seventh cervical vertebra, the bony prominence at the base of the neck. The prominence below is that of the spine of the first thoracic vertebra. The spines of the lower thoracic and of the lumbar vertebrae are less easily felt.

The muscle mass forming the lateral portion of the posterior aspect of the neck and extending inferiorly and laterally from the skull to the shoulder is due largely to the trapezius muscle. "Stiff neck" is usually an inflammation of this muscle (see Fig. 17-2).

A finger tracing laterally the subcutaneous superior border of the clavicle will encounter the acromioclavicular joint as a slight elevation at the lateral end of the clavicle. About one fingerbreadth beyond this is the lateral border of the acromion, which forms the tip of the shoulder Just inferior to the acromion the greater tubercle of the humerus can be felt moving beneath the overhanging acromion when the arm is rotated medially or laterally. If the finger is placed near the lateral end of the clavicle and then brought straight downward for about 2.5 cm, the tip of the coracoid process may be felt in the groove

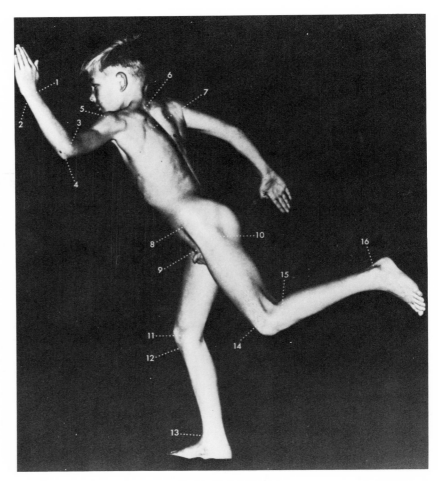

Fig. 17-1. Numbers indicate some of the most common visible and palpable bony landmarks. The approximate corresponding locations are marked on skeleton on opposite page. (From Royce, J.: Surface anatomy, Philadelphia, 1971, F. A. Davis Company.)

1. Styloid process (radius)
2. Styloid process (ulna)
3. Epicondylus lateralis humeri
4. Olecranon (ulna)
5. Acromion (scapula)
6. Spinal process (seventh cervical)
7. Medial border of scapula
8. Crista iliaca anterior superior

9. Pubic arch
10. Greater trochanter
11. Epicondylus medialis femoris
12. Tuberositas tibiae
13. Medial malleolus
14. Epicondylus lateralis femoris
15. Head of fibula
16. Lateral malleolus

between the deltoid and pectoralis major muscles. The entire margin of the acromion and the spine of the scapula are subcutaneous. The medial (vertebral) border of the scapula is palpable, but the superior and lateral (axillary) borders are covered by muscles (Fig. 17-2).

ARM

The bulging belly of the biceps brachii muscle, a flexor and supinator of the forearm, is evident on the anterior part of the upper arm when the elbow is flexed with the palm upward. On the lateral side of the arm the deltoid muscle is readily traced to its insertion on the humerus. When a thin, muscular person contracts a deltoid muscle, the component muscle bundles and the intervening septa of fascia are clearly visible. Just below this it is possible to feel the radial nerve as it passes around the humerus in the radial groove. On the medial side of the arm there is a shallow groove just posterior to the biceps muscle. Along this groove the brachial artery may be felt as it passes inferiorly toward the cubital fossa. This groove is the place to apply pressure in case of severe arterial hemorrhage in the forearm or hand.

At the elbow three bony prominences should be located: the medial and lateral epicondyles of the humerus and the olecranon of the ulna.

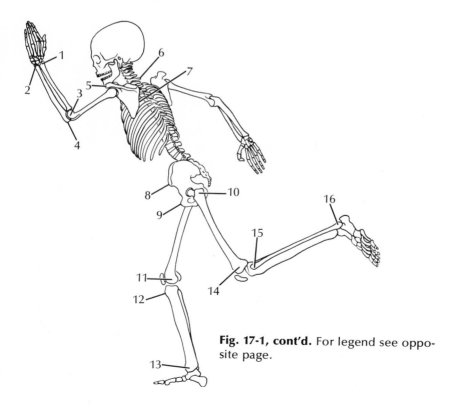

Fig. 17-1, cont'd. For legend see opposite page.

451

When the elbow is extended, these three lie in a horizontal line; when the elbow is flexed, they form the points of a triangle. The ulnar nerve can be felt in the groove posterior to the medial epicondyle. It is the so-called "crazy bone" or "funny bone" of the elbow.

When the elbow is extended, pressure in the dimple posterior and inferior to the lateral epicondyle reveals two bony parts. The proximal one is the distal portion of the lateral epicondyle of the humerus, and the other is the head of the radius. If one presses gently on the head

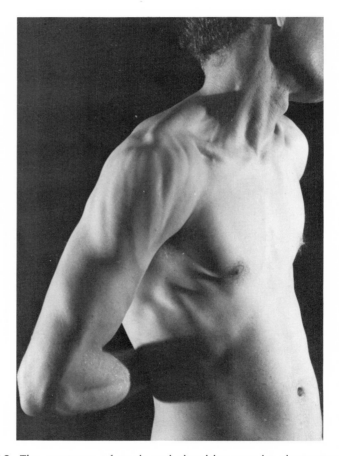

Fig. 17-2. The contours of neck and shoulder may be demonstrated by hooking the fingers of both hands behind the back and pulling against each other. With the head turned sideways and the shoulders pushed downwards many muscles can be tensed so as to become clearly visible. The deltoid shows its many distinctive strands. (From Royce, J.: Surface anatomy, Philadelphia, 1971, F. A. Davis Company.)

of the radius and then slowly supinates and pronates the forearm, the head of the radius may be felt turning beneath the skin.

On the anterior aspect of the elbow the median cubital vein can be seen, except in obese persons, and usually the superficial veins of the forearm can be identified. The median cubital vein is the vien of the choice in transfusions and intravenous therapy (Fig. 17-4).

Numerous muscle tendons are visible at the wrist. Let us study those on the anterior aspect of the wrist, starting on the radial, or thumb, side. First, palpate the inferior end of the radius. The tendon passing directly over the end (styloid) of the radius out to the base of

WRIST

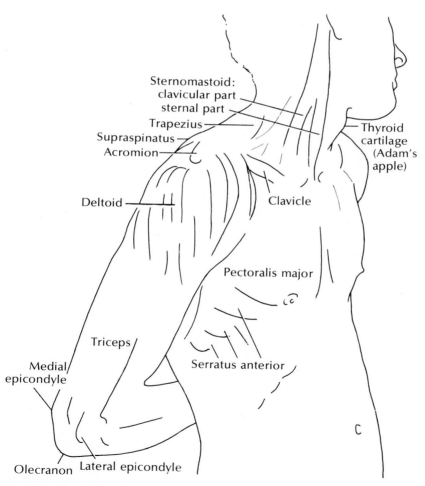

Fig. 17-2, cont'd. For legend see opposite page.

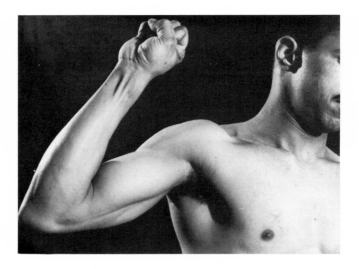

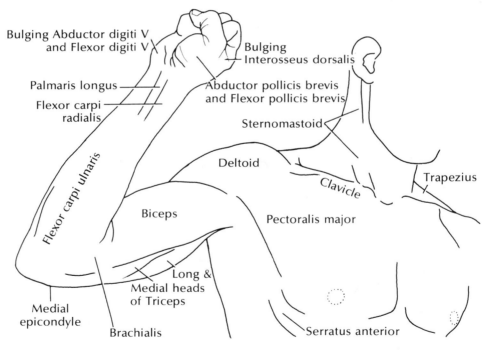

Bulging Abductor digiti V
and Flexor digiti V

Bulging
Interosseus dorsalis

Palmaris longus

Abductor pollicis brevis
and Flexor pollicis brevis

Flexor carpi
radialis

Sternomastoid

Flexor carpi ulnaris

Deltoid

Clavicle

Trapezius

Biceps

Pectoralis major

Long &
Medial heads
of Triceps

Medial
epicondyle

Brachialis

Serratus anterior

Fig. 17-3. In this subject the relationship between neck, shoulder, chest and arm muscles is clearly visible. Note the lateral end of the pectoralis major, which runs over the biceps and disappears underneath the anterior deltoid. The biceps muscle is in an elongated position since the insertion on the radius is moved away from the origin due to the pronation of the forearm (From Royce, J.: Surface anatomy, Philadelphia, 1971, F. A. Davis Company.)

454

the thumb is that of the abductor pollicis longus muscle. Let us now pass a finger across the front of the wrist toward the ulnar, or little finger, side. First is felt the radial artery as it lies on the surface of the radius. This is the artery usually used in taking the pulse. Next in order may be felt the tendons of the flexor carpi radialis and palmaris longus and, on the ulnar side, the flexor carpi ulnaris. If the tendon of the flexor carpi ulnaris is traced inferiorly, it can be followed to its insertion on the pisiform bone, a small seedlike structure in the heel of the palm. When the palm is strongly cupped, the prominent tendon in

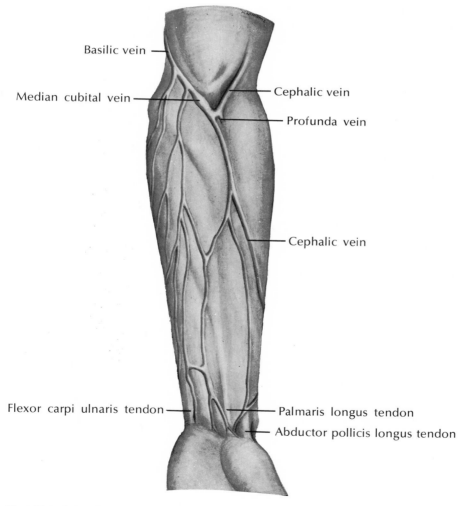

Fig. 17-4. Superficial veins of volar aspect of left forearm.

455

the middle of the wrist is that of the palmaris longus. In about one out of ten persons this muscle is absent. The tendons lying deeper than the palmaris longus belong to the flexor digitorum superficialis (sublimis). The median nerve runs parallel to, and immediately on the radial side of, the tendon of the palmaris longus. The ulnar artery and nerve lie just lateral to the tendon of the flexor carpi ulnaris, and it is often possible to feel the pulsation of the vessel in this location.

On the posterior aspect of the wrist the well-marked tendon of the extensor pollicis longus is seen passing to the distal phalanx of the thumb.

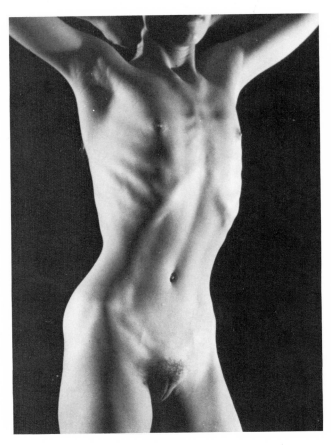

Fig. 17-5. The subject is pulling the elbows back and pressing with the hands against the neck. With a full inspiration and a controlled flattening of the abdomen the anterior trunk muscles become clearly outlined. Supporting the weight on one leg brings out the position of the gluteus medius. (From Royce, J.: Surface anatomy, Philadelphia, 1971, F. A. Davis Company.)

The pit between this tendon and that of the abductor pollicis longus is the "anatomical snuffbox." In the bottom of the pit the radial artery may be felt passing over the scaphoid bone. The artery then turns around the first metacarpal into the palm to form the deep palmar arch, through which it anastomoses with the deep branch of the ulnar artery.

The other extensor muscles are bound to the wrist by a dense fibrous band, the extensor retinaculum (dorsal carpal ligament), but on the back of the hand the tendons of the extensor digitorum communis can be seen going to the fingers.

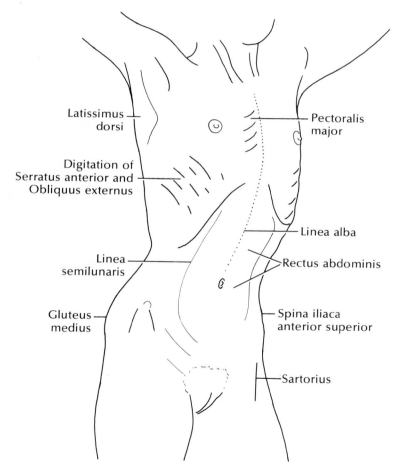

Fig. 17-5, cont'd. For legend see opposite page.

457

**THORAX AND
ABDOMEN**

Just inferior to the medial end of the clavicle the first costal cartilage can be felt as it joins the sternum. The remaining ribs and intercostal spaces can be identified except in obese persons. The apex beat of the heart is palpated usually in the fifth interspace about 8.5 cm to the left of the midline (see Fig. 9-12). Below the apex of the heart, at the costal margin, there is frequently a tympanitic area due to the presence of a bubble of gas in the cardiac portion of the stomach.

In the midline, running from the umbilicus to the symphysis pubis, is the linea alba. This is the site frequently selected by a surgeon for operations on the urinary bladder and the uterus because there are no large blood vessels or nerves to be injured in this line.

The pit of the stomach is the narrow angle between the two costal margins. The tip of the xiphoid cartilage is palpable just at the inferior end of the sternum. Sharp pressure or a blow in the pit of the stomach is very painful because it stimulates the "solar plexus," the collection of visceral nerves about the celiac artery, or the celiac plexus.

For purposes of localization a physician examining a patient may refer to certain vertical lines that are projected inferiorly from various points of the shoulder girdle, such as the midclavicular line, the anterior axillary line, the midaxillary line, and the posterior axillary line. By drawing two imaginary lines at right angles to each other through the umbilicus, the surface of the abdomen is divided into four quadrants (Fig. 17-6). A surgeon frequently refers to pain in the right upper quadrant or right lower quadrant.

By another method the abdominal region may be divided into nine areas. An imaginary horizontal line, the subcostal line, is drawn horizontally across the body at the level of the lowest point of the costal margin (usually the lower edge of the tenth costal cartilage). A second line is drawn through the anterior superior iliac spines. A curved line is drawn along the lateral border of the rectus abdominis muscle on each side. The resulting nine areas are named right hypochondriac, epigastric, left hypochondriac, right lateral, umbilical, left lateral, right inguinal, pubic (formerly hypogastric), and left inguinal (see Fig. 17-8).

The transpyloric plane is quite useful for localization. This is a horizontal plane passed through the body at a point midway between the upper margin of the sternum and the upper margin of the pubic symphysis. It passes through the pylorus of the stomach and the first lumbar vertebra.

THIGH

Except in the obese person, the iliac crest can be felt in its entire length from the anteror superior spine to the posterior superior spine. The inguinal ligament lies in the bottom of a furrow extending from

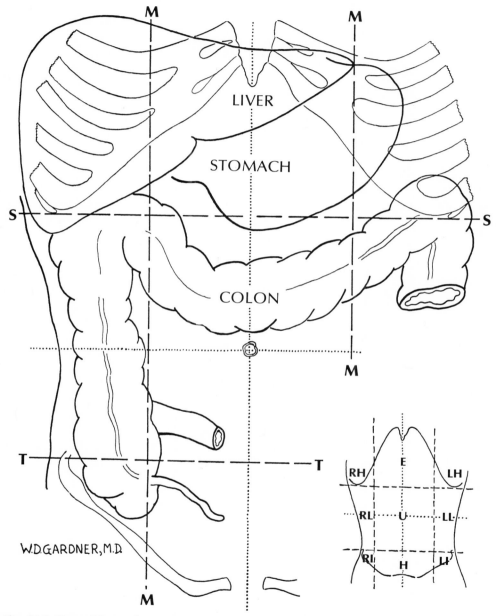

Fig. 17-6. Dotted lines indicate the four quadrants of the abdomen; broken lines indicate the nine regions of the abdomen (From Gardner, W. D.: Diagnostic anatomy, St. Louis, The C. V. Mosby Co.)

459

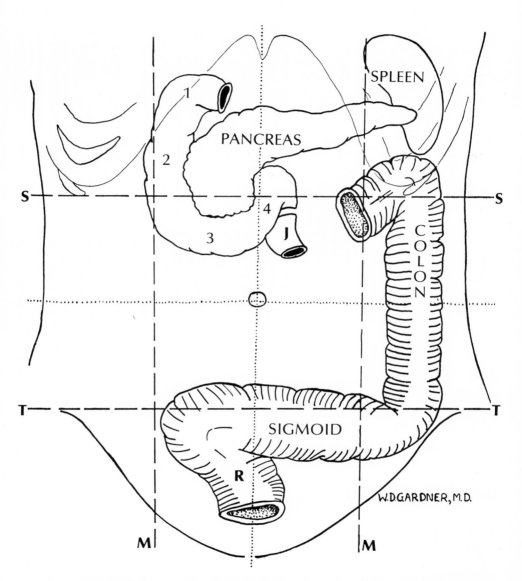

Fig. 17-7. Topographic lines and regions of the abdomen with the projection of certain organs. *M,* Midinguinal line; *S,* subcostal line; *T,* intertubercular line; *J,* jejunum; *R,* rectum. Parts of the duodenum: *1,* superior; *2,* descending; *3,* horizontal; *4,* ascending. (From Gardner, W. D.: Diagnostic anatomy, St. Louis, The C. V. Mosby Co.)

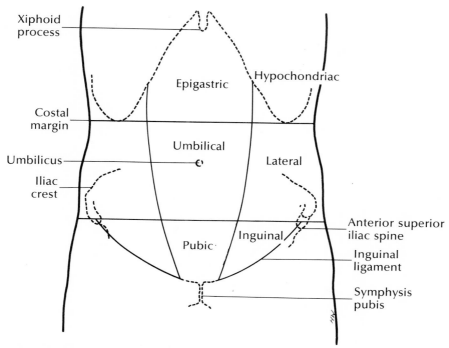

Xiphoid
process

Epigastric

Hypochondriac

Costal
margin

Umbilical

Umbilicus

Lateral

Iliac
crest

Anterior superior
iliac spine

Inguinal

Pubic

Inguinal
ligament

Symphysis
pubis

Fig. 17-8. Diagram of abdominal region.

the anterior superior iliac spine toward the symphysis. The femoral nerve, artery, and vein pass from the abdomen and into the thigh beneath the midpoint of the inguinal ligament and lie in the order named from lateral to medial. Lateral to the femoral nerve the iliopsoas muscle passes beneath the ligament, and medial to the femoral vein is a space, the femoral canal, containing areolar tissue and lymphatic structures. A femoral hernia protrudes through this space (see Fig. 5-46).

The femoral artery passes into the thigh directly toward the adductor tubercle of the femur. The pulsations of the femoral artery can be felt only in the upper part of the thigh, where it is not heavily overlaid by muscles. If the artery is pressed against the shaft of the femur, it is possible to control an arterial hemorrhage occurring inferiorly.

In infants and young children the superficial lymph nodes of the inguinal region are easily palpable. In the adult they are usually too small to be distinguished unless they are diseased.

The greater trochanter can be felt on the lateral aspect of the thigh about 20 cm below the highest point of the iliac crest. The ischial

461

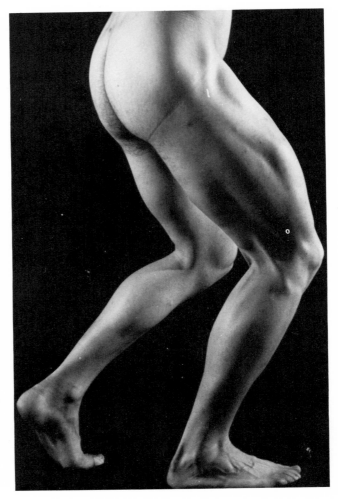

Fig. 17-9. Years of training and competition have developed the leg muscles of this bicycle racer. Although the circumference of the thigh was much greater than that of the average male of the same age, the subject had little subcutaneous fat.

The hamstrings (semitendinosus, semimembranosus, and biceps femoris) are contracted to provide extension in the hip joint, whereas the quadriceps (rectus femoris, vastus lateralis, intermedius and medialis) extend the knee joint. The hamstrings also flex the knee, whereas the rectus femoris also flexes the hip joint. This contrary action is neutralized because of certain mechanical advantages in the total lever system so that both muscle groups can contract to act against gravity. (From Royce, J.: Surface anatomy, Philadelphia, 1971, F. A. Davis Company.)

tuberosity is the bony prominence in each buttock. In a person who is seated the weight of the body is borne on the ischial tuberosities. Just inferior and lateral to the ischial tuberosity the sciatic nerve may be palpated.

At the knee the medial and lateral condyles of the femur and tibia **KNEE** can be identified, as well as the head of the fibula and the patella. The patella glides over the end of the femur in movements of the knee joint. The distance from the patella to the tubercle of the tibia does not change, and the patella articulates only with the distal end of the femur.

On the lateral side of the knee the tendon of the biceps femoris

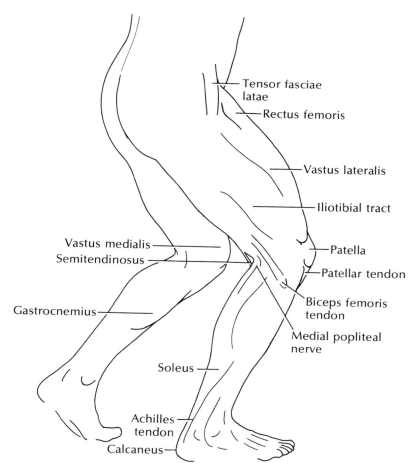

Tensor fasciae latae

Rectus femoris

Vastus lateralis

Iliotibial tract

Vastus medialis

Semitendinosus

Patella

Patellar tendon

Gastrocnemius

Biceps femoris tendon

Medial popliteal nerve

Soleus

Achilles tendon

Calcaneus

Fig. 17-9, cont'd. For legend see opposite page.

463

muscle can be followed to its insertion on the head of the fibula. Just inferior to the head, the neck of the fibula can be felt, and the peroneal nerve rolled beneath the finger as it comes around the neck to enter the leg; the nerve is often injured here in fractures of the superior end of the fibula. On the medial side of the knee the tendons of the gracilis and semitendinosus muscles can be felt at their insertion into the tibia. The tendon of the gracilis is the more superficial. Anterior to these the tendon of the adductor magnus can be traced to the adductor tubercle.

ANKLE AND FOOT   The medial and lateral malleoli are easily identified. The bones of the medial longitudinal arch of the foot have a definite relation to the medial malleolus; one fingerbreadth inferior and anterior to the distal end of the malleolus, the terminal portion of the sustentaculum tali may be palpated, two fingerbreadths inferior and anterior is the tubercle of the navicular, and three fingerbreadths anterior is the base of the first metatarsal. On the anterior aspect of the ankle the tendons of the tibialis anterior, extensor hallucis longus, and the extensor digitorum longus muscles lie in that order from the medial to the lateral margin of the ankle. Just posterior to the medial malleolus the tendon of the tibialis posterior muscle enters the sole of the foot, and immediately lateral and posterior to it may be palpated the terminal portion of the posterior tibial artery. The dorsalis pedis artery, the termination of the anterior tibial, can usually be palpated on the superior surface of the foot between the first and second metatarsal bones. On the lateral side of the foot the tendon of the peroneus brevis muscle passes posterior to the lateral malleolus to be inserted on the base of the fifth metatarsal.

The beginning of the great saphenous vein on the medial side of the ankle is usually visible, and the vein may be traced up to the knee and often to its termination in the femoral vein in the thigh. The beginning of the small saphenous vein on the lateral side of the ankle can usually be seen.

Only a few of the more obvious landmarks are mentioned in this chapter to show how much knowledge of living anatomy may be obtained from one's own body. The observing student should be able to pick out and identify many other strucutres. Good power of observation indeed is essential for the devleopment of a practical knowlege of human anatomy.

REVIEW QUESTIONS

1. Where would you palpate for the following arteries: superficial temporal, brachial, radial, femoral, posterior tibial, and dorsalis pedis?

2. Identify by palpation the following structures: lower border of the mandible,

zygomatic arch, mastoid process, supraorbital ridge, and external occipital protuberance.

3. When you clench your teeth firmly, you are able to feel a bulging beneath the skin over the angle of the lower jaw and in the temple. What muscles produce these bulgings?
4. Name three structures that may be palpated in the anterior midline of the neck.
5. What bony structure forms the tip of the shoulder?
6. Identify by palpation the medial and lateral epicondyles of the humerus, the shaft of the ulna, and the lower end of the radius.
7. What is the usual place for palpation of the apex beat of the heart?
8. Identify the crest of the ilium, the ischial tuberosity, and the greater trochanter of the femur.
9. Name three bony prominences that may be palpated at the knee.
10. Name three bony prominences that may be palpated at the ankle.
11. Try to palpate your ulnar nerve posterior to the medial epicondyle of the humerus and the peroneal nerve just inferior to the head of the fibula.
12. Why is a blow in the pit of the stomach painful?
13. In the event of a severe arterial bleeding from a cut in the hand, where would you apply pressure? Why?
14. Where would you look for the median cubital vein?
15. Where is the epigastric region of the abdomen?
16. A surgeon says that he intends to enter the abdominal cavity through a lower midline incision. Why did the surgeon pick this location.

GLOSSARY

abdomen portion of the body between thorax and pelvis; *abdominis*, "of the abdomen."

abducent drawing away from. The sixth cranial nerve supplies the lateral rectus muscle, which draws the eye from the midline; *abducens*, Latin adjective.

abduct to draw away from the midline; opposite of adduct.

abduction the act of drawing away from the midline; opposite of adduction.

abductor a muscle performing the function of abduction.

abscess localized collection of pus.

absorption passage of a substance through a membrane.

acetabulum "little vinegar cup"; the cavity in the os coxae into which the head of the femur fits.

Achilles tendon tendon of the calcaneus; in Greek mythology Achilles' mother held him by the heel when she dipped him as an infant in the river Styx to make him invulnerable.

acoustic pertaining to the sense of hearing.

acromegaly literally "great extremity"; a chronic disease due to overfunction of the pituitary gland characterized by overgrowth of the extremities and face; also spelled *acromegalia*.

acromion bony process of the scapula forming the point of the shoulder.

acute severe and of short duration; opposite of chronic; used in speaking of duration and severity of disease.

adamant extremely hard, as enamel of a tooth.

adduct to draw toward the midline; opposite of abduct.

adduction the act of drawing toward the midline; opposite of abduction.

adductor a muscle performing the function of adduction.

adenoid resembling a gland.

adenoma a benign tumor of glandular origin.

adipose fatty; the Latin adjective is *adiposus*.

adolescence youth; period between puberty and maturity.

adrenal near the kidney; same as suprarenal.

adventitia outer coat of a vessel or tube; also called *externa*.

afferent carrying or bringing to the center from the periphery; opposite of efferent.

ala wing; plural, *alae*.

alar pertaining to a wing, or winglike.

alba white.

albicans   white.

albuginea   a white fibrous tissue (layer).

alveolus   small cavity; *alveoli* is the plural, and *alveolar* the adjective.

ampulla   a flasklike dilatation; dilated end of a tube or duct.

anastomosis   a communication; plural, *anastomoses*.

anconeus   pertaining to the elbow.

angina   any disease or symptom having sudden suffocative attacks. In angina pectoris there are sudden attacks of severe pain, shortness of breath, and collapse.

ankylosis   the abnormal fixation of a joint.

ansa   literally a handle; any looplike structure.

anteflexion   a forward curvature; a condition in which the upper part of an organ is bent forward; opposite of retroflexion.

anterior   placed in the front or forward part; same as ventral; opposite of posterior or dorsal.

anteversion   a forward turning; a condition in which an entire organ is tipped forward; opposite to retroversion.

antrum   a cavity, or chamber; plural, *antra*.

anus   lower end of large intestine; *ani*, "of the anus."

aorta   the great artery carrying blood from the left ventricle.

apex   top or summit.

aponeurosis   a flat sheet of white fibrous tissue, usually serving as an attachment for a muscle. Plural, *aponeuroses; aponeurotica*, Latin adjective.

appendectomy   removal of the appendix; also termed *appendicectomy*.

appendiceal   pertaining to an appendix.

appendicular   having the nature of an appendix; attached; opposite of axial.

appendix   an appendage; a part attached to a larger portion; plural, *appendices*.

aqueduct   a canal for the conduction of fluid; Latin noun, *aqueductus*.

aqueous   watery.

arachnoid   resembling a spider web.

arbor vitae   "tree of life."

arciform   bow-shaped.

areola   (1) any very small space; adjective *areolar*; (2) the ring about the nipple.

arrector pili   "raiser of a hair"; plural, *arrectores pilorum*.

arteriole   a very small arterial branch.

arteriosus   pertaining to an artery.

artery   a vessel carrying blood from the heart.

arthritis   inflammation of a joint.

arthrosis   a joint; from the Greek.

articular   pertaining to a joint.

articulation   (1) a joint; from the Latin; (2) the mechanics of speaking.

arytenoid   shaped like a jug or pitcher; a cartilage of the larynx.

aspect   position, surface, or face.

aspera   rough.

aspirate   to remove by means of suction.

atlantic   pertaining to the atlas; *atlanto*, combining form.

atlas   the first cervical vertebra; in Greek mythology, Atlas held the earth on his back.

atrium   the first chamber of an organ; Latin word for hall.

atrophy   a wasting away of tissue.

auditory   pertaining to the sense of hearing; see acoustic.

Auerbach   German anatomist (1828-1897).

auricle   (1) portion of external ear attached to the side of the head; (2) an ear-shaped appendage of each atrium of the heart.

auricular   pertaining to the ear or earlike; pertaining to an auricle.

autonomic   being self-controlled; independent.

axial   pertaining to the axis, or line, about which a body turns, therefore pertaining to the trunk; opposite of appendicular.

467

axilla   the armpit.

axon   process of a nerve cell carrying impulses from the cell body; also spelled *axone*.

azygos   unpaired.

barium   a chemical element; barium sulphate is used in visualizing the gastrointestinal tract in x-ray examination.

Bartholin   Danish anatomist (1616-1680).

basal   pertaining to the base or lower part; basilar; *basalis*, Latin adjective.

basilic   important or prominent.

basophil   staining with basic dyes; also spelled *basophile*.

biaxial   turning about two axes.

biceps   having two heads.

biconcave   having two concave surfaces.

bicuspid   having two cusps or points.

bifid   divided into two parts.

bifurcate   forked; divided into two branches.

Bigelow   American surgeon (1816-1890).

bipennate   double feathered; sometimes spelled *bipinnate*.

bipolar   having two poles or processes.

blood   a fluid tissue circulating through heart, arteries, veins, and capillaries.

B.N.A.   Basle Nomina Anatomica; an anatomical terminology accepted at Basle in 1895 by the Anatomical Society.

boss   a rounded eminence.

Bowman   English physician (1816-1892).

brachial   pertaining to the arm.

brachium   (1) the arm; strictly that portion between shoulder and elbow; plural, *brachia*; (2) an armlike process; *brachii*, "of the arm."

brevis   short; opposite of longus.

bronchiole   small subdivision of a bronchus.

bronchus   one of the two divisions of the trachea; plural, *bronchi*.

buccal   pertaining to the cheek.

buccinator   muscle of the cheek, from the Latin word for trumpeter.

bursa   sac or pouch, usually lined with a synovial membrane.

buttock   the breech; the prominence over the gluteal muscles.

calcaneus   the heel bone; also termed *calcaneum*. Adjective may be either *calcanean* or *calcaneal*.

calcarine   spur-shaped.

callosum   thick.

calyx   cup-shaped cavity; plural, *calyces*.

canaliculus   little canal; plural, *canaliculi*.

canine   pertaining to a dog; a fanglike or pointed tooth.

capillary   (1) the smallest blood vessels connecting arterioles and venules; (2) the smallest lymphatic vessels.

capitate   bone of the wrist having a head-shaped process.

capitulum   little head.

capsule   fibrous or membranous envelope.

caput   head; *capitis*, "of the head."

cardia   the esophageal opening of the stomach.

cardiac   pertaining to the heart.

carneae   "fleshy."

carotid   chief artery of the neck, from the Greek meaning "deep sleep." Pressure on the artery may produce unconsciousness.

carpal   pertaining to the wrist.

carpus   the wrist; *carpi*, "of the wrist."

catalyst   a substance that accelerates or retards a chemical reaction without being permanently altered in the process.

catheter a slender tubular instrument for drawing off fluid from a body cavity or for distending a passage.

catheterize to use a catheter; to remove fluid from a body cavity by means of a hollow tube; particularly to remove urine from the bladder.

cauda tail.

caudal pertaining to the tail; opposite of cephalic.

caudate having a tail, or taillike.

cava a cavity; plural, *cavae*.

cavernous containing hollow spaces.

cecum (1) pouch at the beginning of the large bowel; (2) any blind pouch; also spelled *caecum*.

cele suffix meaning a swelling or distention; see hydrocele and varicocele.

celiac pertaining to the abdomen; also spelled *coeliac*.

cementum a layer of bony tissue covering the root of a tooth; also known as *cement*.

central situated in the midportion as opposed to peripheral.

cephalic pertaining to the head; opposite of caudal.

cerebellum literally "the little brain"; a division of the brain posterior to the cerebrum and superior to the pons and medulla; *cerebelli*, "of the cerebellum."

cerebrum the two great hemispheres forming the upper and larger portion of the brain; adjective, *cerebral*; *cerebri*, "of the cerebrum."

ceruminous pertaining to a waxlike secretion.

cervix a neck; adjective, *cervical*; *cervicis*, "of the neck."

chiasm an X-shaped crossing; also spelled *chiasma*.

choana a funnel-shaped cavity or opening; plural, *choanae*.

cholecystectomy surgical removal of a gallbladder.

choledochus the common bile (duct).

Chopart French surgeon (1743-1795).

chorda a cord; plural, *chordae*.

chorda tympani nerve running across the middle ear.

choroid resembling skin; also spelled *chorioid*.

chromaffin having an affinity for chrome salts.

chromatin that portion of the nucleus of a cell that is more easily stainable.

chronic of long duration; opposite of acute.

chyle a milky fluid; lymph containing fat in the lacteals of the intestine; *chyli*, "of chyle."

cilia hairlike processes; plural of *cilium*.

ciliary pertaining to cilia.

cinguli "of the girdle"; so named because the gyrus encircles the corpus callosum.

circumduction the act of moving along the surface of a cone, the joint being at the apex.

circumflex bent or turned about.

cirrhosis a degeneration of liver cells with concurrent decrease in liver function.

cisterna Latin word for cistern, reservoir.

clavicle the collar bone.

cleido pertaining to the clavicle; from the Greek.

clinoid "resembling a bed"; the four processes bear a resemblance to four bedposts.

clitoris erectile genital organ of the female, homologous with the penis; *clitoridis*, "of the clitoris."

coccyx last portion of vertebral column; named from the Greek word for cuckoo, whose bill the bone somewhat resembles; *coccygeum* and *coccygeus*, Latin adjective forms.

cochlea a snail shell; therefore a structure having a similar form.

collagen the main organic constituent of connective tissue.

collateral secondary or accessory.

colliculus a small elevation; plural *colliculi*.

collum the neck; *colli*, "of the neck."

colon portion of large intestine between cecum and rectum; *coli*, "of the colon."

columnae carneae "fleshy columns," bundles of muscle in the ventricles of the heart.

commissure a joining together.

communis common.

concave having a depressed surface; center is at a lower level than edge; opposite of convex.

concha a shell; a shell-like structure; plural, *conchae*.

condyle a rounded knob on the end of a bone; a knuckle.

condyloid resembling a knuckle.

congestion an excessive amount of blood or other fluid.

conjunctiva a delicate membrane lining the eyelids and covering the anterior surface of the eyeball.

conjunctivum connecting.

convex having a rounded elevated surface; opposite of concave.

convoluted rolled together or coiled.

coracoid like a crow's beak; variant of coronoid.

corium the true skin; see cutis.

cornea transparent portion of eyeball anterior to the pupil and iris.

corniculate hornlike; a cartilage of the larynx.

cornu a horn; plural, *cornua*.

coronal pertaining to the crown of the head.

coronary encircling like a crown; as the arteries of the heart.

coronoid see coracoid.

corpus body; plural, *corpora*.

corpus callosum body of fibers joining the two cerebral hemispheres.

corpuscle a small body.

corrugator a "wrinkler," a muscle that wrinkles the forehead.

cortex the bark, rind, or outer layer; *cortical*, pertaining to the cortex; *cortico*, combining form.

Corti Italian anatomist (1822-1876).

costal pertaining to a rib or ribs.

costarum "of the ribs."

Cowper English surgeon (1666-1709).

coxa the hip; *coxae*, "of the hip."

cranial pertaining to the cranium.

cranium the skull or brain pan.

cremaster from the Greek to suspend.

cretin a person who is a dwarf due to underactivity of the thyroid gland.

cribriform sievelike; *cribrosa*, Latin form of adjective.

cricoid ring-shaped.

crista galli "cock's comb."

cruciate shaped like a cross.

crus a leg or a part resembling a leg; plural *crura*.

cubital pertaining to the space anterior to the elbow joint.

cuboid resembling a cube.

cuneatus wedge-shaped.

cuneiform wedge-shaped.

cupula a small cup.

cusp (1) a pointed projection of a tooth; (2) a valve with a pointed segment.

cutaneous pertaining to the skin.

cuticle the outer layer of skin.

cutis the skin; see corium.

cyanosis a condition in which skin appears blue due to poor oxygenation of the blood.

cyst a closed sac containing a fluid or semisolid.

cytoplasm protoplasm of a cell exclusive of the nucleus.

dartos smooth muscle of scrotum.

deciduous that which is shed; temporary; same as first or milk teeth; opposite of permanent; *decidua*, Latin noun.

decussation   a crossing in the form of an X.

deferens   carrying away.

deltoid   triangular; resembling the Greek letter, *delta*.

dendrite   a branched or treelike process of cytoplasm of a nerve cell; the process carrying impulses to the cell body; also called *dendron*.

dens   a tooth.

dentate   toothlike.

dentin   main substance of a tooth, surrounds the pulp and is covered by enamel; also spelled *dentine;* formerly called ivory or substantia eburnea.

dentition   the teeth as a group; the milk dentition; the permanent dentition.

depolarization   change in direction of polarity.

dermis   Greek word for skin; also called *derma*.

descendens   descending.

diaphragm   a cross wall; a septum.

diencephalon   the "between" brain.

digestion   the process of changing food into materials that may be absorbed and assimilated by the body.

digiti   "of a digit."

digitorum   "of the digits."

diploë   from the Greek, a fold.

distal   remote; opposite of proximal.

diverticulum   a small pouch leading from a larger cavity.

dorsal   toward the back; opposite of ventral.

dorsiflex   to turn toward the back; opposite of plantar flex.

Douglas   Scottish anatomist (1675-1742).

duct   a passage or tube; *ductus*, Latin for tube.

duodenum   the first part of the small intestine; literally twelve (fingerbreadths).

dura mater   "strong" or "hard mother"; the outer covering of brain and spinal cord.

eburnea   like ivory; substantia eburnea, an old name for dentin.

efferent   carrying from; opposite of afferent.

effusion   escape of fluid into a part or tissue.

ejaculatory   pertaining to a sudden act of expulsion.

elastin   the essential organic constituent of elastic connective tissue.

embolism   blocking of a blood vessel by material in the blood stream.

embryo   the early stages of the fetus; particularly before the end of the second month.

embryology   the science that deals with the development before birth.

emesis   vomiting.

emissary   affording an outlet.

empyema   pus in a cavity; particularly within the chest.

enamel   the very hard, white substance covering the dentin of the teeth.

endocrine   secreting into the blood or lymph; opposite of exocrine.

endolymph   fluid within the membranous labyrinth of the inner ear; see perilymph.

endosteum   tissue surrounding the medullary cavity of bone.

endothelium   simple squamous epithelium lining blood vessels and lymphatics.

eosinophil   a white blood cell readily stained by eosin; also spelled *eosinophile*.

eparterial   above an artery.

epi   a prefix meaning "on" or "above"; opposite of hypo.

epicolic   "on the colon."

epicondyle   a prominence on a bone above or upon a condyle.

epicranius   "above the cranium."

epidermis   outermost layer of skin.

epididymis   on the testis, a structure attached to the back of the testis; plural, *epididymides*.

epiglottis   cartilage of the larynx; the cartilage "above the glottis."

epinephrine   hormone from suprarenal medulla.

471

epiphysis   a part of or process of a bone that ossifies separately before making osseous union with the main portion of the bone.

epiploic   pertaining to an omentum.

epistropheus   a pivot.

epithelium   the covering tissue of the body; plural, *epithelia.*

epitrochlear   above the trochlea (of the humerus).

equina   pertaining to a horse.

erythrocyte   a red blood corpuscle.

esophagus   the gullet; portion of digestive tract between pharynx and stomach; also spelled *oesophagus.*

ethmoid   sievelike.

eustachian   named after Eustachio, Italian anatomist (1520-1574).

eversion   the act of turning outward; opposite of inversion.

evert   to turn out; to turn the sole of the foot outward; opposite of invert.

exhalation   the act of breathing out; opposite of inhalation.

exocrine   secreting into a duct; opposite of endocrine.

extension   a movement at a joint bringing the two parts into or toward a straight line from a flexed position; opposite of flexion.

external   on the surface or outer side; opposite of internal; Latin adjective, *externus,* or *externa.*

extra   prefix meaning "outside of"; opposite of intra.

extrinsic   external; not pertaining exclusively to a part.

exudate   material found in tissue spaces or on surfaces in inflammation.

facet   a small, plane surface.

falciform   sickle-shaped.

fallopian   named after Fallopius, Italian anatomist (1523-1562).

falx   a structure shaped like a sickle.

fascia   a sheet of connective tissue; plural, *fasciae.*

fasciculus   a small bundle; plural, *fasciculi.*

fauces   a passageway.

femur   thigh; bone of the thigh; *femoral* is the adjective; *femoris,* "of the thigh."

fetal   pertaining to a fetus.

fetus   the child, from the end of the second fetal month until full term; also spelled *foetus.*

fiber   a long, threadlike structure; also spelled *fibre*; adjective *fibrous*; Latin adjective, *fibrosa* or *fibrosus.*

fibril   a minute fiber; Latin form *fibrilla.*

fibula   smaller bone of leg; the splint bone.

filament   a delicate thread or fiber.

filiform   thread-shaped.

filum   a threadlike structure.

fimbria   a fringe or fringelike structure; plural *fimbriae.*

fissure   a cleft or groove.

flavum   yellow.

flexion   a movement in which the anterior surfaces of two segments are brought closer to each other; opposite of extension. In knee flexion the posterior surfaces are approximated.

flexure   the curved or bent part of a structure.

fluoroscope   an instrument for holding a luminous screen during a roentgenoscopic examination.

follicle   (1) a very small sac or gland; (2) a lymphatic nodule.

fontanelle   unossified area of cranium of an infant; word literally means "little fountain"; also spelled *fontanel.*

fonticulus   same as fontanelle.

foramen   a hole; plural, *foramina* or *foramens.*

472   **foreskin**   the prepuce.

fornix vaultlike space.

fossa a pit or hollow; plural, *fossae*.

fourchette a fold of mucous membrane joining the posterior ends of the labia minora.

frontal pertaining to the forehead.

fundus the portion of a hollow organ farthest from the outlet.

fungiform shaped like a fungus or mushroom.

funiculus (1) a bundle of nerve fibers; (2) a cord; the spermatic cord.

fusiform spindle-shaped.

galea a helmet.

Galen Greek physician (130-200).

ganglion a group of nerve cells, usually placed outside the central nervous system; plural, *ganglia* or *ganglions*.

gasserian named after Gasser, Austrian surgeon (1505-1577).

gastric pertaining to the stomach.

gastrocnemius "belly of the leg"; a muscle in the calf of the leg.

gemellus twin; plural, *gemelli*.

genial pertaining to the chin.

geniculate bent like a knee.

genioglossus pertaining to chin and tongue.

genitalia the reproductive organs.

genu Latin word for knee; *genus*, "of the knee."

Gerota Roumanian anatomist (1867-1939).

gland a secretory organ.

glans Latin word for gland or acorn.

glenoid resembling a pit or pocket; the glenoid cavity of the scapula is very shallow.

Glisson English physician and anatomist (1597-1677).

globule a small spherical mass.

glomerulus a little tuft or cluster.

glomus a tuft or ball; plural, *glomera*.

glossal pertaining to the tongue.

glossopharyngeal pertaining to the tongue and pharynx.

glottis space between the vocal folds.

gluteal pertaining to the buttocks; *gluteus*, Latin adjective.

goiter enlargement of the thyroid gland; also spelled *goitre*.

Golgi Italian histologist (1844-1926).

gonad essential sex gland, either testis or ovary.

graafian named after Graaf, Dutch physician and anatomist (1641-1673); ovarian follicle.

gracilis slender.

granule a small particle; a little grain.

groin the lowest portion of the lateral anterior abdominal wall, near the thigh.

gustatory pertaining to the sense of taste.

gyrus a convolution of the brain; plural, *gyri*.

hallux the great toe; *hallucis*, "of the great toe."

hamate the "hooked" bone; this carpal bone has a hooklike process.

hamstring a tendon of the back of the knee; the muscles sending tendons to this area.

hamulus a little hook.

haustra sacculations of the colon; plural of *haustrum*.

haversian named after Havers, English anatomist (1650-1702).

hemoglobin coloring matter of red blood corpuscles containing iron; also spelled *haemoglobin*.

hemopoiesis the formation of blood; also called *hematopoiesis*.

hemopoietic pertaining to the formation of blood; also called *hematopoietic*.

hemorrhoidal pertaining to dilated veins.

473

Henle   German anatomist (1809-1885).

hepar   the liver, *hepatic* is the adjective; *hepatis*, "of the liver."

hernia   abnormal protrusion of an organ or tissue through an opening.

herniorrhaphy   operation to repair a hernia.

Highmore   English surgeon (1613-1684).

hilus   a depression or pit, place of entrance or exit of vessels supplying an organ; also termed *hilum*; adjective *hilar*.

hippocampus   literally a "sea horse"; a curved structure in the floor of the middle horn of the lateral ventricle of the brain; not the hippocampal gyrus.

His   German anatomist (1831-1904); and Wilhelm His, Jr., German physician (1863-1934).

histology   science of the minute structure of tissues.

hormone   the product of a gland of internal secretion.

humerus   the arm bone; *humeri*, "of the humerus."

humor   any fluid or semifluid of the body.

Hunter   English anatomist and surgeon (1728-1793).

hyaline   glasslike.

hydrocele   a circumscribed collection of fluid, particularly in the scrotum; also spelled *hydrocoele*.

hymen   a membrane; specifically a fold that may practically occlude the external opening of the vagina.

hyoid   U-shaped.

hyper   prefix meaning superior to; opposite of hypo.

hyperplasia   increase in the size of a tissue or organ due to an increase in the number of cells.

hypertrophy   increase in the size of a tissue or organ due to an increase in the size of its constituent cells.

hypo   a prefix meaning below or inferior to; opposite of *epi* or *hyper*.

hypoglossal   placed below the tongue; *hypoglossi*, Latin adjective.

hypophysis   from the Greek, meaning "growing under"; an endocrine gland growing from the inferior surface of the brain.

hypothenar   the mound of the palm over the bones of the medial (ulnar) metacarpal bones.

ileum   the distal part of the small intestine; from a Latin word meaning "twisted"; adjective is *ileac*; *ileo* is the combining form.

ilium   the bone of the flank; adjective is *iliac*; *ilio* is the combining form.

incisive   pertaining to the incisor teeth.

incisor   a tooth used for cutting; from the Latin verb "to cut."

incus   an anvil; an anvil-shaped bone of the middle ear.

index   referring to the forefinger or "pointing" finger.

inferior   situated or placed below; opposite of superior; *inferioris*, a Latin form of the adjective.

infra   a prefix meaning "beneath"; opposite of supra.

infraclavicular   below the clavicle.

infrahyoid   beneath the hyoid.

infraspinous   below the spine (of the scapula).

inguinal   pertaining to the groin.

inhalation   the act of breathing in; opposite of exhalation.

innominate   literally "nameless"; *innominatum*, Latin adjective.

inscriptiones   literally "writings"; the *inscriptiones tendineae* have a certain resemblance to a line of script.

inter   a prefix meaning "between."

intercellular   situated between cells.

intercostal   situated between ribs.

474   **interdigital**   situated between digits.

interosseous situated between bones; *interosseus,* Latin adjective.

intima innermost.

intra a prefix meaning "within"; opposite of extra.

intracellular situated within a cell.

intravenous within a vein.

intrinsic situated entirely within or pertaining exclusively to a part; opposite of extrinsic.

intubation the insertion of a tube, particularly into the larynx.

inversion the act of turning inward; opposite of eversion.

invert to turn in; to turn the sole of the foot inward; opposite of evert.

involuntary performing without the will; opposite of voluntary.

iris from the Greek word meaning "rainbow" or "halo"; the colored disc of the eye.

ischium bone of the hip; adjective is *ischiatic, ischial,* or *sciatic.*

ivory a bonelike covering of the teeth, now called dentin.

jejunum portion of small intestine between duodenum and ileum; literally the "empty" (gut).

jugular pertaining to the neck.

Keith English physician (1862-1855).

Krause German anatomist (1833-1910).

Kupffer German anatomist (1829-1902).

labium a lip; plural, *labia.*

labyrinth a system of complicated passages or channels.

lacertus literally "torn."

lacerum torn.

laciniate fringelike.

lacrimal pertaining to tears; also spelled *lachrymal.*

lactation secretion of milk.

lacteal (1) pertaining to milk; (2) an intestinal lymphatic containing chyle.

lacuna a small hollow or space; plural, *lacunae.*

lambdoid shaped like the Greek letter, *lambda.*

lamella a small leaf or sheet; plural, *lamellae.*

lamina a leaf or sheet; plural, *laminae.*

Langerhans German pathologist (1847-1888).

larynx the voice box; adjective, *laryngeal.*

lata wide.

lateral pertaining to the side; opposite of medial.

latissimus dorsi the widest (muscle) of the back.

leukemia a fatal disease characterized by a great increase in the white blood cells; also spelled *leucemia.*

leukocyte a white blood cell, also spelled *leucocyte.*

levator a lifting or raising muscle.

lien the spleen.

ligament a band; *ligamentum,* Latin noun.

linea a line; plural, *lineae.*

lingual pertaining to the tongue.

lipoid fatlike.

lobe a portion of an organ separated from the rest by fissures or septa.

lobule a little lobe.

loin part of back between thorax and pelvis.

longissimus longest.

longus long; opposite of brevis; *longum* is neuter adjective.

lumbar pertaining to the loin; *lumborum,* "of the loins."

lumbrical wormlike.

lumen space within a tube or organ.

475

lunate a bone of the carpus shaped like a crescent moon.

lutein a yellow pigment found in corpus luteum, fat cells, and egg yolk.

luteum yellow.

lymph a transparent, slightly yellow fluid filling lymphatic vessels.

lymphocyte a variety of white cells; such cells are also found in large numbers in lymph nodes and lymphatic tissue.

lymphoid (1) resembling lymph; (2) tissue containing many lymphatic cells enmeshed in reticular tissue.

magnus large; *magnum* is neuter adjective.

major larger; opposite of minor; *majus* is neuter adjective; *majora*, plural.

malar pertaining to the cheek.

malleolus a little hammer; a hammer-shaped process.

malleus a hammer; a hammer-shaped bone of the middle ear.

malpighian named after Malpighi, Italian anatomist (1628-1694); (1) any lymphatic nodule of the spleen; (2) any glomerulus of the kidney; (3) layer of epidermis.

mammary pertaining to the breast.

mammillary like a nipple; also spelled *mamillary*.

mandible bone of lower jaw.

manubrium a "handle"; uppermost portion of the sternum.

marrow soft central part of a bone.

masseter a "chewer"; a muscle of mastication.

mastication chewing.

mastoid nipple-shaped.

mastoiditis inflammation of mastoid air cells.

matrix the groundwork or substance in which anything is cast or placed.

maturation the process of ripening or becoming adult.

maxilla a jawbone; particularly the bone of the upper jaw.

maximus largest; opposite of minimus; Latin genitive and plural, *maximi*.

meatus a passageway.

media middle.

medial pertaining to the center; opposite of lateral.

median pertaining to the middle, that is, between two other structures; see mesial.

mediastinum a median septum or partition.

medulla (1) marrow; (2) the central portion of an organ as opposed to the periphery or cortex; (3) *medulla oblongata*, the portion of the brain between the pons and the spinal cord.

meibomian named after Meibom, German anatomist (1638-1700).

Meissner German physiologist (1829-1905).

membranacea membranous.

membrane a thin layer or sheet; *membrana*, Latin noun.

meninges membranous coverings of the brain and spinal cord.

meninx Greek word for membrane; plural, *meninges*.

meniscus a crescent; plural, *menisci*.

menstruation the monthly flow of blood from the uterus beginning at puberty and ceasing at the menopause or "change of life."

mental (1) pertaining to the chin; (2) pertaining to the mind.

mesencephalon the midbrain.

mesenchyme undifferentiated embryonic tissue.

mesentery a fold of peritoneum attached to an abdominal organ; specifically the fold of peritoneum attaching the small intestine to the posterior abdominal wall.

mesial situated in the middle; see median.

meso (1) a prefix meaning pertaining to the middle; (2) a prefix meaning pertaining to a mesentery.

mesothelium epithelium lining certain serous cavities.

metacarpus "after or beyond the wrist"; the five bones of the hand.

476

metastasis the shifting of a disease from one part of the body to another.

metatarsus "beyond the instep"; the five bones of the foot between the toes and tarsal bones.

metopic pertaining to the forehead.

micturition urination.

minimus least; opposite of maximus; Latin plural and genitive, *minimi.*

minor smaller or lesser; opposite of major; *minus* is neuter adjective; *minora,* plural.

mitral similar in shape to a miter; valve of heart between left atrium and left ventricle.

modiolus a small central pillar or hub.

molar pertaining to the grinding teeth.

Moll Dutch physiologist (1849-1914).

moniliform shaped like a string of beads.

Monro English surgeon (1697-1767).

mons a mound or prominence; the mons pubis is also called the mons veneris, "the mound of Venus."

mucosa mucous.

mucus a viscid watery secretion; adjective, *mucous.*

multangular having many angles.

multifidus split into many parts.

multilocular having many small cavities or cells.

multipolar having more than two poles or processes.

myelin a fatlike substance forming a sheath around myelinated (medullated) nerve fibers.

myeloid related to bone marrow.

mylo prefix donoting molar.

N A approved anatomical nomenclature.

naris a nostril; plural, *nares*; *naris,* "of the nostril"; *nasi,* "of the nose."

navicular boat-shaped.

neurilemma nerve sheath.

neuroglia supporting structure of the nervous system.

neuron a complete nerve cell including its processes; also spelled *neurone.*

neutrophil staining with neutral dyes; also spelled *neutrophile.*

node a swelling, protuberance, or knob.

nodule a little swelling or mass.

nucha nape of the neck; *nuchae,* "of the nape."

nuchal pertaining to the nape of the neck.

Nuck Dutch anatomist (1650-1692).

nucleolus a little nucleus.

nucleus (1) a spherical body within a cell, forming the vital part; (2) a group of nerve cells in the central nervous system.

obese fat.

oblique slanting; between horizontal and vertical in direction; Latin adjective, *obliquus.*

oblongata oblong.

obturator Latin word for a plate covering an opening.

occiput the back of the head.

oculi "of the eye."

olecranon from the Greek word for elbow.

olfactory pertaining to the sense of smell.

omentum from a Latin word for cover, a fold of peritoneum (mesentery) attached to the stomach; plural, *omenta.*

omo prefix meaning pertaining to the shoulder.

ophthalmic pertaining to the eye.

opponens opposing.

opposition the act of opposing one part to another.

optic   pertaining to vision.

orbicular   circular.

orbital   pertaining to the orbit.

organ   a portion of the body having a special function.

os   Latin for mouth; plural *ora*; *oris*, "of the mouth."

os   Latin for bone; plural *ossa*.

osmosis   passage of fluid across a membrane from a less to a more highly concentrated solution.

ossicle   a little bone.

ossification   formation of bone.

otic   pertaining to the ear.

ovale   oval.

ovalis   oval.

oviduct   passageway for ovum.

ovum   egg; plural, *ova*.

pacchionian   named from Pacchioni, Italian anatomist (1665-1726).

pacinian   named for Pacini, Italian anatomist (1812-1883).

palate   roof of the mouth; adjective, *palatine*; *palatini*, "of the palate."

palm   the hollow of the hand.

palpebra   eyelid; plural, *palpebrae*.

pampiniform   shaped like a tendril.

pancreas   "all flesh"; a digestive gland.

panniculus   a layer or membrane.

papilla   a small nipple-shaped elevation; plural, *papillae*.

papillary   pertaining to a nipple, or nipplelike.

para   prefix meaning "beside," "accessory to," or "near."

paracolic   lying along or near the colon.

paralysis   loss of motion or sensation in a living part.

parathyroid   near the thyroid.

parenchyma   the functional elements of an organ as distinguished from its framework.

parietal   pertaining to the walls of a cavity; see visceral.

parotid   situated near the ear.

parturition   the act of giving birth to a child.

patella   "little pan"; the kneecap.

pectinate   shaped like a comb.

pectineal   pertaining to the pubic bone; Latin adjective, *pectineus*.

pectoral   pertaining to the breast or chest; Latin adjective, *pectoris*.

pedal   pertaining to the foot; *pedis*, "of the foot."

pedicle   a process connecting the lamina of a vertebra with the centrum.

peduncle   a stem or supporting structure.

pelvis   a basin or basinlike structure.

pendulous   pendent; hanging.

penis   erectile genital organ of the male.

pennate   shaped like a feather; same as penniform.

peri   prefix meaning "around."

pericardium   sac surrounding the heart.

perichondrium   membrane covering the surface of cartilage.

perilymph   fluid within bony labyrinth of the inner ear, but outside the membranous labyrinth; see endolymph.

perimysium   sheath of connective tissue surrounding a muscle bundle.

perineorrhaphy   operation on perineum to repair lacerations or relaxation.

perineum   space bounded by coccyx, pubic arch, and the rami of the ischium.

periodontal   around a tooth; formerly peridental.

periosteum   a tough fibrous membrane surrounding a bone.

peripheral   pertaining to the periphery, the surface, or outer margin; opposite of central.

peristalsis   a wave of contraction passing along a muscular tube.

peritoneum   serous membrane lining the abdominal cavity and covering the viscera in that cavity.

peroneus   "of the fibula"; variant, *peroneal.*

pes   the foot; *pedis,* "of the foot."

petrous   resembling a rock; the dense portion of the temporal bone.

Peyer   Swiss anatomist (1653-1712).

phagocytosis   the engulfing of particles by a cell.

phalanges   plural of *phalanx,* which refers to any bone of finger or toe.

pharynx   the Greek name for space posterior to the nose and mouth; adjective, *pharyngeal.*

phrenic   pertaining to the diaphragm.

pia mater   "tender mother"; innermost covering of brain and cord, which is thin and delicate.

pilomotor   mover of a hair.

pineal   shaped like a pine cone.

piriform   pear-shaped; *piriformis,* Latin adjective.

pisiform   pea-shaped.

pituitary   the hypophysis.

placenta   a circular, flat organ by which the fetus is attached to the inner wall of the uterus.

plantar   pertaining to the sole of the foot; *plantaris,* Latin adjective; *plantae,* "of the sole of the foot."

plaque   a flat area or plate.

plasma   fluid portion of the blood.

platysma   a platelike muscle.

pleura   serous membrane lining the thoracic cavity and covering each lung.

plexus   a braid or network; plural, *plexus* or *plexuses.*

plica   a fold; plural, *plicae.*

pollex   the thumb; *pollicis,* "of the thumb."

polymorphonuclear   having nuclei of many shapes.

pons   a bridge; *pontis,* "of the bridge."

popliteal   pertaining to the ham or posterior aspect of the knee; *popliteus,* Latin adjective.

porta   gateway; *portal,* pertaining to a gateway.

posterior   situated behind or toward the back; opposite of anterior.

postganglionic   beyond a ganglion; see preganglionic.

Poupart   French anatomist (1661-1709).

preganglionic   before a ganglion; see postganglionic.

premolar   anterior to a molar tooth.

prepuce   the foreskin; a fold of skin covering the glans of the penis (or the clitoris).

preputium   same as prepuce.

procerus   stretched out or long.

process   a slender projecting point; Latin *processus.*

profundus   deep; opposite of sublimis or superficialis.

prolapse   a falling down or sinking of an organ.

pronate   to turn palm inferiorly.

prone   lying with face downward.

propria   proper.

proprius   belonging to one only.

prostate   a gland in the male surrounding the neck of the bladder and first part of the urethra.

prostatectomy   surgical removal of prostate gland.

protoplasm   living matter; the essential material of all plant and animal cells.

protract   to pull forward; opposite of retract.

protraction   the act of pulling forward; opposite of retraction.

479

proximal   nearest; opposite of distal.

pseudo   a prefix signifying "false."

psoas   pertaining to the loin.

pterygoid   shaped like a wing.

puberty   the age at which the reproductive organs become functional.

pubic   pertaining to the region of the pubic bone.

pubis   the pubic bone; plural, *pubes*.

pudendal   pertaining to the pudendum.

pudendum   the external genitalia; espeically of the female.

pulmonary   pertaining to the lung.

punctum   a point; plural, *puncta*.

Purkinje   Hungarian physiologist (1787-1869).

pylorus   opening from stomach into duodenum.

pyramidalis   shaped like a pyramid.

quadrate   four-sided; having a square or rectangular shape.

quadratus   four-sided.

quadriceps   four-headed.

quinsy   an acute inflammation outside the capsule of the tonsil with formation of pus.

quinti   pertaining to the fifth.

racemose   resembling a bunch of grapes.

radius   a spoke; a bone of the forearm.

ramus   a branch; plural, *rami*.

Ranvier   French pathologist (1835-1922).

raphe   a seam or ridge.

rectum   straight; the portion of the large intestine between the colon and the anus; it is not straight in man but is in many animals.

rectus   straight.

renal   pertaining to the kidney.

restiform   shaped like a rope.

rete   a net.

reticular   netlike.

retina   innermost coat of eye.

retinaculum   a halter; a structure that retains an organ or tissue in its place; plural, *retinacula*.

retract   to pull back; opposite of protract.

retraction   the act of pulling back; opposite of protraction.

retro   prefix meaning behind.

retroflexion   a backward bending of one part of an organ on another portion; opposite of anteflexion.

retroperitoneal   posterior to the peritoneum.

retropharyngeal   posterior to the pharynx.

retroversion   a backward turning; the entire organ is turned posteriorly; opposite of anteversion.

rhinencephalon   the olfactory portion of the brain.

rhomboid   shaped like a kite; *rhomboideus*, Latin adjective.

risorius   pertaining to laughing or grinning.

Roentgen   German physicist (1845-1923).

roentgenogram   a photograph made by means of roentgen rays, or x-rays; the rays are named in honor of their discoverer.

roentgenoscopy   examination by means of a fluoroscope.

rotation   the act of turning about a centrally located length axis.

rotundum   round.

480   **ruga**   a ridge or fold; plural, *rugae*.

INDEX

487

497